# Disability in Pregnancy and Childbirth

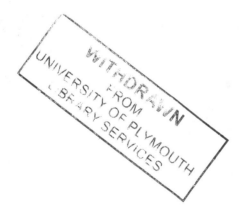

*Commissioning Editor:* Mairi McCubbin
*Development Editor:* Sheila Black
*Project Manager:* Anne Dickie
*Illustration Manager:* Bruce Hogarth
*Designer:* Gene Harris
*Illustrators:* Barking Dog

# Disability in Pregnancy and Childbirth

Edited by

## Stella McKay-Moffat
**MPhil BA(Hons) RN RM ADM CertEd**
**Family Planning Certificate**

*Senior Lecturer – Midwifery and Women's Health, Faculty of Health,*

*Edge Hill University, Liverpool, UK*

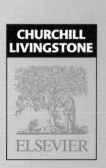

CHURCHILL
LIVINGSTONE

ELSEVIER

Edinburgh   London   New York   Oxford   Philadelphia   St Louis   Sydney   Toronto   2007

2013 → Phym

# CHURCHILL LIVINGSTONE

CHURCHILL LIVINGSTONE
An imprint of Elsevier Limited

First published 2007

978-0-443-10318-6

**British Library Cataloguing in Publication Data**
A catalogue record for this book is available from the British Library

**Library of Congress Cataloging in Publication Data**
A catalog record for this book is available from the Library of Congress

**Notice**
Knowledge and best practice in this field are constantly changing. As new research and experience broaden our knowledge, changes in practice, treatment and drug therapy may become necessary or appropriate. Readers are advised to check the most current information provided (i) on procedures featured or (ii) by the manufacturer of each product to be administered, to verify the recommended dose or formula, the method and duration of administration, and contraindications. It is the responsibility of the practitioner, relying on their own experience and knowledge of the patient, to make diagnoses, to determine dosages and the best treatment for each individual patient, and to take all appropriate safety precautions. To the fullest extent of the law, neither the Publisher nor the Author assumes any liability for any injury and/or damage to persons or property arising out of or related to any use of the material contained in this book.

*The Publisher*

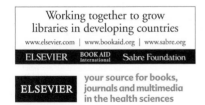

Printed in China

# Contents

# Contributors

**Stella McKay-Moffat** MPhil BA(Hons) RN RM ADM CertEd FPCert
*Senior Lecturer – Midwifery and Women's Health, Faculty of Health, Edge Hill University, Liverpool, UK*

**Pam Lee** MA BA(Hons) RN RM MTD DipN FETC
**DipAppSocSci ENBNO7 PGDip Psychosexual Therapy**
*Senior Lecturer – Midwifery and Women's Health, Faculty of Health, Edge Hill University, Liverpool, UK, Nurse Therapist, Wirral Primary Care Trust, Wirral, UK*

**Linda Moss** MA BA(Hons) RNLD RN CertEd
*Senior Lecturer – Health, Faculty of Health, Edge Hill University, Ormskirk, UK*

**Jackie Rotheram** BA(Hons) RN RM DPSN HealthEdCert NVQ Assessor
*Specialist Midwife in Disability/Disability Advisor, Liverpool Women's Hospital, Liverpool, UK*

# Foreword

This book for midwives will make a real contribution to ensuring that disabled women receive the care that they need and deserve.

Good midwifery support from the start can make all the difference to the experience of pregnancy, birth and the early days of life with a new baby for disabled women. In practice, however, midwives have little opportunity to gain enough experience to be confident in supporting disabled women in the way that they would like. With a broad range of impairments it may be that individual midwives may only meet with one or two clients with particular impairments through their whole careers. This comprehensive volume will go a long way towards addressing this problem.

The midwife is likely to be the key worker for disabled women who are usually keen to be treated as expectant mothers with particular support needs, rather than as disabled women who are pregnant.

Midwives are in an ideal position to act as advocates when this is wanted. They can pass on information concerning a mother's individual requirements to everyone involved in the woman's maternity care, including specialist obstetric staff. They can also ensure that other relevant services work together to ensure any necessary support systems can be in place in advance of the birth. They can also signpost to people who can advise on appropriate equipment or adaptive approaches to baby care, giving the woman the reassurance that she is well-prepared for life with a new baby.

For disabled women, to have midwives who understand their conditions and concerns can be affirming. As an information service frequently approached by midwives anxious to provide such care, we applaud the publication of this book.

**Rosaleen Mansfield**
*Chair of Trustees*
*Disability, Pregnancy and Parenthood International*

# Preface

Women with disabilities are increasingly choosing to become mothers. Key themes in the available literature indicate that this growing minority of women may not be receiving maternity services from professionals with adequate experience, knowledge and skill to provide effective care. Furthermore, there is evidence that some of the women have experienced negative attitudes because of their disability. This book aims to raise the awareness of disability issues in general, and specifically in relation to service provision for women accessing maternity care.

Issues concerning people with disabilities have increasingly become prominent in political and public arenas at local, national and government levels. Disability studies, which began in the 1950s, burgeoned from the 1980s and have contributed to the instigation of the increased interest. Much of this attention has been due to the contribution of both academic and non-academic people with disabilities. However, considerable literature has been from non-disabled academics with an interest in the subject. It could be argued that this has been (and will continue to be) a positive contribution because of their objectivity and ability to see issues from different perspectives. Conversely, it could be contended that they cannot really understand the problems when they have not lived them. In an attempt to harness a diversity of knowledge and understanding, the authors of this book have contributed a wealth of their expertise and experiences from academic, professional and personal events.

Women's disability studies evolved from general disability studies that commonly focused on men. Women-related issues have increasingly become prominent, as evidenced by the availability of specific literature. These issues frequently revolve around the right to have their sexuality recognised and the freedom to choose to have a family in the same way as non-disabled people. Literature related to pregnancy and childbearing for women with a disability has slowly become available. Some of this literature has come from outside the UK and whilst it is often very informative, it may not always meet the learning needs of midwives and other professionals associated with pregnancy and childbearing working in the UK.

To understand factors that influence the lives of people with disabilities today, a broad spectrum of issues needs to be considered. Historical events influence present day situations, which in turn will influence future developments. Over time, theoretical exploration and advancement raises awareness of real-life concerns and offers potential guidance for change. Part of the theory building relates to language and terminology clarification, while another area is concerned with perceptions of disability reflected in personal and societal models of disability. Clear definitions may help to avoid misconceptions and confusion.

Theory alone is not sufficient. The lived experience of people with disabilities must be considered, as should events with the potential to have a profound influence on an individual's life. It must be remembered, however, that people with disabilities are not passive recipients of what is happening around them. Individually and collectively they, and their advocates, have become increasingly proactive in bringing about change from sociological, psychological and political standpoints. Midwives, too, have the potential to have a major influence on the experiences of women in their care.

There are many different types of disability. Some are congenital while others are acquired at any age after birth. These can be subdivided into physical or mental conditions, although they are often interlinked. Disabilities may be visible or invisible and caused by disease or injury. An individual with a disability may not consider themselves 'disabled'. Someone with a medical condition such as diabetes may be disabled by the condition or its effects but not be considered 'disabled' by society. The focus of this book relates to women with a motor or sensory impairment or learning disability that has the potential to cause them problems during pregnancy, during labour and childbirth, or during self care or infant care following the birth.

The themes highlighted here are important elements to aid midwives' understanding of the complexity of factors that may influence the life of a woman with a disability receiving maternity services. The issues will be explored and discussed within the text with the discourse enhanced in places by the experiences of mothers and midwives. Combined with the factual information there will often be suggestions for how to improve the services offered to women.

Chapter 1 focuses on the sociological construction of disability and motherhood and includes discussion about terminology, beliefs, models of disability and parenthood. As no book for midwives about women should be without a chapter on women's health, chapter 2 addresses this topic in relation to the health of women with a disability. Topics range from sexuality and body image, relationships and sex education and contraception, to domestic abuse and the desire for motherhood. All of the subjects in these first two chapters help to underpin an appreciation of the factors that may influence women's health and wellbeing and, in short, their lives.

Chapter 3 explores the maternity experiences of women using the services. The author's experience as a midwife, a mother with a disability, and a disability advisor in one of the largest women's hospitals in Europe offers a depth of understanding that, it could be argued, is second to none. The experiences of the women for whom she has provided a service enhance the quality of the information in the chapter and ensure the information is grounded in practice. Three case scenarios are used to illustrate pertinent points of discussion.

Although there is of necessity a little overlap between chapter 4 and the preceding chapter, the earlier themes are developed and the focus is moved towards professional issues. These include significant issues related to effective communication, advocacy and the promotion of women-centred services. Issues linked to ante-natal, intra-partum and post-natal care are discussed.

Chapter 5 concentrates on women with learning disabilities. Here the reader is taken from historical perspectives to issues of concern to women of today, and the service and support concerns that professionals need to bear in mind. The theme of service provision is further developed and explored in chapter 6 in general terms for women with disabilities. The focus is directed towards standards of care, attitudes and how midwives can be influential in improving both. Midwives' learning needs are identified. The experiences of a small group of women who had used maternity services, and the experiences of midwives who had provided services for women with disability are used to emphasise the issues discussed. This again helps to ensure that the information is meaningful and grounded in real life.

Chapter 7 explores the needs of people with sensory loss and issues that need to be considered by midwives when providing maternity services for women in such situations. Communication with deaf women causes midwives concern and ineffective attempts at information exchange can result in frustration for all and substandard care for women. With this in mind, general principles are offered to improve communication and some basic signs from British Sign Language are given.

Midwives need a sound understanding of some of the disabling conditions women may have. This will enable an appreciation of some of the daily challenges women need to overcome, and the often greater issues they face when undertaking pregnancy and childbearing. Therefore chapter 8 contains an overview of some of those conditions, their manifestations and how pregnancy may interact with the conditions.

Each of these chapters will end with key points to act as an *aide memoir* and reinforce the focus of the chapter. It must be remembered, however, that there will inevitably be some overlap with the different chapters as no topic can be considered in isolation.

The final chapter contains a list of potentially useful resources. Although not an exhaustive list, it contains details of some resources and organisations that offer information and/or support to people with certain conditions, their families and professionals that may be offering services. Contact details are given for the organisations, including postal and internet website addresses. It must be remembered that the best resource to aid midwives' understanding of a mother's situation is a mother herself. A list of suggested further reading is provided that will aid learning. The final section of this chapter contains handouts on contraception, sexual health and pre-conception care that may be copied and given to women, as these are issues that women highlight in the literature as not readily available to them.

**Stella McKay-Moffat**
Liverpool, 2007

# Acknowledgments

I would like to acknowledge two people who have, probably unknowingly, had considerable influence on my disability awareness. Firstly Jackie Rotheram (one of the contributors) who, over 10 years ago, prompted me to consider my own knowledge about, attitudes towards, and experience of providing care for women with disability. Reflecting on all of these issues at the time I realised that I had much to learn.

Second, my husband of six years, David Moffat, who received an industrial injury resulting in the loss of most of one hand long before we met. Living with someone with a disability has taught me many things. It is extraordinary how adaptability can be developed to cope with every day living, but conversely how help must sometimes be sought for things that prove too challenging. Additionally, that there may frequently be a need to minimise or hide a disability to outwardly appear as normal as possible and to avoid the public's concerns or aversion when they see part of the body that is not normal. Finally, there is a need to balance seeing a person before the disability, and forgetting that some things are difficult or impossible to do, with seeing the disability first and wanting to be helpful, and consequently disempowering an individual. It's not easy to always get that balance right so people with disability sometimes have to have patience with, and forgiveness of, the rest of us.

I must also acknowledge Martin Baxter, Senior Media Resources Officer in the Faculty of Health at Edge Hill University, for taking the photographs, Liverpool Women's Hospital for permission to photograph equipment and Adam Rouilly for permission to photograph anatomical models purchased from them.

# 1 The social construction of disability and motherhood

## Pam Lee

## INTRODUCTION

Disability is difficult to define, depending on the different and conflicting constructions regarding its 'nature' and 'meaning'. Society is increasingly self-regulating; with more closely focused definitions of what is 'normal' and what is not, and disability is still a stigmatised condition (Hughes 1998). Feminists argue that women generally are oppressed by the society we live in today. So to be a disabled woman in that society is doubly oppressing. There is a prevailing view that women are the carers, the nurturers and the stalwart of family life. However, if you are a disabled woman then how could you possibly cope with being a mother, would you be a suitable person to bring up a child and could you possibly do this without the intervention of the state? The aim of this chapter is to try and 'unpick' some of these stereotypical responses to disabled women as mothers and put forward a more positive view.

## DEFINITIONS

The Collins English Dictionary—21st century Edition (Trevvy 2000) defines disability as:

1. The condition of being unable to perform a task or function because of a physical or mental impairment;
2. Something that disables; handicap;
3. Lack of necessary intellect, strength, etc;
4. An incapacity in the eyes of the law to enter into certain transactions (p 444).

This definition seems focused on issues of inability and lack of something in the individual, with a legal implication that also focuses on the negative.

Hughes (1998) refers to The Concise Oxford Dictionary of Sociology which widens this definition by including how this fits in with society: 'Loss or lack of functions, either physical or mental, such as blindness, paralysis or mental subnormality—which unlike illness is usually permanent. Disabilities are usually stigmatising. Moreover, disabled persons often need extra finances and personal support [which is often inadequate to sustain their rights] and are a key group in social security and welfare programmes'. This definition also focuses on the problem of loss or lack, but adds to that an emphasis on the person requiring extra resources and the 'dependent' nature of many disabled people.

A third definition from the British Disability Discrimination Act 1995 defines physical and mental impairments and reflects on the fact that the disabled person may be unable to cope with 'normal' life: 'A person has a disability if he or she has a physical or mental impairment which has a substantial and long-term adverse effect on his or her ability to carry out normal day to day activities'. This definition takes things further than the previous two in that it places an emphasis on the person with the disability being unable to carry out normal activities, thus suggesting that normality is natural and taken for granted. Examples are given in the Act of activities which may not be able to be achieved by people so defined, thus taking them outside the norm. Examples of these activities are:

- Inability to see moving traffic clearly enough to cross a road safely.
- Inability to turn taps or knobs.

■ Inability to remember and relay a simple message correctly.

The state is therefore required to put interventions in place to assist these individuals to achieve a 'normal' life-style.

Lennard Davis (1997) states that the concept of a norm implies that the majority of the population must or should be part of the norm. The norm pins down that majority of the population that falls under the arch of the typical bell-shaped curve. This is the normal distribution curve and there will always be people at the extremities of the curve that will have different characteristics from the majority. These are considered deviations from the norm and therefore they are open to scrutiny and discrimination by the majority. People with disabilities may be thought of as deviants and effort will be put in by those in power to make them conform to what is considered to be the norm in health, mobility, and the environment.

Swain & Cameron (1999) quote the Union of the Physically Impaired Against Segregation (UPIAS) who define impairment as: 'Lacking all or part of a limb, or having a defective limb, organ or mechanism of the body' (p 69). According to Neville-Jan (2004) people with a disability would prefer to be thought of as physically impaired, rather than disabled as many do not feel disabled in themselves, only by the society they live in. UPIAS also offer an alternative definition of disability: 'The disadvantage or restriction of activity caused by a contemporary social organisation which takes no or little account of people who have physical impairments and thus excludes them from participating in the mainstream of social activities. Physical disability is therefore a form of social oppression' (p 69). This definition supports Neville-Jan's (2004) beliefs.

Language is a powerful tool and the words that we use to describe people with disabilities can stigmatise and insult them. Some of the definitions stress that the person is 'unable' or 'impaired' whilst others point to institutions which 'dis-able' people. There has been much discussion about the correct language to utilise. The innate meaning of some words has been challenged, whilst others are no longer readily acceptable or felt to be 'politically correct' for example: to label someone as 'spastic' is seen as derogatory and offensive. Negative attributes are often associated with different terms depending on the sociological philosophy at the time. The way society is organised determines the meaning of disability (Vernon & Swain 2002). Corker & French (1999) refer to Susan Peters, who went even further by maintaining that labels and language prevent the development of a positive identity by damaging self-image, giving what she called a false consciousness.

All the definitions appear to ignore the idea that non-disability/disability may be seen as a continuum rather than as discrete states. Many people have a disability which occurred as a result of an accident and as such they will have perceived themselves as 'normal' in the first instance and may not perceive themselves as 'abnormal' following their change in status. Jenny Morris (1993) describes the events following her spinal injury, acquired whilst attempting to rescue a child from a railway embankment. She was generally viewed negatively as it was thought she had attempted suicide and due to her acquired disability was now considered to be an unsuitable person to look after her 1-year-old daughter.

## BELIEFS

Definitions have changed over time and beliefs about disability have also changed. There are passages in the Old Testament that determine people with 'blemishes' or physical defects, for example, blind or lame, as impure or tainted. Hughes (1998) discussed earlier work by Carol Thomas, who had argued that in most pre-modern societies, disability has been religiously explained as divine punishment. Women in the Old Testament were also seen as impure and this therefore increases the stigma attached to being a disabled woman. In the New Testament there are examples of healing the disabled and a moral call to do 'good works' and show pity to those 'less fortunate than ourselves'. Disability has been seen as a 'curse' or a 'Cross to bear' in the Christian faith and it has been surrounded by ignorance, fear and superstition (Hughes 1998).

Historically there was a movement that believed that disability was a form of pollution, the evidence of sin. There was a belief that people with a disability or the 'feeble-minded' should not reproduce for fear of contaminating society (Hubbard 1997). The eugenics movement did not start with the Nazis; they only took it to extremes (Hubbard 1997). The idea of having a 'perfect' race developed in Britain in the late 19th and early 20th century. Francis Galton, cousin of Charles Darwin, coined the term 'eugenics' which means 'well born' in Greek, but was taken as a term to improve the stock of the nation. Galton helped found the English Eugenics Education Society and eventually became the Honorary President. Marie Stopes, best known for her work as the pioneering advocate of birth control was a firm believer in eugenics. She wrote a book called 'The control of parenthood' in 1920 and even tried to prevent her son's marriage to a woman who wore glasses on the basis that it would be a crime against his country (Campion 1995). As late as 1941, Julian Huxley, brother of Aldous Huxley, wrote an article arguing that it was crucial for society that 'mental defectives' should not have children and that there should be prohibition of marriage or segregation in institutions, combined with sterilisation for those still 'at large' (Hubbard 1997).

The American eugenics movement built on Galton's work between 1905 and 1935. There was a belief that the families where 'gifted' children were born, were few and far between and that poor, illiterate families were 'breeding' excessively. Charles Davenport was a leading exponent of eugenics and in 1904 he became the director of the 'station for the experimental study of evolution' (Hubbard 1997, p 190). His aim was to collect large amounts of data on human inheritance and store them in a central office. He managed to persuade many rich and influential people to sponsor the movement and the office and its staff became major resources for promoting two legislative programmes that formed the backbone of US eugenics: involuntary sterilisation laws and the Immigration Restriction Act of 1924. The first sterilisation law was enacted in 1907, and by 1931 some 30 states had compulsory sterilisation laws on their books. By 1935 some 20 000 people in the United States had been forcibly sterilised, almost half of them in California (Hubbard 1997).

The Nazi movement took eugenics to the extreme with 'racial cleansing' and extermination of the weak, feeble-minded and children and adults with disabilities.

Killing children with disabilities is not that far removed from aborting foetuses with abnormalities. Antenatal screening tests for Down's syndrome or neural tube defects are carried out regularly, the assumption being that the pregnancy will be terminated if an abnormality is revealed.

The front page of The Sunday Telegraph (21st May 2006) carried an article by Beezy Marsh (health correspondent) about pregnant women carrying a Down's syndrome baby being pushed into having late abortions by doctors so that they would not have a 'mentally retarded' child. One mother in the article was offered termination at 35 weeks gestation. However, she refused and the article carried a picture of her 2-year-old son who, according to his mother, is happy and enjoying life. Marsh referred to The Down's Syndrome Association who warn that doctors and health professionals with 'outdated views' on what life is like with a Down's syndrome child are failing to provide a balanced view by encouraging abortion. The Association provides statistics for the article showing that there were 657 live births and an estimated 937 abortions for Down's syndrome babies in 2004. This was a three-fold increase in terminations for this condition over the last 15 years. Marsh used figures from the Department of Health to support his argument. These included 124 late abortions over 24 weeks, every year for all 'disabilities': 18 of them over 32 weeks. Some agencies are now campaigning for the rights of the unborn child to prevent some of these terminations from taking place, but generally in the population there is a belief that every parent has the right to a 'perfect' baby (McLaughlin 2003).

Jenny Morris (1996) discusses the belief that if someone is severely disabled that life 'is not worth living' and that the population of non-disabled people cannot understand how severely disabled people can think that life *is* worth living. She highlights the case of Larry McAfee in the United States in 1989 who was so severely disabled that the Courts considered letting him have his life-support machine turned off because both they and he considered his life not worth living. However, disabled activists wanted to support him to live and argued that with the right degree of support he could have a reasonable quality of life. Unfortunately his health insurance ran out and he ended up institutionalised and extremely depressed and upset. In contrast, compare this case with that of Christopher Reeves who had a good quality of life, was able to travel and encourage other disabled people to make the most of their lives. This was possible because he had the financial resources to do it. Perhaps it is the society we live in and the lack of financial support that is more disabling to people than their physical condition.

## PEOPLE WITH DISABILITIES—VALUING THEIR DIFFERENCE

People without disabilities assume that those affected by disability would want to conform to the norm and do everything in their power to achieve that. This is not the case and people with impairments may value their 'difference'. This perspective was graphically explained in a BBC television programme called 'One life - to see and be seen' (BBC 1 24 May 2006). Tara, a 17 year old with congenital absence of the iris and progressive blindness, was being offered the chance of improving her eyesight through a donation of corneal stem cells from her mother. Everyone, including the doctor, parents and siblings, seemed to think that this was a good idea. But Tara had great misgivings about it, not just the surgery, but the fact that she might regain more sight than she could 'cope with'.

Tara's friends were largely partly sighted like herself. She also plays goalball at an international level. This game is for the visually impaired only and relies on them listening to a bell within the ball and saving goals as the ball is aimed at the goal post. It was obvious that this game was a big part of Tara's life and if her sight was sufficiently improved she would not be able to play it at the same level. Nevertheless, she did agree to the surgery. Her mother said Tara did not know what she was missing, and was impressive in her commitment to help her daughter. However, there was the distinct indication that Tara felt pressured into the surgery. The outcome of the procedure was that Tara's eyesight in one eye was sufficiently improved that she can now see objects held close to her face, but not so improved that she is not considered visually impaired. The programme highlighted some of the pressures put on people with impairments to try and conform to normality.

Similar pressures can be identified when looking at pioneering surgery on cochlear implants. Whilst undertaking a course in British Sign Language (BSL), I met a number of families at a social club for the hearing impaired where they had refused the offer of surgery for their congenitally deaf child. They feel that their lives were shaped by their lack of hearing; they have their own language, culture and social life which they do not feel is valued by the hearing population. Why make their children conform to 'normal' values, to be able to hear; why not accept the difference and diversity of their non-hearing culture?

Deafness and deaf people can be viewed from a medical or socio-cultural perspective. The medical perspective defines them as being disabled and in need of 'treatment' to try and enable them to hear and speak. The socio-cultural perspective is one where it is accepted that some deaf people are born into families where deafness is the 'norm'. The children grow up in an environment where sign language is the favoured method of communication and speech is not part of this: the family is part of the deaf community (Miles 1988).

Historically deaf people have been stigmatised and isolated. 'Deaf and dumb' people were considered to be 'feeble-minded' and legally incompetent. As early as the fourth century, it was recognised that deaf families existed and communicated through 'gestures', however, there is no evidence to suggest that these families had full status in the society at that time. Speech was considered essential in the Roman Code of Justinian in the sixth century; without it individuals had no legal rights because they could not take part in religious ceremonies which demanded that they recited special formulae.

According to Miles (1988), Spain was one of the first countries in the sixteenth and seventeenth centuries to investigate the incidence of deafness overall. Concern arose because there was inbreeding between noble families which resulted in the spread of hereditary deafness. Whereas deafness in the lower classes was not seen as a problem because of their low status, in the upper classes it was viewed as problematic, as Spanish Law forbade anyone without speech from inheriting lands and titles. Juan Fernandez de Navarette (El Mundo— The Mute) was a court painter (1568–1579) from a wealthy family who was born hearing. He became deaf at the age of 3 years following an illness. His religious paintings are said to depict 'signing poses' as he and his tutor had developed signs to aid communication (see the picture 'Adoration of the Shepherds' by El Mundo). Juan Fernandez used signs with King Philip II and other court members and he was able to find interpreters to help him verify formal business dealings.

In England, Richard Carew's survey of Cornwall in the 1580s describes an inhabitant of Saltash, who had been deaf for a long time, who signed to make himself understood and also lip-read as well. A servant called Edward Bone was also mentioned as being deaf 'from the cradle', but was considered 'very alert', religious and clean living and could 'sign' to make himself understood (Miles 1988). At that time communication between the hearing and non-hearing took three forms:

- Mime or mime-like signs understood by hearing people.
- Lip-reading, which some deaf people, and also some hearing people, could understand.
- Sign language—understood by most deaf people in their community but not by most hearing people.

At least there was some attempt to communicate with deaf people rather than just isolating them in their families.

By 1644 a physician called John Bulwer published a book called 'Chirologia: or the natural language of the hand'. He illustrated it with drawings of typical hand shapes, some of which are still used in BSL today. His second book called 'Philocophus, or the deaf and dumb man's tutor' (1648) was dedicated to two deaf brothers from a wealthy family. Bulwer believed that sign language was of a universal nature, but unfortunately that was not the case and signing varies from place to place, both at home and abroad. During the seventeenth century reports came from Spain about signing and lip-reading and together with Bulwer's book, there was a greater interest in communicating with the deaf. One-handed and two-handed alphabets for spelling out English words were devised and there were similar developments in European countries. These alphabets were mainly used for the education of children from wealthy families who also wanted

their children to speak; speech was generally seen to be proof of gentility and intelligence. From this time deaf people with speech were considered more desirable than deaf people who communicated by signing (Miles 1988).

In Britain, by 1760, education of the deaf was quite profitable and Thomas Braidwood set up a school in Edinburgh which taught oral and written skills to the deaf. For the next 80 years or so the Braidwood family had virtual monopoly in the field of deaf education. Braidwood moved from Edinburgh to London and in 1792 the first 'charity' school was opened under the charge of his nephew Joseph Watson. Similar schools developed throughout the country. This helped the development of the deaf community as children were brought together to learn, and sign language could be standardised.

Education of deaf people in France evolved differently and rather than demanding speech as the acceptable form of communication, sign language was accepted instead. However, the emphasis was on using correct French grammar and the signs developed showed every part of it. Teachers went from all over Europe to learn the technique, but eventually it was felt to be too cumbersome as a method of communication and was abandoned.

By the nineteenth century people travelled widely to learn about educating the deaf. Thomas Gallaudet came from Connecticut in 1816 and took back with him to America ideas about communicating and educating the deaf. Together with a Frenchman named Laurent Clerc, he played a major part in establishing the first school for the deaf in America; the work of the Gallaudet school is still influential in the United States today (Miles 1988).

As society developed and there was better education and more acceptance of deaf people, many were able to take up good positions of employment and found comradeship with the deaf community. The legal status of non-hearing people had improved, but there was still discrimination against the deaf community and an anxiety about a deaf variety of the human race evolving (following Charles Darwin's book published in 1859). It was noticed that they met together, communicated in a way that hearing people did not understand and had their own clubs and newspapers. Alexander Graham Bell, who had just invented the telephone, was a Scottish-born American who himself was married to a deaf woman. He held eugenic views that hereditary deafness should not be passed on to future generations. He did not like sign language and felt that all deaf people should have speech so that they would integrate better with the hearing population. Bell was strongly influenced in his eugenic theories by research he conducted on a remote island off the coast of Massachusetts, USA. One in 55 of the population were deaf which was much higher than the mainland. The island had been settled in 1640 by men who came from Maidstone, Kent and the deafness had come from one of those men. Intermarriage had occurred and a large deaf community had developed. Bell wanted to eradicate deafness by forbidding deaf people from marrying. He wanted to break away from sign language as a form of communication and insisted on 'oralism' being taught in schools instead so that the deaf would have speech and be able to be understood by the hearing population. This belief, for which he actively campaigned, led to 'oralism' being reintroduced into schools and signing being banned. The ideal quickly spread through Europe at the expense of sign language. By the twentieth century BSL gradually disappeared from the classroom and deaf children were taught to speak. Deaf teachers were considered unfit for this task as their speech may have been limited and so they also disappeared from deaf schools.

Deaf children rebelled, however, and would sign amongst themselves when the teachers were not present. George Taylor and Juliet Bishop, editors of 'Being deaf, the experience of deafness' (1991) collected some harrowing accounts of how deaf children were forced to speak even when they were profoundly deaf. If they did not comply with trying to speak, they had their hands tied behind their backs to stop them from signing and were not given things until they vocalised that they wanted them. The aim was to try and make the child 'normal' i.e. speak so that they would 'fit in' with the hearing population. Attempts were made to use powerful hearing aids, which were often uncomfortable to wear and increased extraneous sounds rather than audible speech. The children and their parents were told that they were not deaf, just unable to hear very well (Fletcher, in Taylor & Bishop 1991).

However, there are still parents of deaf children who argue for 'oralism' i.e. wanting their child to speak even though they cannot hear. They feel that integration is the key to success for their children and want them to be accepted by the hearing population as they see speech as being the way forward. Heather MacDonald, a mother of three deaf children who have all learnt to speak, has put this case forward eloquently in Chapter 6 in Taylor & Bishop (1991). Perhaps the way forward is for 'Total Communication' which includes both 'oralism' (speech) and signing being encouraged as acceptable methods of communication.

Standards of deaf education had been causing concern for a number of years and in 1979 the first ever comprehensive survey of school leavers was carried out. Sadly the results revealed that deaf school leavers had a reading age of 8.75 years on average and their speech was mostly unintelligible (Ladd in Miles 1988). These findings led to a movement in the mid to late 1980s to reintroduce BSL into deaf schools and also hearing schools so that everyone had a chance to learn to sign.

BSL has survived because its users do not have any other reasonable means of communication. Although many young people were educated under the 'oralist' regime, they reverted back to signing in their own homes. Deaf clubs have formed in cities and towns up and down the country and there are often rallies and conventions where members meet together. As many deaf children are sent to boarding school away from where they live, they often meet up with old school friends at these events and exchange thoughts and ideas about their community.

Deaf children may have hearing parents and vice versa so hearing people also attend the clubs. They learn BSL and teach it to others so that more people can use it to communicate. BSL is accepted as a language in its own right and is the fourth language in Britain, the other three being English, Welsh and Scottish Gaelic. In 1988 the European Parliament called on member nations to recognise their own sign language as an official language of their country, yet BSL is still not fully recognised as a language in Britain (Smith 1996). The deaf community have their own authors, poets, musicians, entertainers and leaders and it is time they were recognised and valued for their differences.

Deafworks is an organisation campaigning to provide greater access for the deaf and hard of hearing to arts, cultural and tourism venues. The conference: 'Opening Up!' was a joint venture between Deafworks and the London Borough of Camden, Arts and Tourism which aimed to encourage greater access to these areas for the deaf (Deafworks 1999). Speakers from interested agencies discussed how best to facilitate the deaf community and proposed how they could be accommodated alongside hearing people, for example in theatres, cinemas and art galleries. A directory was published as a result of the conference so that deaf people could see what services were available to them in these areas.

## STEREOTYPES

Multiple stereotypes about people with disabilities abound. Gordon Hughes (1998) suggests the following:

- Feel ugly, inadequate and ashamed of their disability.
- Lives are a burden to us and barely worth living.
- 'Crave' to be 'normal' and 'whole'.
- Naïve and lead sheltered lives.
- Cannot ever accept their condition—if they are cheerful and fulfilled, they are just putting on a brave face.
- See daily living as a challenge and want to 'prove' themselves.
- They are asexual or at best sexually inadequate.
- Any able-bodied person who marries them must have had a special reason for doing it—but not love.
- If a relationship fails, it is because of the disability.

There are many more stereotypes of a similar nature; generally they are very negative and serve to reinforce the belief that disability in some way is deviant and that stigma is attached to it. These stereotypes do not take into account the lives of prominent disabled people who have achieved great things in their lives, for example Tanni Gray Thompson (paralympic gold medallist), David Blunkett (politician), Alison Lapper (artist—a sculpture of her pregnant torso is in Trafalgar Square). Unfortunately, disabled people are frequently viewed as a homogenous group and are not recognised as individuals with their own aspirations.

## MODELS OF DISABILITY

To aid understanding and explain the world and specific concepts within the world, individuals formulate ideas and beliefs into what are often referred to as frameworks or models. These are sets of ideas or constructs which help the individual to make sense of their perceptions and thoughts. Models which are frequently used in the disability debate are shaped by society and life events experienced by the individual.

The traditional approach to disability is a medical model: our bodies are viewed as a machine; if a part is not functioning, then medical opinion is sought, the impairment is diagnosed and management is determined (Hughes 1998). The impairment is seen as 'the problem', the individual's problem not societies' problem, and the disabled person has to cope as best they can with the 'special services' that the state can provide. The doctor is the person who decrees whether the individual needs a disabled sticker for their car, whether they need a home help and what financial and other benefits they can apply for. The fact that a doctor is responsible for these things pathologises the condition and ensures that 'the problems' are maintained at an individual level (Cunningham & Davis 1985).

Unfortunately for individuals born with a disability, from an early age they are often investigated, examined, photographed and discussed by medical practitioners in such a way as to be made to feel like an object. Hughes (1998) refers to Michelle Mason's graphic description of her experiences in hospital when she was a child. She thought it was going to be good having her photograph taken and was surprised to be told to take everything off so that 'bits' of her could be photographed rather than a whole picture. She was even more alarmed to find that the photographs were going to be put in a book, her permission was not sought and she considered the process to be a violation of her rights and a gross invasion of her privacy (p 78, 79). The medical professionals probably felt that the photographs provided better understanding of the condition for people reading the book. They had obviously not considered that they should have sought permission. This just reinforces the belief that disabled people cannot make decisions for themselves.

Disabled activist groups locate 'the problem' of disability within society as opposed to the individual i.e. the social model of disability. The disability which does not allow the individual to lead a full life is more a failure of society to make appropriate provision than the fault of the individual. What is needed from society is better housing, access to public places, transport systems, financial benefits and a view that 'able-bodied-ness' is not the 'norm'. Social policies should be geared to the integration of disabled people into society and not their marginalisation (Hughes 1998).

Neither model is entirely satisfactory at explaining the lived experience of people with disabilities. The World Health Organisation (WHO 2001) published the International Classification of Functioning, Disability and Health (ICF) designed to conceptually integrate the medical and social models of disability. However, Shakespeare & Watson (2002) took a more radical view and suggested that it was time to move away from both models and start again. There have been criticisms of the impairment/disability distinction and perhaps there is an argument for constructing a sociology of impairment that recognises physical, emotional and sexual dimensions of disability (Neville-Jan 2004).

## HISTORICAL DEVELOPMENT OF CHARITIES

The early history of charities for disabled people links with the beliefs mentioned previously and residential care was provided by religious orders or church organisations. With the philanthropic movement of the nineteenth century, many charities developed to improve the lives of children, the poor and the disabled. The type of care provided was based on the medical model i.e. that of disabled people needing 'treatment', if not to cure their condition, then to help them live with it. Institutions were built and people who could not be looked after at home were 'hidden away'. Life was often hard with regimentation, discipline and cleanliness being the 'norm' and with loss of identity and control (Hughes 1998).

Hiding the disabled away in these charitable institutions continued into the twentieth century and with two world wars, more 'care homes' developed for the disabled victims. In the 1960s the 'thalidomide tragedy' raised the public's awareness of the difficulties faced by parents endeavouring to bring up children with multiple disabilities. The Thalidomide Society was formed in 1961 to support families and children and to encourage research into people living with severe disabilities. It still operates today ensuring that the long-term health problems/needs of those affected by thalidomide are being met/kept in public focus.

Disabled children were segregated, institutionalised and disciplined until the 1970s. Since then there has been a gradual decline in charitable regimes. Many charities still work for people with disabilities, but they may also be responsible for the negative imagery associated with the disability (Hughes 1998). However, for children with severe physical disabilities, residential institutions still exist. Alison Lapper, born in 1965 with phocomelia, gives a graphic description of what it was like for her spending 19 years of her life in such care (Lapper 2005). The regime may have changed from that of the Victorian era; nevertheless, care was regimented and harsh at times with no thought for modesty and dignity or the needs of the individual. There was still the belief that the children had to conform to 'normal' values by using prosthetic limbs to help them to eat in a more 'normal' manner and to stand upright. Normality was standing on two legs, even though it may not have been in the children's best interests. Alison Lapper 'threw away' her prostheses when she became independent and is mobile in her own way now, walking on her shortened limbs, using a wheelchair, or driving her car.

## COMMUNITY CARE

Changes in policy brought about a shift to community care with the Community Care Act 1990. The major change here was the introduction of 'homes' in the community for people with learning disabilities. These are houses where people can live as a 'family' group with paid carers to help with daily activities. It is interesting that similar improvements for people with physical disabilities came on the back of policy changes for people with learning problems (Hughes 1998).

Stephen Baldwin (1993) argues that 'community care' is based on an inappropriate 'speciality model' of provision focused on traditional beliefs about segregation of clients into specialist groupings including rehabilitation and learning disabilities. He sees people filtered into specialist groups according to 'diagnostic' categories by virtue of age, impairment, disability, chronic condition, sex and handicap. Although 'in the community', they are segregated from mainstream life and marginalised. They may end up being less able to access special needs services because they are thought to have them already, for example mobility aids, prostheses, large-print books and befriending services. Although some disabled people may have achieved physical integration by living in the community, they may have simultaneously failed to achieve social integration due to absence of human contact outside their carers.

There is no single solution to the challenge of social integration; it is a two-way process involving reciprocal relationships. If people with disabilities and impairments can be assisted to experience social integration, this process should enable them to offer reciprocal relationships to others, as well as to receive contact from them. Care in the community meant that the general public were more exposed to people with disabilities, but in some cases there was opposition to having social services houses in residential areas.

## DISABILITY AND DISCRIMINATION

Legislation to provide equal opportunities developed from the 1970s with the Equal Opportunity Act 1975 and Race Relations Act 1975. The ensuing years brought employment rights through legislation to ensure that 'normal' people i.e. the non-disabled, would be free from discrimination. The major legislation for the disabled was the Disability Discrimination Act of 1995, parts of which did not come into force until 2000. The Act covers definitions and many activities of daily living for people with disabilities, for example:

- employment;
- access to goods, facilities, services and premises;
- letting or selling land or property;
- education;
- public transport vehicles.

The Disability Act was complemented by the Disability Discrimination Act—Special Educational Needs 2001 which reinforced the requirement of schools, colleges and higher education institutions to integrate pupils/students into their place of learning. However, there was nothing in the legislation that specifically met the needs of girls and women.

A European Disability Forum was set up with a Working Group on Women and Disability, and a Manifesto by Disabled Women in Europe was adopted in Brussels on 22nd February 1997 and launched by the European Parliament on 4th December 1999. The Manifesto should ideally form a base for political activity to improve the situation for disabled girls/women wherever European Union (EU) policies are involved. It recognises that cultural differences exist not only in relation to other countries, but also within the EU. The ideological basis for the Manifesto is the notion of human rights and equal opportunities. Non-discrimination is an important concept and a 'social' model of disability should be adopted rather than a 'medical' model, although the needs of the individual and medical differences should not be ignored.

The manifesto focuses on the specific situation of disabled girls/women, looking at it both as a biological construct i.e. sex differences, and a social construct i.e. gender differences. A view is given that women with disabilities are doubly oppressed by gender and disability. Disabled women are disadvantaged compared with non-disabled women or with disabled or non-disabled men. Further discrimination also occurs according to age, ethnic background, sexual orientation and socio-economic background. The Manifesto makes recommendations related to the following factors:

1. Human rights, ethics.
2. National and European legislation.
3. Conventions and other international legal instruments.
4. Education.
5. Employment, vocational training.
6. Marriage, relationships, parenthood, family life.

7. Violence, sexual abuse and safety.
8. Empowerment, leadership development, participation on decision-making.
9. Disabled women with different cultural backgrounds.
10. Awareness-raising, mass media, communication and information.
11. Independent living, personal assistance, technical needs and assistance, counselling.
12. Social security, health and medical care, rehabilitation.
13. Public buildings, housing, transportation, environment.
14. Culture, recreation, sport.
15. National focal point on women with disabilities.
16. International focal points.
17. Regional and sub-regional activities, project funding.
18. Statistical information, research (p 1).

The Manifesto looks at each of these headings in depth and makes recommendations to ensure that disabled girls/women are not discriminated against in all areas. Certainly, with some of the areas: education, employment, marriage, relationships, parenthood, family life, violence, sexual abuse and safety, many non-disabled women would welcome non-discrimination as well.

## POVERTY AND INEQUALITY IN HEALTH

The income of disabled people is likely, on average, to be less than half that of non-disabled people and therefore they are more likely to live in poverty and have more housing problems. Nine out of 10 families with disabled children are affected in this way (Prime Minister's Strategy Unit 2005). However this is not new as it has been well documented over the years, and clearly in the Black Report in 1979, that low income results in lower standards of living, which result in inequalities in health (Acheson 1998, Townsend 1992). If someone is already disadvantaged by having a disability then the problems are compounded: low income equals poorer housing, poorer access to services, poorer health and social exclusion. The government has set up a Social Exclusion Unit to deal with disadvantaged

members of the community so that inequalities could be addressed, but it has not significantly improved the lives of disabled people.

A government committee chaired by Sir Donald Acheson, formerly Chief Medical Officer of Health, produced a report called the 'Independent inquiry into inequalities in health' (Acheson 1998). Chapter 7 reported on mothers, children and families and covered issues related to the improvement of health (Box 1.1). Each of these areas included discussion on inequality, evidence, benefit and recommendations. It is a comprehensive report and provided evidence for changing policies to lessen inequalities generally, but not specifically for disabled people, their families or for parents of disabled children.

More recently the government, through the Prime Minister's Strategy Unit, has developed a strategy for 'Improving the life chances of disabled people' published in a final report in January 2005 (The Prime Minister's Strategy Unit 2005). The report was produced in conjunction with the Department for Work and Pensions, the Department of Health, the Department of Education and Skills and the Office of the Deputy Prime Minister. The report redefined disability as an encompassing disadvantage experienced by an individual that resulted from barriers to independent living or educational, employment and other opportunities that impact on people with impairments and/or ill health. The report went on to look at the type of barriers faced by disabled people (Box 1.2). In the foreword by the Prime Minister, Tony Blair states that the aim of the Strategy Unit was to look at what the Government can do to 'improve disabled people's opportunities,

---

> **Box 1.1 Issues in the Acheson report (1998) for health improvement**
>
> - Reducing poverty in families.
> - Improving the health and nutrition of women and children.
> - Promoting breast-feeding.
> - Fluoridating the water.
> - Reducing the prevalence of smoking in pregnancy.
> - Social and emotional support of parents.
> - Promoting the health of 'looked-after' children.

**Box 1.2   Types of barriers to independent living (Prime Minister's Strategy Unit 2005)**

- Attitudinal—disabled people themselves may have a negative attitude about their ability to get a job and employers, health professionals and service providers may also have a negative attitude.
- Policy design and delivery may not take disabled people into account.
- The environment might put up physical barriers such as poor transport systems or poor design of the building for wheelchair access.
- Barriers may be around empowerment with the providers of services not consulting the disabled person about preferred service provision.

**Box 1.3   The key points in the Executive Summary of 'Improving the life of disabled people' (Prime Minister's Strategy Unit 2005)**

- Helping disabled people to achieve independent living by moving progressively to individual budgets for them, drawing together the services to which they are entitled and giving the disabled person more choice over the support they receive.
- Improving support for families with young disabled children by ensuring that they benefit from child-care and early education provided to all children: meeting the extra needs of families with disabled children and ensuring services are centred on them.
- Facilitating a smooth transition into adulthood by putting into place improved mechanisms for planning the transition to adulthood and the support that goes with this. There should be a more transparent and appropriate menu of opportunities and choices.
- Improving support and incentives for getting and staying in employment by ensuring that support is in place long before a claim for benefits is made. There should be work-focused training and improved access to work.

to improve their quality of life and strengthen our society' (The Prime Minister's Strategy Unit 2005).

The report is an ambitious vision for improving the life chances of disabled people (Box 1.3). Disabled people should have full opportunities and choices to improve their quality of life, and they should be respected as equal members of society. The centrepiece of this new government strategy is to promote independent living and this means providing disabled people with choice, empowerment and freedom. This does not mean that disabled people are expected to do everything for themselves, but they have the biggest say in what they do and how they live their lives. One of the problems for many disabled people is that they are unable to find suitable employment and therefore have to rely on benefits for income. Whilst the DDA 1995 and Disability Discrimination Commission sought to address this by putting in legislation to encourage employers not to actively discriminate against disabled people, the reality is that many employers do not provide suitable working conditions for this to occur. Although there has been some progress, it has been recognised that disabled people are more likely to be living in poverty, to have fewer educational qualifications, to be out of work and experience stigma and abuse. They still find themselves experiencing poorer services which are organised to suit the providers, rather than personalised around the needs of disabled people (Prime Minister's Strategy Unit 2005).

Assessing the population of disabled people is difficult as many of them, for example elderly people, do not identify themselves as such. It is estimated that there are 11 million adults and 77 000 disabled children in the UK: one in five of the total population. The population of disabled people is distinct from and much larger than the 3 million people in receipt of disability-related benefits. The population of people with disabilities is highly diverse and constantly changing. People with different impairments, different socio-demographic backgrounds and facing different barriers will have very different day-to-day experiences.

Only one out of two disabled people are currently in employment compared with four out of five non-disabled people. People need adequate budgets and disabled people and parents of disabled children should be able to choose whether they want their budgets in cash, in some combination of cash and services, or as entirely commissioned services.

The budget should be used to get the individual what they need to allow them to live independently and this may include transport to and from work, special equipment, housing adaptations or something else entirely.

The Prime Minister's Strategy Unit envisages a staged approach in the short-term with the focus on working with local authorities, and where appropriate with Local Strategic Partnerships taking forward Local Area Agreements. The aim should be to build a coherent evidence base, without adding to local authority burdens, and also to build up an invest-to-save fund to provide up-front resources to introduce the changes required by the new system. There should be direct involvement of disabled people through local Centres for Independent Living so that they can play an effective part in planning services and supporting other disabled people to achieve independent living.

The government is also committed to abolishing child poverty and intend to target support to families with disabled children so that they can have a better start to life. When asked, children from lower income families are more likely to report long-standing illness or disability and mental health issues, reflecting a two-way link between low income and disability. Families of children with disabilities should also be able to access budgets to allow them to meet the individual needs of the child and home-based support if required. Families with disabled children and the child itself will benefit from the new proposal to give support during the transition to adulthood. Any advantages gained during the early years will be lost if this is not addressed. There are three key issues:

- Planning for transition focused on individual needs.
- Continuous service provision.
- Access to a transparent and appropriate menu of opportunities and choices.

Over time, individualised budgets should mean a seamless transition to adulthood.

The government have already introduced some significant improvements regarding employment for disabled people. These include the New Deal for Disabled people, extensions to the DDA 1995, the national minimum wage and Pathways to Work. Whilst these have improved incentives to get disabled people off benefits and back into work, much more still needs to be done. Future government policy should be designed to ensure that in 20 years any disabled person who wants a job and needs support to get and keep a job should, wherever possible, be able to do so. Assessments for incapacity benefit entitlement should be moved closer to the claim, and should be used to assess what support that person would need to get a job, rather than just to assess them for entitlement to benefit.

If all the report's recommendations are accepted and implemented, then by 2025 disabled adults who wish to work should be able to gain employment, achieve independent living and improve their quality of life. This should then reduce the amount of poverty and health inequalities that currently affect many disabled people.

## PARENTHOOD AND DISABILITY

With the implementation of the Disability Discrimination Acts and the European Manifesto, there is a greater awareness of the rights of the disabled woman. Yet awareness does not necessarily mean acceptance and disabled girls/women may still be marginalised by the non-disabled population. Section 6.1 of the Manifesto sets out: 'The right to have a family, relationships, sexual contacts, to be a mother, should be guaranteed for disabled women, in accordance with Standard Rule No 9' (p 8). (Standard Rule No 9 is part of the UN Standard Rules on the Equalisation of Opportunities for persons with Disabilities and the Beijing declaration and Platform for Action from the 4th World Conference on Women.) However, there is strong evidence to suggest that the 'normal' population does not think that disabled women should become mothers (for instance Asch & Fine 1997, Campion 1995, Morris 1991 and Neville-Jan 2004). Asch & Fine (1997) quote a 35 year old who had polio at the age of 5 years: 'Each time I announced I was pregnant, everyone in the family looked shocked, dropped their forks at the dinner table—not exactly a celebration' (p 241). There seems to be a belief that disabled women should not become mothers. In order to see where this view has come from the social construction of motherhood needs to be considered.

## MOTHERS/WIVES/LOVERS

If anyone in our society is asked what a mother is, the response is likely to be stereotypical. Apart from being someone who has given birth, she is usually associated with someone who cares, nurtures, looks after others, is often self-sacrificing and will always put the family first: very positive beliefs. If someone says they are a mother, it tells people a lot more about them than if a man said he was a father. Media images reinforce society's view of what a mother should be and when media headlines read 'the "home-alone" children left to fend for themselves by a terrible mother': no-one asks where the father is. If then, this imagery of what a mother should be is true, how can a disabled woman possibly be a mother? She needs caring for, possibly needs bathing, changing and feeding, so how can she do this for someone else? The opportunities of women with disabilities to nurture and be nurtured, and to be lovers and to be loved are constrained. They are less likely to fulfil their 'womanly' role, although it must be acknowledged that some women have no desire for this, disabled or not. If a disabled woman chooses to become pregnant, is she fit to be a parent? As recently as 1974, Sir Keith Joseph stated that a high proportion of children were being born to mothers who were unfit to bring them up, especially those who were single, teenage and lower socio-economic class (Campion 1995). The choice of parenthood is withheld from many disabled people through the disapproval of others, and there is less likely to be support for them if they cannot conceive naturally.

Disabled women generally are less likely to be married: in the 1980s only 49% of disabled women were married (Asch & Fine 1997). However, marriage is on the decline generally and today nearly half of babies born are to mothers not married. Interestingly, a woman with a learning disability is more likely to be married than one with a physical disability. Is this because she fits in with the criteria to be a good wife i.e. docile, passive and loyal?

Asch & Fine (1997) quoted the work of Brownmiller, who characterised nurturance when applied to women as 'warmth, tenderness, compassion, sustained emotional involvement in the welfare of others, and a weak or non-existent competitive drive' (p 221–222).

This sort of belief leads to the question: can a disabled woman minister to a man's needs? Partners of disabled women are often viewed with curiosity with questions posed such as, 'what did they see in the disabled woman in the first place'? There is a public assumption that this woman is a burden, her husband must be a 'saint' and that if she has a child, then he will do the entire extra care.

The media reinforces the prejudice as they only report on negative cases where children have had to be removed from disabled parents rather than positive stories that show how well everyone is coping.

More children born with disabilities are surviving now and living to child-bearing age and beyond. Their quality of life is better; they socialise, have sex and marry: things which years ago would have been seen as impossible (Campion 1995). They live independently and can determine their own life-style, but as parents, they remain 'invisible'. Is this because they do not want any interference or adverse comments about their disability? They may not be able to access popular places where families go to relax and meet other families, for example local parks, mother and toddler groups and family centres. Conversely, some disabled parents do make headlines, but this is often around 'how brave they are', not that they are perceived like 'normal' parents.

In order to become a parent, one assumes that individuals have to have been in a relationship first. This can prove difficult for some disabled people, particularly if they are dependent on carers looking after them. Sian Vasey (1996) writes about the problems of being a wheelchair user and her need for 'ongoing facilitation' with activities of daily living. This means that for a large part of her day there is a 'third person' present. However, the cover is not seamless but piecemeal which does allow her times when she is able to take 'risks' and act independently. She describes how her main problem is centred on how to have a sexual relationship when needing help getting to bed, turning over in bed, and getting up in the morning. Before anyone even thinks about intimacy there is the issue of everyday privacy, or lack of it, to consider. Sian found it difficult to separate friendship and what friends would do for her, from paid help and how much friendship was part of that. This confirms that any relationship can be difficult for someone dependent on other people for everyday living.

Taleporos & McCabe (2003) conducted a research study titled 'Relationships, sexuality and adjustment among people with physical disability'. It was a large study which recruited disabled people from different countries: United States of America, Australia, United Kingdom, Canada, New Zealand and a few from other parts of the world. Of the 1196 people who participated and completed a questionnaire, 748 identified themselves as having a physical disability and 448 without disability. Questions related to disability were only completed by those with a disability. Other questions related to self-esteem, general depression and anxiety, sexual esteem, sexual depression, sexual activity and sexual satisfaction.

The findings were interesting as, contrary to popular belief, many of the disabled participants reported an active and satisfying sex life. One of the main determinants of this was whether they were single or married, or in a stable relationship but living apart. The latter group reported the highest levels of satisfaction. The married group, both disabled and non-disabled reported the lowest levels of sexual satisfaction. Single disabled people often found it difficult to form sexual relationships, although this was age-related to some extent as disabled adolescents seemed to have as good a sexual relationship as their non-disabled counterparts. Women generally fared better at forming relationships than men and sexual adjustment appeared to be easier for disabled women. This is possibly because they have traditionally placed more emphasis on interpersonal aspects of sexuality, such as tenderness and emotional sharing. Some of the dissatisfaction reported by the married disabled participants was attributed to the difficulties of having a partner who was also a full-time carer. Disabled people who are in a relationship outside of marriage may be more likely to be together because they are fulfilled by the relationship, rather than as a result of obligation.

Overall the study indicated that physical disability and its severity are related to decreased opportunities for the formation of relationships. In terms of their psychological adjustment, single people with physical disabilities were not seriously disadvantaged when compared to their non-single counterparts. However, they were clearly disadvantaged in relation to their sexual esteem and their opportunities for sexual activity (Taleporos & McCabe 2003).

The authors conclude that perhaps interventions are required to increase the social interactions of people with physical disabilities. One hopes that with the integration of children with physical disabilities into state schools in the United Kingdom, then social interaction between disabled and non-disabled people will become the norm. The results also suggest that married couples where one of the partners is disabled may need more support if marital relationships are to be improved.

Once in a relationship it may not be very straightforward for a disabled woman to become pregnant. This may be because of physical difficulties having intercourse or because the woman may have problems with fertility, as many non-disabled women do. If she should require assisted conception, all sorts of problems may arise. Mukti Campion (1995) describes some of the problems faced by women needing 'the medical gift' of a child. In-vitro fertilisation (IVF) is available on the National Health Service (NHS) but certain criteria have to be met. These may vary from hospital to hospital but generally would also fulfil adoption criteria. These conditions relate to age, marital status, sexuality and residence, existence of other children, general health and normal range for body mass index (BMI). With the rationing of NHS resources and the desire for 'designer babies', disabled women may be disadvantaged by these criteria. At the end of the day, fertility consultants have the power to decide who they will treat and although some consultants may say that they will look at each request individually, disabled women may not be a high priority, particularly when resources are scarce. If the disability is due to a genetic disorder, then genetic counselling will be offered, but pregnancy may be discouraged if the risk of having an affected child is thought to be high.

## ADOPTION AND FOSTERING

If a disabled woman is unable to conceive and not considered a 'good' candidate for assisted reproduction, where to next in her bid to become a parent? It is not clear if the couple would be considered suitable to adopt a child by the adoption agencies. Adoption is a legal process whereby parental rights are transferred from the birth mother/father and invested in another person/couple. The Adoption Act 2004 has updated who may adopt and there is mention of same-sex couples being entitled to apply for adoption, but it does not specify whether people with disabilities can or cannot apply. However, there may be some clues from the Office of Public Sector Information (OPSI). On their website can be found The Adoption Agencies Regulations 2005 which clearly state that the adopter's medical practitioner should be contacted by the adoption agency, and in part 2 of Schedule 4 that agencies must report on the adopter's health including any serious disability or any mental health problems.

Adoptions are usually processed through adoption agencies with social workers who go out to the potential adopter's homes to ascertain whether they meet 'the criteria' for adoption. Whilst the law deals with age and residency, each agency constructs its own requirements for suitability. As there are fewer babies available for adoption these days, older children may be offered instead. But if someone uses a wheelchair or has learning disabilities they may not be considered suitable. Nevertheless, it is increasingly difficult to look for the traditional 'ideal' couple for many of the children now available for adoption. 'Suitable' parents are becoming scarce and the need to find 'unusual parents for unusual children' means that the assessment criteria may be broadened (Campion 1995). In other words a disabled couple might be considered 'fit' to adopt a disabled child.

The Children Act 1989 puts the welfare of the child as paramount and therefore alternative care must be in the child's 'best interests'. However, who determines what the child's best interests are and do stereotypical ideas about people with disabilities prevent them from being considered as adoptive or foster parents? No one is denying that being an adoptive or foster parent is difficult; there is no pregnancy during which to get to know the baby and to be psychologically prepared; and there may be emotional issues associated with being unable to conceive. There is only uncertainty about what is going to happen. Despite these caveats many parents and children come through the procedure to their mutual satisfaction. Anyone who did not feel able to give a child a warm and loving environment would not apply to adopt, therefore disabled couples should be able to apply for the same reasons.

In spite of this, there is a lot of pressure on social services to 'get it right' when looking at child-care and child protection. Campion (1995) argues that it may be this outside pressure that discourages agencies from placing children for adoption with disabled people.

## SEPARATION/DIVORCE

Divorce is common in our society with a divorce rate of 14 in 2003, i.e. the number of couples divorcing per 1000 married couples (Office for National Statistics 2006). Legislation is available to ensure that both parties and any children are dealt with fairly and equitably. In custody disputes (now called residency disputes) the issue becomes one not just of parent's rights versus children's rights, but also between the individual parents' rights (Campion 1995). The usual outcome for couples who parted was for the mother to gain residency and the father to be granted reasonable access (unless child abuse or domestic abuse was proven).

For many women with disabilities this has not always been the case as there is great concern as to whether they can look after the child or children on their own. The breakdown of the marriage may be considered to be her 'fault' because of her disability, particularly if her husband is able-bodied. However, Nosek et al's (2001) National Study of Women with Physical Disabilities indicates that more than half the women interviewed believed that disability was not a major cause of the marriage or relationship ending. The report also found that women with disabilities were significantly more likely to stay in a bad marriage for fear of 'losing' the child or children. If the disabled woman wanted residency, there would be many investigations by social workers into her ability to care for the child appropriately and there would also be concerns that the child would become a 'carer' for its mother.

## TOWARDS AN ENABLING SOCIETY?

In this chapter, I have explored how disability and motherhood have been socially constructed. Some negative perspectives have been put forward but some positive aspects have also been included. To emphasise these, the lived experiences of women with disabilities need to be appreciated. Nosek (Nosek et al 2001) introduces the National Study of Women with Physical Disabilities: Final Report with an account of her own feelings as a disabled woman, brought up with all the negative stereotypes and beliefs about being disabled. She explains that in undertaking the research, she found out that many women with those stereotypes have overcome their effects and have had 'wonderful success' (p 6) in developing relationships, families and satisfying lives. Many of the women who have achieved this were not meant to survive; they have beaten the odds and achieved their potential, despite the society they live in and not because of it. In this chapter some such women have been included: Mukti Champion, Alison Lapper, Jenny Morris and Ann Neville-Jan. By making the lives of women with disabilities more visible, challenging common thoughts and beliefs and encouraging other women to not just accept their lot but fight for their rights, these authors have shown how a positive outlook on disability can improve self-esteem, the ability to form relationships and the chance of becoming mothers, if so desired.

Ann Macfarlane (1996) offers insight into the key issues in daily practice when dealing with people with disabilities and formulating care. If these points are followed by healthcare planners, it might make the lives of people with disabilities more fulfilling. Below is a synopsis of the key points she makes:

- Having knowledge and balanced information gives the individual the power to make decisions and choices, and experience leads to confidence.
- Professionals need to work in partnership with individuals in formulating plans and setting aims and objectives, and not assume they know best. Roles and responsibilities should be clearly defined and agreed and the uniqueness of an individual's life-style recognised and respected.
- Mutual trust and respect develop from effective communication, transparency, honesty and confidentiality.

- Needs may be perceived differently by individuals and carers, therefore priorities should be identified through effective communication and reference to influencing factors. Creativity and innovative ideas may be required to meet needs.

Legislation is in place and the UK Disability Forum's manifesto by Disabled Women in Europe (1999) gives hope for the future rights of women with disabilities. However, unless the prevailing stereotypes can be overcome, it is going to be some time before there is a definite change for the better and women with disabilities will become more visible.

---

## CONCLUSION—KEY POINTS

- Disability is difficult to define and means different things to different people—the term impairment may be more acceptable to someone who does not feel disabled.
- Language is a powerful tool—words can stigmatise, insult and prevent the formation of a positive identity.
- Non-disabled people often believe that life for disabled people is not worth living.
- The concept of 'norm' and multiple stereotypes serve to marginalise and give a negative perspective but people with disabilities value their difference.
- The powerful medical model of disability expects conformity but the social model may not reflect the lived experience of disability. Non-disability and disability are a continuum rather than discrete states.
- Charities may have perpetuated disability stereotypes and do not always provide sensitive care. Community care may actually prevent access to available services.
- Disabled women have a right to relationships, sexual contacts and to be mothers. But marriage and forming sexual relationships are challenging. Assisted conception is not always available if needed.
- Integrating young people into normal schools improves their chances of forming relationships.

■ Discrimination exists despite legislation—women are particularly vulnerable. The Manifesto by Disabled Women in Europe hopes to address discrimination yet separated/divorced women may find it difficult to get residency of their children if their partner is non-disabled.

■ A positive outlook on life can help disabled women achieve their potential.

## References

Acheson D 1998 Independent inquiry into inequalities in health report. HMSO, London

Adoption Act 2004 HMSO, London

Asch A, Fine M 1997 Nurturance, sexuality and women with disabilities: the example of women and literature. In: Davis L J (ed) The disabilities studies reader. Routledge, London, p 241–259

Baldwin S 1993 The myth of community care: an alternative neighbourhood model of care. Chapman & Hall, London

BBC 1 2006 One life — to see and be seen. BBC television, channel 1, 24 May 2006

Campion M J 1995 Who's fit to be a parent? Routledge, London

Children Act 1989 HMSO, London

Community Care Act 1990 HMSO, London

Corker M, French S 1999 Disability discourse. Open University Press, Buckingham

Cunningham C, Davis H 1985 Working with parents: a framework for collaboration. Open University Press, Milton Keynes

Davis L J 1997 The disability studies reader. Routledge, London

Deafworks 1999 'Opening Up' in association with London Borough of Camden, Arts & Tourism, Deafworks, London

Disability Discrimination Act 1995 HMSO, London. Online. Available: http://www.drc-gb.org 12 Sept 2005

Disability Discrimination Act—Special Educational Needs 2001 HMSO, London

Equal Opportunity Act 1975 HMSO, London

European Disability Forum 1999 Manifesto by Disabled Women in Europe. UK Disability Forum Women's Committee. Online. Available: http://www.edfwomen.org.uk/manifesto.htm 10 Sept 2005

Hubbard R 1997 Abortion and disability. In: Davis L (ed) The disability studies reader. Routledge, London, p 187–202

Hughes G 1998 Constructions of disability. In: Saraga E (ed) Embodying the social: constructions of difference. Routledge with the Open University, London, p 44–88

Lapper A 2005 My life in my hands. Simon and Schuster, London. Extracts Online. Available: http://www.alisonlapper.com 9 June 2006

Macfarlane A 1996 Aspects of intervention, consultation, care, help and support. In: Hayes G (ed) Beyond disability towards an enabling society. Sage Publications with The Open University, London, p 6–18

McLaughlin J 2003 Screening Networks: shared agendas in feminist and disability movement challenges to antenatal screening and abortion. Disability and Society 18(3):297–310

Marsh B 2006 As toll of Down's victims leaps, the boy doctors wanted to abort at 35 weeks. The Sunday Telegraph May 21st front page

Miles D 1988 British Sign Language — a beginner's guide. BBC Books, London

Morris J 1991 Pride against prejudice. The Women's Press, London

Morris J 1993 Women confronting disability. In: Clarke J (ed) A crisis in care? Challenges to social work. The Open University, London, p 122–131

Morris J 1996 Pride against prejudice: 'Lives not worth living'. In: Davey B, Gray A, Seale C (eds) Health and disease: a reader. 2nd edn. Open University Press, Buckingham, p 107–110

Neville-Jan A 2004 Selling your soul to the devil: an autoethnography of pain, pleasure and the quest for a child. Disability and Society 19(2):113–127

Nosek MA, Howland C, Rintala DH et al 2001 National study of women with physical disabilities: final report. Sexuality and Disability 19(1):5–39

Office for National Statistics 2006 Divorce rates for the year 2003. Online. Available: http://www.statistics.gov.uk 17 June 2006

Office of Public Sector Information (OPSI) 2005 Statutory instrument no.389. The adoption agencies regulations. Online. Available: http://www.opsi.gov.uk 9 June 2006

Prime Minister's Strategy Unit (2005) Improving the life chances of disabled people. Online. Available: http://www.strataegy.gov.uk 9 November 2006

Race Relations Act 1975 HMSO, London

Shakespeare T, Watson N 2002 The social model of disability: an outdated ideology? Research in Social Science and Disability 2:9–28

Smith C 1996 Sign language companion — a handbook of British signs. Human Horizons

Series. Souvenir Press (Educational and Academic), London

Swain J, Cameron C 1999 Unless otherwise stated: discourse in labelling and identity in coming out. In: Corker M, French S (eds) Disability discourse. Open University Press, Buckingham, p 68–78

Taleporos G, McCabe MP 2003 Relationships, sexuality and adjustment among people with physical disability. Sexual and Relationship Therapy 18(1):25–43

Taylor G, Bishop J 1991 Being deaf: the experience of deafness. Pinter in association with Open University Press, London

Townsend P 1992 Inequalities in health: the black report and the health divide. Penguin, London

Trevvy D (editorial executive) 2000 Collins English Dictionary. 5th edn. Collins, London

Vasey S 1996 The experience of care. In: Hayes G (ed) Beyond disability towards an enabling society. Sage Publications with the Open University, London, p 82–87

Vernon A, Swain J 2002 Theorising divisions and hierarchies. In: Barnes C, Oliver M, Barton L (eds) Disability studies today. Policy press with Blackwell Publishers, Cambridge, p 77–97

World Health Organisation (WHO) 2001 ICF: International classification of functioning, disability and health. World Health Organisation, Geneva

# 2 Women's health and disability

*Stella McKay-Moffat, Pam Lee*

## INTRODUCTION

The promotion of health and a healthy life-style, and the availability of health promotion strategies or intervention plans to rectify any lack of well-being are very much on political, health professional and societal agendas. Issues related to all elements of health and well-being form as much of a concern to a woman with a disability as they are to any other woman. However, these have not always been recognised by the providers of health services, therefore requirements have often gone unmet. Whilst the majority of issues can be addressed via the usual channels, some alternative or additional strategies may need to be considered.

In this chapter we will discuss some health issues pertinent to women and aim to raise the reader's awareness of the needs of women with a disability related to those topics, and how those needs may be met. For midwives knowledge of the relevant issues and the impact they may have on women has an important influence on their ability to provide holistic care during the whole of women's childbirth experience. Of equal or even greater importance is the need to understand how those issues may influence the well-being of women with a disability to ensure that care provision is sensitive to an individual woman's situation.

## GENERAL HEALTH ISSUES

The health concerns of women with a disability are no different to those of all women. This includes the need for general information about nutrition, weight, mental health and health screening services (Welner & Temple 2004), as well as matters specifically pertinent to women's health including reproduction, contraception, cervical and breast screening. At the same time physical access to services must be ensured. Once there, appropriate equipment needs to be available to enable examinations to be undertaken as comfortably as possible and with privacy and dignity. Additional time is commonly needed for history taking and to enable preparation for examination when mobility is limited. For women with sensory impairment this latter aspect will need additional thought, for example guidance to an examination couch may be needed, and the practitioner must be in a position to ensure that communication with women who are hard of hearing is possible during the examination. Furthermore, when health services are offered to women with a disability other medical issues and challenges with physical and cognitive ability may need to be taken into consideration.

## WOMEN'S HEALTH ISSUES

The health needs of women with a disability related to specific 'women's' issues are increasingly being acknowledged as not being adequately met, for example Jackson & Wadley (1999) report that women with spinal cord injury were less likely to have a routine mammogram. This discrimination goes against the 'equal opportunities for all' ethos and legislation of a civilised society (for example in the UK the Disability Discrimination Act 1995, in the USA the Americans with Disabilities Act 1990 and the Manifesto by Disabled Women in Europe (UK Disability Forum 1999)) that stipulates that all public services should be available to *everyone,* which of course includes health services.

Factors influencing women's experiences of accessing health services were clearly demonstrated in two American studies (Becker et al 1997, Nosek et al 1995). These included the women's previous encounters with medical care, their own knowledge about reproductive health, and inaccessibility to reproductive health services. This latter factor not only included physical access to facilities but related to service policies, and the attitudes of the professionals providing those services. Insensitive practitioners often appeared surprised that the women were sexually active. As a result of all of these factors, women tended to avoid gynaecological visits.

Women's disability studies and discourse have done much to bring the inadequacy of women's health services to the forefront of understanding. Lonsdale (1990) presented a feminist perspective on the experiences of women with disabilities related to issues of gender and sexuality. She identified the key points as those concerning the lack of information about sexual activity, contraception and childbirth. Murphy & Young's (2005) review of American literature and research from the late 1990s and early 2000 found that young people with disabilities continued to be less likely to have received information about reproduction and contraception.

Morris (1995) had earlier identified these themes from her study of questionnaires from 205 women paralysed by spinal cord injuries. In her chapter on sexuality and child-bearing she highlighted the prejudice women experienced towards their sexuality, and the lack of research and advice on contraception. Additionally, the deficit of information on sexually transmitted infections (STIs) has been highlighted (for example Becker et al 1997, Kallianes & Rubenfeld 1997). Much of this may be associated with the opinion of professionals and society that people with a disability are asexual (Becker et al 1997, Kallianes & Rubenfeld 1997, Lonsdale 1990). But women and adolescents with a disability are just as likely to have sexual desires and needs as their non-disabled peers as Choquet et al's French study (1997) and Sawin et al's American study (2002) revealed.

However, historically the stigma of disability and the common misconception that disability is hereditary fuelled the belief in the past (and possibly still today) that women with a disability should not have children. Demonstration of society's disapproval has come from the lived experiences of the women. Campion (1990) and Shackle (1994) reported the negative attitudes women had received had related to their sexuality and parenthood, often manifested as distaste and overt discussed towards them. This, it could be argued, had occurred because of society's attraction to individuals they perceive as beautiful, and the belief that anyone 'less than normal' is unattractive.

At the same time as people with physical disability were perceived as asexual the potential sexuality of people with learning difficulties had been recognised and caused concern. Clarke & McCree (1986) and Whitman & Accardo (1990) pointed to the Eugenics Society in Britain and America during the late nineteenth and early twentieth centuries when it was believed that the nation's intelligence would be diluted if people with learning difficulties were 'allowed' to reproduce. Institutionalisation and gender segregation became the accepted 'remedy' for this 'problem'. Forced sterilisation (Whitman & Accardo 1990) and automatic termination of pregnancy (Gates 2001) have been other methods of denying women with disabilities the opportunity of motherhood. These actions may have resulted from family and professionals' concerns about a woman's ability to cope with pregnancy and a child, fears of producing a child with a disability, or an endeavour to protect the family and society from the burden of caring for a child.

In contrast, the feminist perspective of women with disability is the right to have children and not to have a pregnancy automatically terminated. However, this is a direct contradiction to traditional feminist thinking that women should have the right to abortion on demand (Kallianes & Rubenfeld 1997, Morris 1991). Indeed, Morris (1991) argued that 'quality-of-life' issues had not been addressed by these feminists and she contended that no one should make value judgements on another person's life.

## SEXUALITY

### Models

Disability activists advocate a social model of disability rather than a medical model although both models have been challenged with the more holistic model from the World Health Organisation (WHO): the International Classification of Functioning, Disability and Health (ICF). Tom Shakespeare (1996) expanded the social model of disability, by proposing that it should encompass sexuality and replace the predominant medical model that relates a lack of sexuality to physical incapacity. He also feels that society's expectation of asexuality is linked to the perception of people with a disability as child-like because of their dependence on help. However, Blackburn (2003) postulates that asexuality may have been perpetuated by failure of researchers to publish study results that revealed the reality that refuted asexuality. She argues that this is either because they lacked solutions to identified issues or because of concerns about society's response to their findings. Yet for some women, being viewed as asexual may be an advantage as the pressure to marry and have children as a 'societal norm' may be absent (Swain et al 2003).

## Body image

Everyone is influenced by their life experiences, inter-actions with others and personal expectations. These help to build up an individual's perception of self and 'fit' within society. The challenges of everyday life to fulfil personal expectations for someone with a physical or cognitive disability may need not only a positive attitude, but alternative solutions or different ways of thinking to overcome social, psychological and emotional barriers.

Body image has a powerful influence on an indi-vidual's behaviour. People with a congenital disabil-ity who see the disability as part of who they are may or may not be happy with their body. A person with an acquired disability may have held strong nega-tive attitudes towards people with a disability before becoming disabled. This may then lead to negative feelings about self and how others see them, includ-ing partner, family and friends. The resulting loss of self-esteem could affect their whole perception of self including body image and sexuality. Psychosexual consequences may result.

## Psychosexual issues

Practically every chronic or debilitating condition has the potential to cause sexual dysfunction (Goodwin & Agronin 1997). Healthcare professionals do not often ask questions about sex during routine exami-nations; there is a stereotypical view that if you have a disability then you are not interested in sex and so the subject is not raised. However, this is not the case and sexual function is an important part of all our lives. Disability is a term encompassing a vast number of issues; people with disabilities are not a homogenous group any more than people without disabilities are and it is therefore difficult to say what sexual problems may be encountered.

One of the main aspects of physical disability/illness that are likely to cause problems is pain. The body shuts down thoughts of sexual desire if the person is feeling pain. Acute pain can also shut down the sexual response cycle and when an individual has pain that is chronic and debilitating, then desire and arousal shut down on a long-term basis (Goodwin & Agronin 1997). Normal sexual response is dependent on normal brain and periph-eral nervous system function, intact genital nerve pathways and adequate supplies of sex hormones (Bancroft 1989). Depending on the type of disabil-ity, there may be a disturbance in the nerve path-ways, endocrine function and blood supply to the reproductive tract which can have an adverse effect on sexual response. Add to these problems the nega-tive effects of poor body image and low self-esteem, general lack of confidence and performance anxi-ety and it becomes obvious why some people with disabilities have psychosexual problems.

Muscle spasm may be another area of concern; if there is some spasticity of the lower limbs then full penetration may be difficult. The couple need to experiment with different positions and aim to be as relaxed as possible. There is a lot more to sexual pleasure than just penetration, and caress-ing, kissing and mutual masturbation can produce orgasm and sexual satisfaction without full inter-course. Catherine Kalamis (2003) in her self-help book 'Women without sex' describes a variety of exercises including fantasizing which can improve love-making techniques.

Another problem which may be encountered is vaginismus. This is the involuntary contraction of the muscles which support and surround the vagina and when they go into spasm, penetration becomes impossible and attempting it is very painful. Fear of penetration can then make the situation worse and the vaginismus increases, thus setting up a vicious circle: fear of penetration, fear of pain, increased vaginismus, and so on. A factor to additionally consider is a history of childhood sexual abuse as this is one of the potential causes of vaginismus. But often there is no such history and the cause may be unclear, although it is usually psychological in origin. Perhaps a strict upbringing, negative views of sex within the family, fear of pregnancy, religious and cultural influences all have a part to play.

Psychosexual therapy includes looking at a sexual growth programme for a woman, increasing her sense of self as a sexual person and her knowledge about normal sexual response which may help to alleviate some of the fear and tension. Vaginal trainers can be used to try and overcome the vaginismus: small trainers the size of a little finger can be used initially with a lubricant to help insertion. A woman will be taught relaxation exercises to assist her during the insertion of the trainer. Gradually, and in her own time, a woman will be encouraged to use trainers of increasing diameter until a 'penis-sized' one can be inserted. Then she and her partner should be encouraged to try penetration, preferably with her in the superior position so that she has the control (Hawtin 1985).

If the partner is aware of the pain and anxiety suffered by the disabled person, he may also develop sexual dysfunction and put up barriers to sexual activity. Another issue is that he may be the disabled person's main carer; if he is attending to the personal hygiene and toileting needs, he may not find that person 'sexy' or desirable. Sian Vasey (1996), a wheelchair user dependent on a 'care package' to enable her to live independently, describes the problems faced when trying to form employment relationships (her carers) and sexual relationships. One of the issues she highlights is how difficult it is to have a sexual relationship when there is often a 'third party' present as well, attending to other personal needs. She also emphasises the problems of determining what friendship is, how much help can friends be expected to give (like helping her to the toilet) and where does this fit in with paid carers? She concludes that forming close and intimate relationships can prove difficult and quite daunting. Despite some of these negative aspects, however, many disabled women have perfectly adequate/satisfactory sex lives and good relationships with their partners (Taleporos & McCabe 2003).

Whilst there has been little research into sexuality and women with disabilities generally, one area that has been investigated is sexual response in women with spinal cord injuries. Tepper et al (2001) and Whipple & Komisaruk (1997), researchers at the Kessler Institute for Rehabilitation in West Orange New Jersey, conducted a survey into the sexual responses of women with spinal cord injuries. Over half the women in the trial were able to achieve orgasm regardless of the pattern or degree of neurological injury. Those women who achieved orgasm also had a higher sex drive and a greater sexual knowledge. However, some women in another study said that they shut down all thoughts of sexual activity as they felt that they could not achieve orgasm due to loss of sensation in the genital area (Kalamis 2003, p 50). Research now shows that sexual activity can be resumed and enjoyed despite grave injury, as the vagus nerve, thought to be responsible for transmitting sexual pleasure sensations, can be stimulated from other parts of the body and not just from the genitalia (Whipple & Komisaruk 1997).

Loss of desire is a symptom of depression and some people with chronic and debilitating pain can become depressed. Sometimes the anti-depressants used for treatment can have an adverse effect on sexual function; they can suppress sexual desire and make the situation worse rather than better. Good management of the physical condition, prevention of anaemia and other conditions which may cause fatigue can help improve sexual function and alleviate the feelings of depression (Kalamis 2003).

Women with disabilities are as much at risk of gynaecological problems as any other woman. If dyspareunia (painful intercourse) is a problem, the assumption should not be that it is part of the disability; a woman needs a full pelvic examination to exclude pelvic pathology such as endometriosis. If there is gynaecological pathology, then appropriate treatment should be given, but add to that general advice about positions for love-making, taking into account mobility issues. Sometimes just changing the position to female superior can help alleviate deep dyspareunia. If superficial dyspareunia is the problem, advice about foreplay to increase arousal and lubrication or the use of added lubricants to ease penetration may help improve sexual function.

Continence problems can interfere with sexual activity and advice may be needed about bowel evacuation and emptying of the bladder prior to intimacy and how to manage if there is an indwelling catheter. Again, there may be problems with lack of lubrication and a water-based lubricant may be all that is required to improve the situation. Women with stomas may have body image concerns and be anxious about the response of a partner to the stoma.

Women must be their own advocates regarding sexual activity. If they have pain which is interfering with their engagement in love-making, then they need to seek help and obtain more adequate pain control (Goodwin & Agronin 1997). There should be more easily accessible information about sexual function as knowledge about the normal sexual response can help the couple develop a more satisfactory sexual relationship. Support groups may be able to offer advice regarding sexual activity for people with specific disabilities such as multiple sclerosis or spina bifida.

Sexual awareness is important and it is helpful for a woman to know her own limitations, strengths and weaknesses. Couples should focus on sexual activities within these boundaries and avoid unrealistic expectations, for example if it is not physically possible then it should not be tried. Women can build up their physical strength with exercises so that sexual activity becomes a possibility. Prior to sexual activity, women should make sure that they are well rested and could try relaxation exercises, setting the scene, e.g. using candles or aromatherapy, and plan for the event by introducing some romance. Different positions could be tried and there is no need to rush; sensuous stroking and caressing and time spent on finding out what pleases each other can be beneficial to the couple (Heiman & LoPiccolo 1992). Attitude is very important; women need to remember that they are a person first, and disabled or physically compromised second. With a little preparation and planning, sexual activity can be very rewarding and a lot of fun.

## Relationships

Women who have congenital disabilities may have been segregated during childhood and have had a lack of opportunity to form relationships. If the disability occurred during adolescence, which is a major time of physical and psychological upheaval, the individual may have found it hard enough to come to terms with the disability without having to worry about sexual identity and forming relationships. Young people may not have been given sex education or adequate information about where to seek help and advice as they are considered 'asexual'. There is an emphasis on sexual behaviour being all about penetration and there is not enough emphasis on sexual pleasure being gained through touching, caressing and warm, loving and intimate relationships. Young people are often under pressure from their peers to have full penetrative sex, but it is up to the individual and they need advice, counselling and support to empower them to make their own decisions.

Teenagers often meet parental disapproval and financial constraints when trying to meet others and initiate relationships. For the teenager with a disability, challenges with mobility, personal acceptability and incontinence may need solutions. A lack of self-identity and independence may be compounded by isolation from peers and an inability to develop relationships (Blackburn 2002). This limited social experience and any medical conditions may delay the acquisition of sexual knowledge. But this is not only true for the teenage years. For all people with disabilities inhibited access to leisure and social events or exclusion from the workforce due to physical, psychological and social barriers lessens opportunities to meet others, make friends and develop close and intimate relationships (Shakespeare 1996). Nevertheless, Murphy & Young (2005) found that young people were just as likely to experience sexual activity at a similar age as their non-disabled peers although generally on fewer occasions.

Blackburn (2002) found that people with spina bifida had normal sexual needs and drive. Ann Neville-Jan (2004) gives a graphic account of the problems she faced when trying to have a loving and satisfying sexual relationship with her husband. Normal sex drive was present, but pain and depression, treated with anti-depressants, meant that there was loss of pleasure as anorgasmia developed. As her husband commented: 'It seems to me like selling your soul to the devil, trading relief of pain for loss of pleasure' (p 113). Changing medication can sometimes improve the outlook by giving adequate pain relief, whilst still retaining the ability to achieve orgasm.

## Sex education

Sexual activity is still a sensitive topic for discussion for the majority of people despite the apparent openness of society to sexuality. Everyone has the right to information and the opportunity to discuss their own pertinent issues and seek help where required. This should preferably occur in private without the individual's helper unless communication difficulties are present. Nuefeld et al (2002) offer a list of topics for addressing sexuality for teenagers but this is no different from that which should be offered to all teenagers or those denied the opportunity at that time in their lives.

These topics cover the whole spectrum from the basic facts of life to reproduction and parenthood, the right to choose when and if to have relationships, contraception and STIs. This then increases the opportunity for individuals to embark on safe and fulfilling relationships. Therefore, it is not a question of *if* these issues are addressed, but how appropriate information can be effectively offered to aid leaning. However, equity of opportunity for sex education may not always be available.

Blackburn (2002) compared a group of young American people with spina bifida and/or hydrocephalus (SB/HC) with a matched non-disabled (control) group. She found that 80% of the SB/HC group had received some sex education whilst at school compared to 94% of the control group. Few had received any education outside of school. Of greater concern was the fact that only 18% of the SC/HC group had received any specific education about sex and disability. When asked, their main concerns related to sexuality were urinary and faecal incontinence.

Blackburn (2002) discovered that the participants in her study preferred educational media in video format and simple leaflets or magazines which enabled repeated review of the information. Whatever format is utilised it should readily aid and reinforce learning. Making use of appropriate and realistic models, audible and visual/tactile aids with active rather than passive learning will enhance the quality of the learning experience. This may be facilitated either individually or in a group setting depending on the individual's comfort, inhibitions, and levels of perceived embarrassment, as with all people.

## CONTRACEPTION

The key factors for successful contraception for any woman or couple are availability, acceptability and suitability (see Table 2.1 for a summary). But barriers to obtaining contraception may exist for women with a disability because of the attitudes or a lack of knowledge of their helpers or health providers (Welner 1997). These involve inappropriate or negative viewpoints towards their desire or need for contraception and a lack of knowledge about women's potential needs and methods suitable to meet their specific requirements (see Table 2.1). Nevertheless, women with a disability are entitled to access family planning and contraception services which form, as Drey & Darney state '.....part of providers' responsibility to acknowledge the full lives and health needs of people who are disabled' (2004, p 122). However, professionals do not always ask about contraception use; this is perhaps linked to their surprise that women are indeed often sexually active (Becker et al 1997).

Spacing of pregnancies is often an important consideration for women with a disability. The ability to manage a small child may be compromised by the arrival of a second. Recovery time may also need to be considered between pregnancies to allow for maximum health to be regained (Cooper & Guillebaud 1999). For these reasons women may wish to limit their families, therefore effective contraception is essential.

## Availability

In the UK locally based family planning clinics offer counselling, confidential advice and free contraceptives to all clients, including emergency post-coital methods. Generally all of the readily available contraceptives approved for use in the NHS are stocked including intrauterine devices, implants, hormonal methods, cervical caps and condoms. Intrauterine devices (coils) and intrauterine systems (a coil with a progesterone stem) and progesterone implants may not be fitted at all clinics. However, clinic staff can make referrals and appointments for clients to attend clinics offering these services.

Many general practitioners offer contraceptive advice (including emergency hormonal post-coital contraception) and free prescriptions, although these

*Table 2.1* **Contraceptive method availability, suitability and acceptability for women with disability**

| Method | Availability | Failure rate[a] | Ease of use | Advantages | Disadvantages/ possible risks |
|---|---|---|---|---|---|
| Male condom | Free at family planning clinics Readily available for purchase in varied retail outlets | 2% | Application prior to intercourse or any genital contact Requires dexterity for application & removal by the male or his partner | No medical implications except latex allergy—polyurethane available Ease of acquisition Can always have available *Some* protection against STIs[b] & human papilloma virus that causes cervical cancer | May inhibit spontaneity in love-making Incorrect application/ removal may lead to method failure e.g. from condom damage or semen spillage Polyurethane splits more easily Damaged by oil-based creams e.g. petroleum jelly & Gyno-Daktarin |
| Female condom | Purchased at pharmacies | 5% | Insertion prior to intercourse or any genital contact Leg abduction needed Requires considerable dexterity for correct insertion by woman or partner | No medical implications except latex allergy Can always have available Some protection against STIs[b] & human papilloma virus that causes cervical cancer | May inhibit spontaneity in love-making The need to touch genitalia may be unacceptable Poor perineal sensation e.g. due to spinal cord injury, inability to abduct legs, tremor or poor fine movement may inhibit correct insertion/removal Rustles during use which may be 'off putting' Method failure due to penile penetration outside of the condom, or incorrect positioning or removal |
| Combined oral contraceptive pill (COC) (oestrogen & progesterone) | Prescribed at family planning clinics or by GP Free of charge | Less than 1% | Small & easily swallowed 12-hour safety time[c] Cognitive ability & no chaotic life-style to ensure regular/timely use Possibly some joint improvement in rheumatoid arthritis | No inhibition of spontaneity in love-making Menstruation very regular Blood loss light—less hygiene issues & anaemia 3 packs can be taken consecutively to avoid withdrawal bleeding | Reduced reliability with some medication e.g. carbamazepine (Tegretol) used in MS & epilepsy, St John's Wort Increases effects of beta blockers, diazepam & corticosteroids DVT[d] risk if circulation poor or higher coagulation potential due to immobility |

*table continued*

*table continued*

| Method | Availability | Failure rate[a] | Ease of use | Advantages | Disadvantages/ possible risks |
|---|---|---|---|---|---|
| | | | | | Reliability diminishes with a bout of diarrhoea, or broad-spectrum antibiotics e.g. ampicillin (use additional method for at least 7 days after the episode/treatment) Risk of pregnancy with delayed or missed pill Less suitable for women over 35, those obese & smokers Unsuitable if breast-feeding |
| Progesterone only pill (POP) ('Mini pill') | Prescribed at family planning clinics or by GP Free of charge | 1% | Small and easily swallowed 3-hour safety time[c] (New Cerazette has a 12-hour safety time) Cognitive ability & no chaotic life-style *essential* to ensure regular/ timely use | No inhibition of spontaneity in love-making Very reliable if taken promptly every day Suitable in many cases when COC not e.g. with certain conditions, for over 35s, when DVT[d] risk & when breast-feeding Menstrual flow may lessen/cease—less hygiene issues & anaemia | Reliability may be reduced by some medication (see COC above) & body weight over 70 kg Short safety time—high risk of pregnancy with delayed or missed pill Some side effects such as headache & fluid retention may be unacceptable Irregular menstruation possible Long-term use unclear about affects on bone density |
| Depo Provera (long-acting progesterone injection in an oily preparation) | Prescribed & injected at family planning clinics or by GP Free of charge | Less than 1% | One intramuscular injection regularly every 11–12 weeks into buttock/large muscle as more painful in smaller muscle Cognitive ability or guidance from helper to ensure effective uptake | No inhibition of spontaneity in love-making Suitable in many cases when COC not (see POP above) Menstruation may cease after initial irregularity/heavy loss—less hygiene issues & anaemia | Reliability may be reduced by some medication (see COC above) Injections may be unacceptable or large muscle not available/accessible Side effects as with POP—weight gain—may affect mobility Irregular menstruation possible Return of fertility may be delayed after discontinuation |

*table continued*

*table continued*

| Method | Availability | Failure rate[a] | Ease of use | Advantages | Disadvantages/ possible risks |
|---|---|---|---|---|---|
| Skin implants (slow-release progesterone) e.g. Implanon | Prescribed & inserted/ removed at family planning clinics (some GPs) under local anaesthetic Free of charge | Less than 1% | Single 'rod' inserted under skin of the underside of upper arm Changed every 3 years (see Fig. 2.2) | No inhibition of spontaneity in love-making Infrequent attendance at clinics needed Small but constant daily dose released = less side effects Fertility may return more readily after removal than with Depo Provera Suitable when COC not (see POP above) Menstruation benefits (see Depo Provera above) | Reliability may be reduced by some medication (see COC above) Insertion procedure may be unacceptable Removal may be difficult Skin may initially be uncomfortable Side effects as with POP above Long-term use possible loss of bone density |
| Combined patch (Evra) progesterone & oestrogen | Some family planning clinics & GPs | 1% | 5 cm × 5 cm skin patch 3 patches in total—1 patch lasts 7 days then changed These 21 days followed by 7 days patch-free Withdrawal bleed in this time Repeat cycle (see Fig. 2.1) | Lower overall dose than COC Steady blood levels of hormones Useful in a chaotic life-style/difficulty remembering a daily pill/reminder from a helper Reliable when broad spectrum antibiotics taken 3 cycles can be used without a break to avoid withdrawal bleeds | See COC above Reliability reduced if weight over 90 kg Skin sensitivity in some women Spotting during first 1–3 cycles |
| Emergency contraception (high dose of progesterone) (see intrauterine system & IUCD below for alternative method) | Free at family planning & STI[b] clinics Prescribed by GP (free) Purchased from some prescribing pharmacists at approximately £26 | 5% within 24 hours 15% 25–48 hours 42% 49–72 hours | 1 pill taken within 72 hours of unprotected intercourse or failed method e.g. condom split | Prevention of fertilization & implantation Can have a supply in as back-up for failure of method— more effective with minimal time delay | See POP above |

*table continued*

*table continued*

| Method | Availability | Failure rate[a] | Ease of use | Advantages | Disadvantages/ possible risks |
|---|---|---|---|---|---|
| Intrauterine system e.g. Mirena (a coil with progesterone) (see Fig. 2.3) | Prescribed & inserted/ removed at family planning clinics (few GPs) with local anaesthetic often to cervix Free of charge | Minimal | Chlamydia screening prior to insertion Replaced every 5 years Leg abduction needed for insertion | No inhibition of spontaneity in love-making Infrequent attendance at clinics needed 2 contraceptives in one raises reliability Small but constant daily progesterone released—less side effects Fertility may return more readily after removal than with Depo Provera Suitable in many cases when COC not (see POP above) Menstruation benefits (see Depo Provera above) Used as emergency contraception within 5 days of unprotected intercourse/failed method | Progesterone efficiency may be reduced by some medication (see COC above) Insertion may be unacceptable to woman Leg abduction needed for fitting—may be difficult with arthritis/leg spasms with MS[e] or cerebral palsy Less easy/more painful to fit if woman not had a child Risk of autonomic dysreflexia on insertion when woman has spinal cord lesion (see Chapter 8) May initially cause heavy periods/excess pain Unrecognised pain of PID[f] if pelvic sensation poor e.g. with spinal lesion, or poor under-standing e.g. with learning disability |
| Intrauterine contraceptive device (IUCD) (coil) (see Fig. 2.3) | Fitted at family planning clinics & a few GPs Free of charge | Less than 1% | Chlamydia screening prior to insertion Replaced approx. every 5 years— higher copper content increases time Leg abduction needed for insertion | No inhibition of spontaneity in love-making Infrequent attendance at clinics needed May also be used as emergency contraception within 5 days of unprotected intercourse/failed method | Procedural difficulties & complications (see Mirena system above) |

*table continued*

*table continued*

| Method | Availability | Failure rate[a] | Ease of use | Advantages | Disadvantages/ possible risks |
|---|---|---|---|---|---|
| Diaphragm (cap) with spermicide (see Fig. 2.4) | Size measured & cap supplied at family planning clinics & some GPs (free) Pack of different sizes purchasable at some large pharmacies | 2–8%— higher with FemCap & non-fitted varieties | Insertion prior to intercourse or any genital contact Leg abduction needed Considerable dexterity for correct insertion by woman or her partner Remains in place for min. 6 hours after intercourse Less effective 3 hours after insertion unless additional spermicide added | No medical implications apart from latex allergy —silicone available (FemCap) Can always have available *May* offer protection against transmission of the human papilloma virus that causes cervical cancer | Poor perineal sensation e.g. due to spinal cord injury, inability to abduct legs, tremor or poor fine movement may inhibit insertion The need to touch genitalia may be unacceptable Damaged by oil-based creams e.g. petroleum jelly & Gyno-Daktarin (see Fig. 2.5) |
| Natural methods i.e. predicting date of ovulation/'safe' days for intercourse using calendar, body temperature or urine test with Persona device | Ideally, specialist family planning advice | 6% but depends on comp-liance/ mens-trual regularity Persona 4% | Requires considerable cognitive ability & commitment from woman & partner Dexterity to collect & test urine with Persona | No medical implications Under woman's control & once understood no need for professional advice | Predictability of ovulation may be inhibited by condition or medication Low reliability may be unacceptable Persona & disposable test sticks expensive |
| Female sterilisation (tubal ligation) | Waiting list for NHS procedure Private surgery possible | 0.5% (specific proce-dures may increase reliability) | Hospital stay for procedure If laparoscopic procedure recovery relatively quick Immediate contraception Informed consent may be an issue for women with learning disability | Long-term method No medical implications/further intervention | Surgical procedure not without risk especially if general anaesthetic used & in certain conditions of potential compromised breathing e.g. high spinal cord lesions Pain may cause autonomic hyperreflexia if spinal cord injury (see Chapter 8) |

*table continued*

*table continued*

| Method | Availability | Failure rate[a] | Ease of use | Advantages | Disadvantages/ possible risks |
|---|---|---|---|---|---|
| Male sterilisation (vasectomy) | As above | 1:2000 cases | Often done as a hospital day case Recovery within days 3 sperm-free semen specimens needed | As above Partner seen to be taking any risk away from woman | As local anaesthetic normally used there is little surgical risk especially if non-disabled |

[a]Failure rate indicates the number of women out of 100 using the method correctly for 1 year who become pregnant.
[b]STIs = sexually transmitted infections.
[c]Safety time—the number of hours *after* the time the normal daily tablet should have been taken in which the woman can still consider herself safe from pregnancy.
[d]DVT = Deep vein thrombosis i.e. a blood clot in the deep veins, commonly the calf, that may dislodge and travel to the heart, lungs or brain with the potential to cause collapse & death.
[e]MS = Multiple sclerosis.
[f]PID = Pelvic inflammatory disease—less common with IUCD or Mirena since screening/treatment for chlamydia prior to insertion.

are mostly for hormonal methods and cervical caps. Only a few with relevant training and available resuscitation equipment may insert intrauterine devices and implants. They cannot prescribe condoms which must be purchased by the client from a retail outlet. Therefore their service is somewhat limited. They may not match the vast experience of family planning doctors and nurses to be able to discuss in depth the individual needs of women with a disability.

## Acceptability

A woman with a disability is no different to any other woman in this respect. A method that suits one woman or couple may be unacceptable to another. Choice of method may be more limited for women with a disability because of specific issues of suitability. Additionally, policies related to acceptance of contraception use by women with learning difficulties may be influential in whether they actually use contraception, or if used, the method chosen.

## Suitability

Again, as with all women, suitability of method must be considered on an individual basis. Age, smoking, body mass index, medical history and medication e.g. anti-epileptic drugs, must be considered. An irregular or chaotic life-style and the ability to understand the correct method of utilisation will influence compliance and success of contraception.

In addition, for women with a disability, aspects for consideration include peripheral circulation, coagulation potential, dexterity, mobility and sensation (Drey & Darney 2004). Menstruation and associated hygiene may also need to be thought about as well as cognitive ability and consent to the contraception.

For women with learning difficulties cognitive and medical factors may not be the only influence on choice of method. In a Belgium study Servais et al (2002) found that policies related to sleeping environment (institutional or home) and sexual relationships affected contraception use. This resulted in a very different pattern of utilisation to the rest of the population. Over 40% were actually without contraception, 22% had been sterilised, 18% used oral contraception, 17% had received intramuscular Depo Provera and 1% had an intrauterine device fitted.

## Methods

### Hormonal

The combined oral contraceptive (COC) of oestrogen and progesterone (the pill) is known to have a slight risk of causing thromboembolic disorders. If a woman has poor circulation from either a medical cause or from sitting position, or has little or no mobility or sensation, for example from spinal cord injury, she may be at more risk of developing a pain-free deep vein thrombosis that goes undetected. Therefore treatment and prevention of further complications is inhibited.

Taking a pill every day needs a woman or someone else to have a good memory (Cooper & Guillebaud 1999). This memory is not necessarily associated with intellect as someone with learning difficulties may be able to develop a pattern of behaviour with initial support and guidance. In addition there is a need to be able to swallow. An alternative combined method not yet available in the UK (but likely to be so in the near future) is a vaginal ring and an injection (Szarewski 2006). The ring is left in place for 3 weeks followed by 1 week without. The injection is monthly which may be less acceptable.

An option that is now available, although not necessarily readily at all family planning clinics, is the combined skin patch called Evra (see Fig. 2.1). A single patch is worn on the upper outer arm, thigh or buttock and replaced weekly for 3 weeks followed by a patch-free week. It not only has the advantage of increased compliance, but in addition a lower overall dose is needed as the hormones are absorbed via the skin. This is because there is delay in drugs passing through the liver for metabolism. Further advantages include consistent blood levels rather than the peaks and troughs of oral administration, and greater reliability when broad spectrum antibiotics are used because of the lack of gastrointestinal involvement in drug absorption (Szarewski 2006). Some women may have skin sensitivity. Another disadvantage reported by Anne Szarewski (2006) from research evidence in the literature is the slight possibility of spotting during the first two to three menstrual cycles. Reliability of the method appears to be high, although less so for women over 90 kg in weight.

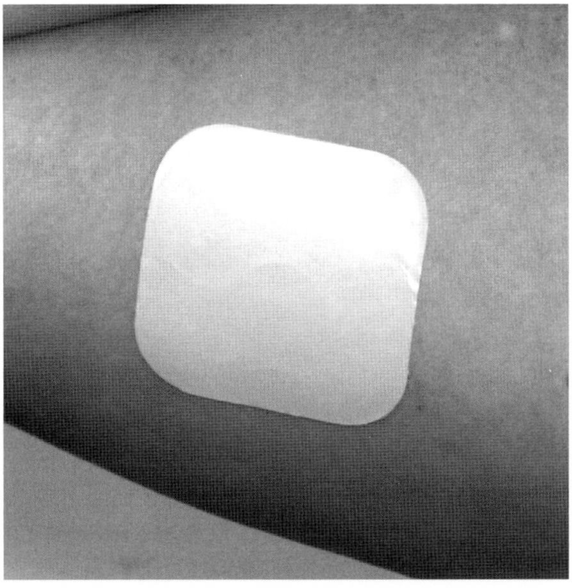

Progesterone alone may be the solution for a woman who chooses hormonal contraception as the potential risk factors associated with oestrogen are not present. However, oral progesterone has only a 3-hour safety time i.e. repeat pills need to be taken within 3 hours of the usual time to maintain effective contraception, therefore regularity is important. A newer tablet of progesterone has recently arrived on the market, Cerazette, which has a 12-hour safety time (Szarewski 2006). Progesterone (Depo provera) that is effective for 12 weeks may be given by intramuscular injection, or it can be administered by an implant (Implanon) under the skin, usually the underside of the upper arm, for longer term action i.e. 3 years (Fig. 2.2). As progesterone alone does not always inhibit ovulation, particularly if plasma levels fall significantly, these two methods have the advantage of sustaining optimal plasma levels thus improving the contraceptive effect and lowering the chance of pregnancy. Additionally, these methods are useful if a chaotic life-style or cognitive ability makes regular oral administration problematic.

*Figure 2.1* An Evra-combined oestrogen and progesterone patch demonstrated on an upper arm. Photograph by Martin Baxter.

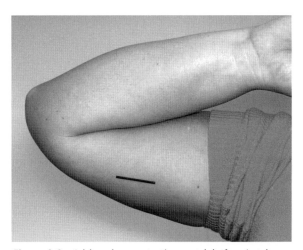

*Figure 2.2* A blue demonstration model of an Implanon (active ones are white) shown on the inside of the upper arm where implantation would be under the skin. Photograph by Martin Baxter.

A further advantage of progesterone is that menstrual loss may be minimal or absent which benefits women if coping with personal hygiene is difficult, and may be useful for this reason even if contraception is not needed. However, progesterone may cause an increase in appetite and the subsequent increase in food intake and weight gain may compromise mobility if this is an issue. If women are aware of this possibility they may be able to avoid the pitfalls (Cooper & Guillebaud 1999). Implants have the disadvantage of requiring a woman to keep still during insertion and removal which may prove difficult for some women.

### Intrauterine devices

The copper intrauterine device (coil) has the advantage of long-term protection: 5–10 years for some types, with few contraindications for use. Again, where compliance with a method is an issue, the coil is effective immediately and insertion is also suitable within approximately 5 days of unprotected intercourse to prevent pregnancy. However, menstrual loss is commonly heavier with more pain initially, therefore it may not be suitable for every woman. The intrauterine system (for example the Mirena) is a coil with a stem that contains slow-release progesterone (Figs. 2.3a, 2.3b). With this

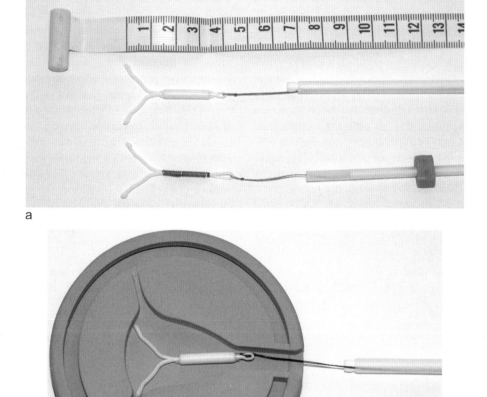

*Figure 2.3* **a)** A copper T coil and a Mirena system. Note the thicker stem of the Mirena and the copper thread on the coil. The ruler helps to show the size. **b)** A coil inserted into a model to demonstrate how it is located in the cavity of the uterus. Photographs by Martin Baxter.

method menstruation often diminishes after an initial irregularity, with subsequent amenorrhoea. Furthermore, as the progesterone acts more locally than systemically the side effects (for example fluid retention and weight gain) are fewer.

The potential advantages of an intrauterine device may be negated by the difficulty of insertion. Women with lack of mobility in hip joints or muscular spasm causing difficulty in abduction of legs may find it impossible to facilitate the position that is needed to view the cervix for insertion. A mutually acceptable position will need to be adopted for both woman and practitioner (Cooper & Guillebaud 1999) which might mean a woman needs too adopt a lateral position.

During insertion women with a spinal cord lesion are susceptible to autonomic dysreflexia due to cervical stimulation resulting in a dramatic rise in blood pressure (Cooper & Guillebaud 1999) (see Chapter 8 for more details about autonomic dysreflexia). Therefore fitting should be carried out in a hospital setting rather than a family planning or general practitioner clinic. Additionally, there is a hypothetical risk that the warning signs of pelvic inflammatory disease or ectopic pregnancy would be missed in women without pain sensation (Drey & Darney 2004). This risk could also be considered in women without the cognitive ability to express their symptoms. However, the risk of infection is much reduced as screening and any necessary treatment for chlamydia and gonorrhoea is routinely undertaken prior to insertion. The risk of infection and ectopic pregnancy reduces with time when the copper device is used and is negligible with the intrauterine system.

### Barrier methods

The condom (male and female) and the cervical cap (diaphragm) act as barriers to sperm: the former should ideally be one with a spermicidal lubricant, and the latter is usually smeared with a spermicide to increase effectiveness. Although contraceptive safety is not as high as hormonal methods or the coil/intrauterine system (Table 2.1), medical safety is high as latex allergy is one of the few side effects. This may be an issue for women with spina bifida (see Chapter 8). Condoms and diaphragms made of polyurethane are available but Murphy & Young (2005) warn that they are not as strong as latex,

and condoms in particular have a higher rate of splitting during intercourse, therefore an additional method may be needed to ensure safety from pregnancy.

Application of the spermicide and insertion of the cap (or a female condom) requires considerable dexterity and mobility to ensure correct placement (Figs. 2.4a, 2.4b, 2.4c). One-handed insertion is possible but does require considerable skill. To enable insertion women commonly lift one leg with the foot resting on a support e.g. the edge of the bed or chair, therefore balance is needed (Fig. 2.5). Insertion whilst lying down is possible if arms are long enough to reach but sitting on the edge of a chair or the bed may be better (not on the toilet in case the cap is dropped). Cap or female condom insertion may be undertaken by the partner if acceptable to both parties. For women with learning difficulties this may prove an asset.

Adequate sensation is needed to recognise that the cap or the female condom is in correctly. If incorrectly positioned the cap in particular may cause bladder neck trauma as well as ineffective contraception. When the cap is used correctly it is considered 92–98% effective (Cooper & Guillebaud 1999) but this may not be adequate if pregnancy must absolutely be avoided. Failure of forward planning to insert the cap prior to intercourse will lead to method failure.

The male condom also needs forward thinking for timely use and two-handed dexterity for correct fitting (Fig. 2.6). Therefore if a woman's partner has upper limb impairment this may not be the most appropriate choice of method, although if her dexterity is adequate in this situation she could fit the condom. Nevertheless, someone used to using one hand for everything may be able to effectively fit a condom. Clear instructions on correct fitting are needed particularly when learning difficulties are the issue. A demonstration of fitting using a model of an erect penis will aid clarity of understanding rather than using a simulation object e.g. a banana (Cooper & Guillebaud 1999).

The female condom has the advantage over the male condom in that it can be inserted a short time prior to intercourse. The two main issues related to acceptability with the female condom are appearance (Fig. 2.7) and complaints from users that it 'rustles' during intercourse.

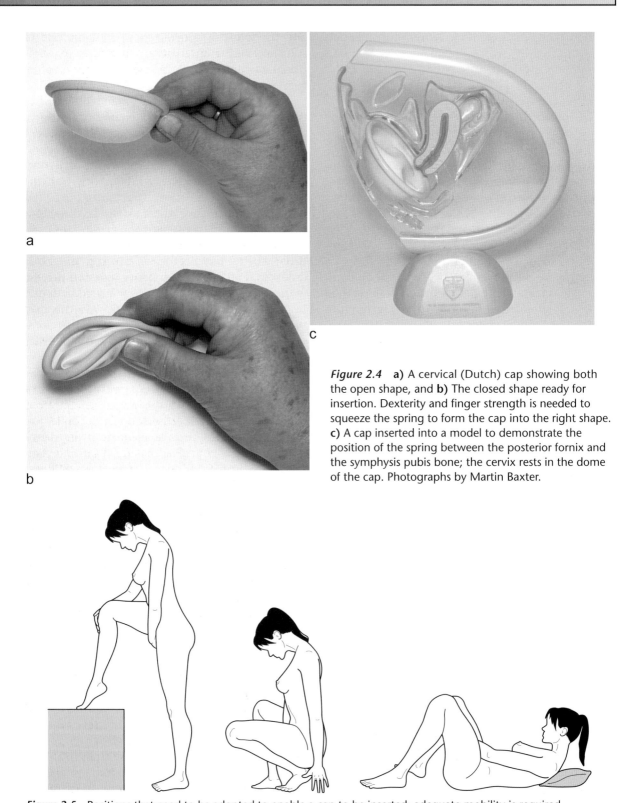

***Figure 2.4*** **a)** A cervical (Dutch) cap showing both the open shape, and **b)** The closed shape ready for insertion. Dexterity and finger strength is needed to squeeze the spring to form the cap into the right shape. **c)** A cap inserted into a model to demonstrate the position of the spring between the posterior fornix and the symphysis pubis bone; the cervix rests in the dome of the cap. Photographs by Martin Baxter.

***Figure 2.5*** Positions that need to be adopted to enable a cap to be inserted; adequate mobility is required.

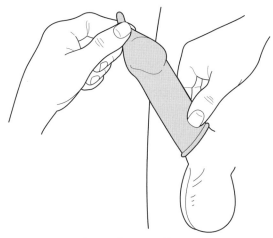

*Figure 2.6* A male condom usually requires two-handed dexterity for ease of application.

Barrier methods may only be suitable for women in whom these issues are unproblematic. Both methods have the added advantage of offering some protection against STIs although only the condom protects against the human immunosuppressant virus (HIV).

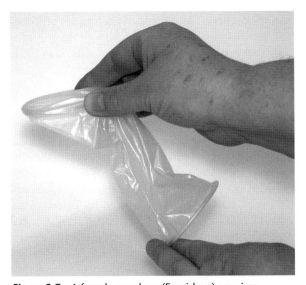

*Figure 2.7* A female condom (Femidom) requires dexterity to squeeze the inner ring for insertion; the outer ring remains at the vulva. Photograph by Martin Baxter.

### Sterilisation

As a method of contraception sterilisation is considered virtually 100% effective and permanent; there is a miniscule chance of pregnancy and limited reversal success. This may be the choice of method for a woman with a disability if she has had the children she wants, or chooses not to have children at all. This latter element may be because of her concerns about her ability to cope with pregnancy, birth or parenthood, worries about inherited conditions, or simply that she does not wish for children in her life. However, even if a woman's wish is never to have children, the removal of her choice to do so may be unacceptable. Informed choice to have the surgery is her prerogative but there may be anaesthetic and post-operative concerns depending on her condition. Another consideration is that if the existing contraceptive causes amenorrhoea and the method is stopped, menstruation is likely to return unless the method continues, following surgery.

Sterilisation as a method of contraception for women with learning difficulties involves a complex minefield of legal and ethical issues. Knifton's (1998) well-balanced discussion offers insight into the elements of UK law that inform carers and health professional of their duty of care. The subjects of informed consent and in whose best interest sterilisation would be considered are under much debate. So too is the definition of 'best interest'. Although the procedure is acceptable as in someone's best interests if performed for therapeutic reasons, the courts may need to rule on the lawfulness of the surgery in other cases. However, defining lawful surgery in no way implies consent by the courts. As Knifton points out, there are still undertones of eugenics in this process. Therefore there is no clear-cut answer to every situation.

### Natural methods

These methods that involve abstinence from intercourse during the fertile period require considerable understanding and motivation. They are only considered suitable for women with very regular menstrual cycles although the Persona device that involves testing urine may be more accurate at predicting fertility. But where pregnancy must be avoided the failure rate of 6% is probably unacceptable (Cooper & Guillebaud 1999).

## GENITAL AND SEXUALLY TRANSMITTED INFECTION

Some women with disability may be more susceptible to genital tract infections because poor mobility, dexterity and continence issues create an area of suboptimal hygiene and thus an environment where microorganisms flourish. Perineal discomfort or pain, vaginal discharge and cystitis are symptoms that may be unrecognised, either because of poor sensation or lack of understanding, for example, in women with learning disabilities, which may then delay action to seek treatment.

Sexually active women with disability are just as vulnerable to STIs as other women. They may possibly be at an even greater risk if they have difficulty in employing safe sexual practices. Those practices may not be utilised because of a lack of understanding of the importance of having safe sex or an inability to obtain condoms; compliance with sexual activity rather than as part of a partnership; or a lack of assertive skills to insist that a partner uses a condom when he chooses not to.

Signs and symptoms of STIs may not be recognised by women and thus diagnosis and treatment are delayed and complications develop (Table 2.2). One common complication of STIs is pelvic inflammatory disease, particularly with gonorrhoea and chlamydia. Welner (2004) postulates that impairment of sensation in the pelvic area and barriers to obtaining medical care may also increase women's chances that pelvic inflammatory disease goes undetected. Women with spinal cord lesions about T6 or above may notice symptoms of autonomic dysreflexia (see Chapter 8) caused by the pain stimulation prior to the acute or chronic awareness of pain.

Table 2.2 summarises the recognition and management of genital tract and STIs while greater detail is given below under specific infections.

### Fungal infections

Fungal infections with monilia i.e. yeasts, may be present as part of normal vaginal and perineal flora. Levels may become exacerbated by incontinence, or when women are taking the combined oral contraceptive pill or during pregnancy. The increased incidence in the latter two situations is because vaginal pH is less acidic and the normal vaginal flora (lactobacilli, usually Döderlein's bacilli which make lactic acid) are less abundant.

Welner (2004) warns that some oral antifungal agents may interact with medication taken by women, for example steroids and some anti-arthritis drugs. Vaginal preparations for treatment are usually inserted as a pessary or by using a syringe-type applicator for a cream. Women with impaired dexterity may find using these forms of medication problematic. In this situation a single-dose preparation that could be inserted by health professionals may be the answer to a longer course of treatment.

### Bacterial vaginosis

This is not a STI. It is caused by anaerobic bacteria, e.g. *Gardnerella vaginalis*, levels of which may fluctuate, and an asymptomatic colonisation is often left untreated. If levels of lactobacilli (see above) increase, anaerobic numbers decrease. Women with poor continence management may develop higher bacterial levels resulting in the need for treatment. Welner (2004) states that metronidazole often used for this condition is not recommended for women with neurological conditions. This is because the drug is associated, in rare cases, with numbness and parasthesia (tingling), therefore any potential to cause an additional challenge to the central nervous system should be avoided. Hay (2001) does offer an alternative treatment with vaginal clindamycin.

### Trichomonas

*Trichomonas vaginalis* is an STI by flagellated (with tails) protozoa that cause an unpleasant, frequently odorous green-yellow vaginal discharge. The condition may cause dysparaunia (painful intercourse), dysuria (pain on micturition) and lower abdominal pain. However Sherrard (2001) points out that 10–50% of women are asymptomatic. Women with impaired pelvic sensation may not perceive symptoms although they may notice the odour and feel generally unwell (Welner 2004). Diagnosis is made on symptoms and visualising the organisms using

*Table 2.2*  **Recognition and management of genital tract and sexually transmitted infections in women with disability**

| Condition & organism | Recognition | Raised susceptibility | Management | Issues with management |
|---|---|---|---|---|
| Fungal (yeasts) e.g. monlia/candida | Thick, white vaginal discharge Perineal irritation Frequency of micturition & cystitis may be present Symptoms may not be perceived by women with poor sensation e.g. spinal cord lesions or those with cognitive difficulties Culture of a vaginal swab | Incontinence Combined hormonal contraceptive Pregnancy | Vaginal creams/ pessaries e.g. clotrimazole (e.g. Canesten) or miconazole nitrate (e.g. Gyno-Daktarin) Oral metronidazole (e.g. Flagyl) | Poor mobility, dexterity and perineal sensation may reduce ability to self-treat—single dose regime applied by health professional/helper Gyno-Daktarin damages condoms & diaphragms Metronidazole: possible interaction with some drugs e.g. steroids and those for arthritis Cautious use during pregnancy & breast-feeding Caution when CNS[a] impairment as may cause numbness & parasthesia (tingling) |
| Bacterial vaginosis (anaerobic organisms) e.g. *Gardnerella vaginalis* | May be asymptomatic Offensive odour Watery vaginal discharge Burning sensation at introitus Poor recognition (as above) Culture of a vaginal swab | Incontinence Combined hormonal contraception Pregnancy | Oral metronidazole (e.g. Flagyl) or oral or vaginal clindamycin | Metronidazole: (see above) Clindamycin: cautious oral use as toxic Application difficulty (see above) & compliance as vaginal preparation a 7-day course |
| Trichomonas (a flagellated protozoa) i.e. *trichomonas vaginalis* | 50% asymptomatic Odorous, green-yellow discharge Dysparaunia (painful intercourse) Frequency of micturition & cystitis Lower abdominal pain | Unprotected intercourse | Oral metronidazole or tinidazole | See above—also relevant for tinidazole |

*table continued*

*table continued*

| Condition & organism | Recognition | Raised susceptibility | Management | Issues with management |
|---|---|---|---|---|
| | Generally feeling unwell Poor recognition (as above) Swab taken & organism visualised on a wet slide | | | |
| Chlamydia (intracellular parasite) | Often asymptomatic Frequency of micturition & cystitis Lower abdominal pain Poor recognition (as above) Cervical swab culture or first pass urine specimen (home testing equipment now available) | Unprotected intercourse | Oral tetracycline or doxycycline or single dose of azithromycin | Drugs contraindicated in pregnancy/breast-feeding Reduced antibiotic effect with some anti-epileptic drugs e.g. carbamazepine (Tegretol) Reduces effect of hormonal contraception especially combined Untreated in pregnancy can result in baby eye infection during birth which may result in blindness |
| Gonorrhoea (a diplococci) i.e. *Neisseria gonorrhoeae* | Asymptomatic in early stages Vaginal discharge Frequency of micturition & cystitis Lower abdominal pain Dysparunia Uterine bleeding/ pelvic pain in later stages Poor recognition (as above) Cervical swab culture | Unprotected intercourse | Single intramuscular injection of amoxicillin with probenecid (which reduces the urinary excretion of the antibiotic) or spectromycin or 4-quinolone if penicillin allergy Ceftriaxone (cephalosporin) as a single dose | See above Untreated in pregnancy can result in baby eye infection during birth which may result in blindness |
| Syphilis *Treponema pallidum* | Primary stage (3 weeks to 90 days after exposure)—single chancre at infection site which rapidly disappears (therefore easily missed by woman | Unprotected intercourse | Intramuscular procaine benzylpenicillin (procaine penicillin) penicillin allergy | See above Untreated by the second trimester of pregnancy will result in congenital syphilis |

*table continued*

*table continued*

| Condition & organism | Recognition | Raised susceptibility | Management | Issues with management |
|---|---|---|---|---|
| | or helper with daily hygiene) Secondary stage— 6 weeks to several months later e.g. fever, myalgia (muscle pain), headache, fatigue (easily blamed on existing condition e.g. MS[b], arthritis), body rash, genital ulcers Latent stage— symptoms disappear (therefore difficult to recognise) but infection persists Tertiary stage— final stage of untreated condition— neurological damage e.g. loss of pain sensation & poor muscle coordination (MS[b] has similar symptoms) Blood tests (routine in pregnancy) | | | |
| Herpes simplex virus | Painful blisters on the external genitalia (vaginal & cervical blisters may also be present)—initial infection often very painful Generally feeling unwell & sweating Condition remains dormant with recurrent episodes Poor recognition (as above) | Unprotected intercourse/ genital contact | Local application of disease-modifying antiviral ointment e.g. acyclovir Early treatment of recurrence limits length of symptoms Topical local anaesthetic gel to reduce risk of autonomic dysreflexia | Poor mobility, dexterity and perineal sensation may reduce ability to self-treat therefore help needed—compliance may be an issue Lesions may be slow to heal when mobility is impaired or incontinence Caesarean section recommended during an active outbreak to avoid a potential life-threatening infection to baby |

*table continued*

*table continued*

| Condition & organism | Recognition | Raised susceptibility | Management | Issues with management |
|---|---|---|---|---|
| | especially early warning of recurrence e.g. skin tingling Painful episodes may initiate autonomic dysreflexia (see Chapter 8) in women with spinal lesions | | | |
| Human papilloma virus | Some strains cause painless fleshy growths (warts) anywhere on genitalia or peri-anal area Easily missed if mobility & dexterity limit tactile exploration of area, especially if growths are small, or missed by helper with hygiene Other strains cause cervical cell changes with a risk of cancer | Unprotected intercourse/ genital contact | Warts: podophyllum solution (e.g. Condyline) painted on twice daily for 3 days on 5 consecutive weeks Cryotherapy (freezing) or laser treatment Cervical smears, colposcopy & relevant treatment | Poor mobility, dexterity and perineal sensation may reduce ability to self-treat—therefore help needed—compliance may be an issue Wart treatment not usually used during pregnancy Abduction of legs for smears & colposcopy e.g. if spasm/pain |
| Pelvic inflammatory disease A variety of organisms e.g. chlamydia gonorrhoea E. coli | Symptoms not always clear Low grade to severe lower abdominal pain, deep pain during intercourse (which may be missed if no pelvic sensation) Pain may cause autonomic hyper-reflexia in women with spinal cord lesions Pyrexia Vaginal discharge | Sexually transmitted infection following insertion of an intrauterine device or surgery Early sexual activity/ multiple partners Sex during menstruation | Laparoscopy, endometrial biopsy, cervical/vaginal swabs & scan to aid diagnosis Exclude tubal pregnancy A combination of 2–3 broad-spectrum antibiotics over 14 days | Reduced antibiotic effect with some anti-epileptic drugs e.g. carbamazepine (Tegretol) Reduces effect of hormonal contraception especially combined Untreated likely to result in blocked tubes & infertility |

[a]CNS = central nervous system.
[b]MS = multiple sclerosis.

fresh material on a wet slide. Metronidazole is an effective treatment (see above) or tinidazole as an alternative. If the condition is present during pregnancy, pre-tem birth and a low birth weight baby is possible (Sherrard 2001).

## Chlamydia

Chlamydia is a very common STI. Horner (2006) states that in the UK 5–10% of women under 24 years of age who are sexually active have the infection. The condition is caused by intracellular parasites and is often asymptomatic. It is a particularly problematic infection in that it is a prime cause of pelvic inflammatory disease: Horner (2006) quotes 10–40% of untreated infection. If present during a baby's birth it may lead to severe neonatal eye infection or pneumonia.

Diagnosis has always been via culture of a cervical swab transported in special medium. However, a simpler test identifying the organism in a first pass specimen of urine has been developed making diagnosis much easier. There are even home testing kits available. For women with mobility issues or difficulty abducting their legs to enable a vaginal swab, this screening test is much more client friendly. Treatment is commonly with tetracycline. Caution is needed to ensure that women are not pregnant or breast-feeding when this drug is used as it is known to damage fetal and neonatal dentition. Newer forms of tetracycline, in the form of doxycycline, which is still contraindicated in pregnancy, or azithromycin, which is conveniently in a 1-g single dose, are available (Horner 2006).

## Gonorrhoea

This gram negative sexually transmitted organism, *Neisseria gonorrhoeae*, is a diplococci, i.e. it is in two sections and looks rather like two halves of a coffee bean linked together. The infection may be asymptomatic in the early stage but vaginal discharge, dysuria and dyspareunia (see above) often develop fairly quickly, with uterine bleeding and pelvic inflammatory disease developing some time later if untreated. Diagnosis is commonly from a culture of the organism from cervical secretions, although Welner (2004) points out that a heavy bacterial colonization with gram negative organisms, which is not uncommon

in women with disabilities, may give a positive result. The first choice of treatment is still with penicillin. However, resistant organisms are increasing and these will need an alternative antibiotic. Untreated infection at the time of a baby's birth will result in severe neonatal eye infection.

## Syphilis

This STI is caused by the organism *Treponema pallidum*. A primary infection often presents as a single painless ulcer or chancre at the infection site. Women with disability may not notice this painless lesion, and if they have helpers giving care with personal hygiene they may not take note of a lesion as they rapidly disappear. Treatment has traditionally been with penicillin but Goh (2002) recommends using tetracyclines, possibly because of organism resistance. Untreated syphilis during pregnancy will result in congenital syphilis which is why a routine blood screening test is offered to all women at the initial booking visit.

Secondary syphilis develops about 6 weeks after an untreated primary infection. Symptoms can be variable in this situation and common ones such as fever, myalgia (muscle pain), headache and fatigue are similar to those of rheumatoid conditions. Skin rash may also appear. Therefore symptoms may easily be missed as those of a STI. Treatment at this stage is the same as for the primary condition. If treatment is not obtained the condition outwardly appears to subside but actually enters the latent stage which is not so easy to diagnose from blood tests.

The latent stage requires treatment with large doses of intramuscular penicillin on several occasions. Home visits by a community nurse may be useful to ensure treatment is completed if mobility difficulty makes attendance at a clinic problematic.

Tertiary syphilis is the final stage of an untreated condition. Although this can be treated with a combination of high doses of intravenous, intramuscular and oral penicillin, neurological damage is one consequence of the long duration of the disease. Neurological symptoms may include loss of energy and pain sensations, headache and shooting pains, paralysis and poor muscle coordination. Similar symptoms can be part of the effects of multiple sclerosis therefore there is the potential for a misdiagnosis and a missed condition (Welner 2004).

## Herpes simplex virus

Genital herpes is a highly infectious STI if sexual contact occurs when someone has an active infection and is therefore shedding viruses. Once infected the virus lies dormant in the affected nerves and reactivates periodically. The condition presents as blisters that are very painful, particularly at the time of the initial infection. However, women with poor sensation may miss diagnosis of the lesions or mistake the pain for pressure area trauma. General symptoms such as malaise and sweating may be mistaken for symptoms associated with a woman's disability. The early sensations that preclude a recurrent infection, often a tingling sensation, and again the general symptoms, may also be missed. Delay in applying the disease-modifying ointment acyclovir may result.

Neurological symptoms may trigger autonomic dysreflexia (see Chapter 8) in women with spinal cord injury. Welner (2004) recommends the application of a topical local anaesthetic gel to inhibit nerve stimulation. Lesions may be slow to heal in someone whose mobility is impaired, e.g. a wheelchair user. Self-treatment may be difficult for women with impaired dexterity.

Pregnant women with an active outbreak of herpes are usually recommended to have a caesarean section at the time their babies are due. This avoids exposing neonates to the highly contagious virus which has potential life-threatening consequences.

## Human papilloma virus

This sexually transmitted virus leads to genital warts. These can be treated locally with topical preparations but have a tendency to recur. Self-treatment is possible for recurrence but some preparations are caustic and care is needed in their use. If a woman's dexterity or coordination is compromised lack of precision application could potentially lead to damage of healthy skin.

Some of the strains of human papilloma virus are implicated in cervical cancer, therefore cervical screening is advisable probably on a more frequent basis than government directives for standard cervical screening policies. For some women with a disability, actually accessing screening services is difficult. Women may also have difficulty in trans-ferring to examination couches which are usually high and non-adjustable, and abducting legs for smears to be taken. The left lateral position may be more suitable. Colposcopy is the best screening procedure when the papilloma virus is present. But this may produce challenges to both women and practitioners to ensure women achieve and maintain a position to enable screening to take place. A very skilled practitioner may be able to work with women in the left lateral position, but a helper will be needed to hold a woman's right leg up.

## Other viral infections

Other viral infections such as Hepatitis B and C and HIV are mentioned here for completeness of the topic. However, the only consideration of note for women with disability is that caution needs to be used to ensure that medication taken for these infections does not interact with those needed for the disabling condition. This could present considerable challenges for specialist practitioners where HIV is concerned because of the complex nature of treatment for this condition.

## DOMESTIC ABUSE

Domestic abuse, categorised as physical, emotional, financial and sexual (Shipway 2004), can occur across the social spectrum, affecting people of all social classes, races, gender, age and culture. To some people it may seem unthinkable that disabled people should face abuse, but it is quite clear that both children and adults with physical and learning disabilities are greatly at risk (Shakespeare 1996). Abuse of children is likely to come from their carers, and investigations show that both men and women are involved in perpetrating the abuse. Following in-depth interviews, Maddie Blackburn (2002) provides case studies of four young men and four young women with varying degrees of spina bifida and hydrocephalus. Physical and sexual abuse was present in half the cases and the potential for sexual exploitation was present in them all. Blackburn comments that these cases highlight the need for recognition that some disabled people may need appropriate and life-long protection from sexual exploitation and harm.

Disability in itself does not cause the abuse and disabled people are the same as other people in this respect: disabled children do not experience different abuse—they experience the same kind of abuse as other children. Shakespeare (1996) says that disabled children are the ones 'chosen' because they cannot speak of the horror. They cannot run away or tell anyone about it, and if they did, who would believe them? There is a prevailing belief in our society that disabled people are asexual and unattractive therefore why would anyone want to sexually abuse them?

It is well documented that domestic abuse in pregnancy is harmful to both the mother and unborn child (Shipway 2004). Healthcare professionals should be aware that abuse may be more prevalent in the disabled child-bearing woman and offer her the opportunity to be interviewed/examined on her own without the partner present, so that the issue can be discussed. If a woman is hearing impaired, it is important that the interpreter used is not a family member as evidence of domestic abuse may be suppressed and the woman is then unable to seek help. Similarly, for a woman with learning disabilities, a 'neutral' person needs to attend the clinic with her to help obtain an appropriate history from her. Unfortunately people with learning disabilities are not only at risk of abuse from their families, but also their carers. Dick Sobsey (1994) gives a graphic account of a case where a young woman was systematically abused by a carer and had not dared to tell anyone as she was told that if she did her mother would die. Someone a woman did not live with, such as a key worker, might be able to support her adequately during the clinic visit and help her disclose any abuse.

During the antenatal period it is important that midwives are aware of the vulnerability of all women during pregnancy to domestic abuse, but particularly to that of women with physical or intellectual disabilities. There should be a protocol of how and where women can seek further help, particularly if they are not able to seek this help out for themselves. Suggestions of abuse should not be ignored but followed through properly.

## ABORTION

There are feminist arguments that all women have the right to choose abortion if they do not wish to be pregnant (Hubbard 1997). Feminists campaigning for abortion rights use the fetus diagnosed with a congenital malformation as one reason why a woman should have this right to choose. But this argument fails to address the rights to life of a person with a disability (McLaughlin 2003). Routine screening is available to all women at 20 weeks of pregnancy when they are offered a fetal anomaly scan with a view to terminating the pregnancy should a malformation be found. Problems may arise for a woman with spina bifida who has a fetus diagnosed with the same condition. How would she feel about her own life if she agreed to a termination? *Changing Childbirth* (DoH 1993) advocated that all women should have informed choice and should be supported when making decisions, but how much information is she given about the positive achievements people with spina bifida can make? Sharpe & Earle (2002) argue that antenatal screening for abnormalities and the subsequent offer of terminating the pregnancy is discriminatory against disabled people. As technology advances and more anomalies can be detected, where do we stop? The greater the ability to identify potential conditions, the greater pressure there is on women to eradicate them (McLaughlin 2003). Unfortunately disability is constructed in a negative way and efforts should be made to stop it from happening.

Another screening test offered to women is the 'Triple test' at approximately 16 weeks of the pregnancy. This test gives a 'probability' of how likely Down's syndrome is of occurring. Abnormal levels of substances are looked for in a woman's blood, and combined with her age and the gestational age, an estimate of the likelihood of Down's syndrome occurring is made. If this is greater than 1:250, women are offered amniocentesis, where fetal chromosomes can be identified. If trisomy 21 (Down's syndrome) is diagnosed, women are often expected to accept the offer of termination. As stated in the previous chapter, this may be when the pregnancy is quite advanced and the fetus capable of independent life, therefore should it be delivered? The decision to end that life is never undertaken lightly, but many women are being offered screening when they do not always understand the ramifications of it and would not have previously been considered 'high risk'.

## DESIRE FOR MOTHERHOOD

Women in today's society are fortunate that they can choose whether to have a baby or not as contraceptive methods are effective if used properly. However, for the person with a disability it is sometimes difficult to get the right advice about planning a pregnancy in order to have a successful outcome (Asch & Fine 1997). Many women with disability do conceive without particularly planning to, and have a healthy baby at the end of pregnancy (for example see Armstead 2000, Lapper 2005). Problems may be encountered in achieving motherhood if natural conception does not occur, or the pregnancy fails. Ann Neville-Jan (2004) who has spina bifida, had the unfortunate experience of having two miscarriages, one a spontaneous pregnancy and the other following assisted conception. However, because no one informed her that miscarriage may occur in one in four pregnancies in women *without* disability, it was made to seem as though her disability had been the cause. Eventually she and her husband decided to adopt a baby from China as the desire for parenthood was so great. Following that process she was treated with immunological drugs, managed to conceive naturally and had a normal child at the end of it. She had been advised by one gynaecologist that it was probably better that she did not have children at all as she would not physically be able to cope; she certainly proved them wrong.

Gillian Beck (Robinson-Walsh 1997) has multiple sclerosis (MS), which was diagnosed before she was married or considering becoming a mother. When she became pregnant she made a conscious decision not to have any prenatal testing as she felt that having a disability herself meant she would be able to support a child with a disability. Gillian actually felt better during her pregnancy as some of the stiffness and muscle spasms lessened, probably because of the natural increase in steroid production which occurs as the placenta develops. Gillian

went on to have a second child, but as her MS had worsened between pregnancies, she decided that two children were enough and her family was complete.

Nosek et al (2001) found in their study that women with disabilities were sexually active, able to use contraceptives and to decide whether or not to try for a pregnancy. It is often other people's negative attitudes that deter them in their decision to have a child and this means that a disabled woman who chooses to get pregnant may be greeted with disbelief from her family. The desire for motherhood is often great amongst women with or without a disability but it may take great willpower and perseverance to achieve it.

## PRECONCEPTION CARE

Any woman planning a pregnancy should be recommended to seek advice prior to conception. Preconception care is aimed at enabling women (and possibly their partners) to reach the optimum physical condition to ensure a successful pregnancy outcome. Probably the most well-known government campaign via the Health Education Authority was the Folic Acid Campaign (HEA 1996). Taking folic acid for 3 months prior to conception and during early pregnancy can reduce the risks of neural tube defects (McKay-Moffat & Lee 2006). Preconception care also aims to ensure that women have sensible eating habits; they give up smoking, avoid hazardous substances, adopt a healthy lifestyle and focus on being calm, relaxed and healthy. If there is a disability or chronic medical condition, then preconception care aims at achieving the best health outcome that is possible. Drug regimes may have to be altered, for example in the treatment of epilepsy, as some drugs may be harmful to the developing embryo and need replacing with other less toxic agents. Three months is usually long enough for changes to be made and it may take the couple another few months to conceive, but when they do so, they are in optimum health to have a child. Preconception care may be given by the general practitioner, midwife, specialist nurse or consultant and it is free of charge, although prescriptions may have to be paid for until pregnancy occurs.

## PSYCHOLOGICAL ISSUES

Women with disabilities may have low self-esteem. Nosek et al's study (2001) identified three important factors that affect the sense of self of women with physical disabilities more so than women without disabilities. These were: 1) work; 2) relationships; and 3) abuse. Noticeably the disability itself did not seem to be a factor. Some of these aspects have been discussed previously, but it is worth noting here that women with disabilities have less opportunity to benefit from being economically independent because of barriers and disincentives to employment. Going out to work not only provides money, but also the opportunity to meet other people and even to form romantic relationships. Little is known about the effects of disability on forming interpersonal relationships, and more research is required here, but what is well established is the notion that we all need to feel wanted and loved if we are to have positive self-esteem (Nosek et al 2001).

Women with disabilities are more likely to have chronic health problems and these may lead to low self-esteem and depression. It would seem that they find it difficult to access services which may give them a better quality of life, such as exercise facilities, day centres and non-discriminatory healthcare (Nosek et al 2001). If the women have good family support or a loving relationship they are less likely to suffer from depression, although Nosek et al (2001) noted that women who were in a relationship, but did not live with their partners all the time, demonstrated more satisfaction in that relationship than women who were married. Perhaps it is about the available time they have to themselves, rather than being at the demand of their partners all the time that really makes the difference. Long-term health problems can certainly be ameliorated by a positive outlook, but this may not be easy to achieve.

### CONCLUSION—KEY POINTS

- The health concerns of women with disabilities are no different to those of all women.
- Physical access to health services must be ensured and sufficient time allocated for examination.
- Good communication is essential when dealing with all women but particularly those with sensory impairment.
- Misplaced beliefs about the hereditary nature of disability means that women with disabilities are being discouraged from having children.
- Disability can lead to psychosexual problems which need referral.
- Women have the right to choose abortion but should not be coerced into it.
- Women with disabilities may want children and should be supported in that decision.
- Preconception care is important for all women planning a pregnancy.
- Low self-esteem and depression are more likely to occur if a woman does not have adequate family/partner support

## References

Americans with Disabilities Act 1990 In: Duprey MM 2004 Americans with Disabilities Act and The Women's Health Provider. In: Welner S L, Haseltine F (eds) Welner's guide to the care of women with disabilities. Lippincott Williams & Wilkins, Philadelphia, p 17–24

Armstead R 2000 Fighting for the support to parent: a personal experience. Disability, Pregnancy and Parenthood 28(32):5–7

Asch A, Fine M 1997 Nurturance, sexuality and women with disabilities: the example of women and literature. In: Davis L J (ed) The disabilities studies reader. Routledge, London, p 241–259

Bancroft J 1989 Human sexuality and its problems. Elsevier Science, London

Becker H, Stuifbergen A, Tinkle M 1997 Reproductive health care experiences of women with physical disabilities: a qualitative study. Archives of Physical Medicine and Rehabilitation 78(12 suppl 5):S26–S33

Blackburn M 2002 Sexuality and disability. Butterworth Heinemann, Oxford

Campion M J 1990 The baby challenge: a handbook on pregnancy for women with physical disability. Routledge, London

Choquet M, du Pasquier F L, Manfredi R 1997 Sexual behaviour among adolescents reporting chronic conditions: a French national survey. Journal of Adolescent Health 20(1):62–67

Clarke D, McCree H 1986 Mentally handicapped people: living and learning. Ballière Tindall, London

Cooper E, Guillebaud J 1999 Sexuality and disability: a guide for everyday practice. Radcliff Medical Press, Oxon

Department of Health (DoH) 1993 Changing Childbirth. Report of the Expert Maternity Group. HMSO, London

Disability Discrimination Act 1995 HMSO, London. Online. Available: http://www/drc-gb.org 1 March 2006

Drey E A, Darney P D 2004 Contraceptive choices for women with disabilities. In: Welner S L, Haseltine F (eds) Welner's guide to the care of women with disabilities. Lippincott Williams & Wilkins, Philadelphia, p 109–130

Gates B 2001 Learning disabilities. 3rd edn. Churchill Livingstone, London

Goh B 2002 UK guidelines on the management of syphilis. British Association for Sexual Health and HIV. Online. Available: http://www.bashh.org 23 June 2006

Goodwin A J, Agronin M E A 1997 Woman's guide to overcoming sexual fears and pain. New Harbinger, Oakland, USA

Hawtin K 1985 Psychosexual therapy. Sage, London

Hay P 2001 National guidelines on the management of bacterial vaginosis. British Association for Sexual Health and HIV. Online. Available: http://www.bashh.org 23 June 2006

Health Education Authority (HEA) 1996 Folic acid and the prevention of neural tube defects: guidance for health service providers. HEA, London

Heiman J, LoPiccolo J 1992 Becoming orgasmic: a sexual and personal growth program. Fireside Simon & Schuster, New York

Horner P J 2006 National guideline for the management of genital tract infection with chlamydia trachomatis. British Association for Sexual Health and HIV. Online. Available: http://www.bashh.org 23 June 2006

Hubbard R 1997 Abortion and disability. In: Davis L (ed) The disability studies reader. Routledge, London, p 187–202

Jackson A B, Wadley V 1999 A multicenter study of women's self-reported reproductive health after spinal cord injury. Archives of Physical Medicine and Rehabilitation 80(11):1420–1428

Kalamis C 2003 Women without sex: the truth about female sexual problems. Self-Help Direct, London

Kallianes V, Rubenfeld P 1997 Disabled women and reproductive rights. Disability and Society 12(2):203–221

Knifton C 1998 Non-consensual sterilization of the adult with learning disabilities. British Journal of Nursing 7(19):1172–1176

Lapper A 2005 My life in my hands. Simon and Schuster, London. Extracts online. Available: http://www.alisonlapper.com 9 May 2006

Lonsdale S 1990 Women and disability: the experience of physical disability among women. Macmillan Education, London

McKay-Moffat S, Lee P 2006 A pocket guide for student midwives. Wiley, London

McLaughlin J 2003 Screening networks: shared agenda in feminist disability movement challenges to antenatal screening and abortion. Disability and Society 18(3):297–310

Morris J 1991 Pride against prejudice: transforming attitudes to disability. Women's Press, London

Morris J 1995 Able lives: women's experience of paralysis. Women's Press, London

Murphy N, Young P C 2005 Sexuality in children and adolescents with disabilities. Developmental Medicine and Child Neurology 47(9):640–644

Neville-Jan A 2004 Selling your soul to the devil: an autoethnography of pain, pleasure and the quest for a child. Disability and Society 19(2):113–127

Nosek M A, Young M E, Rintala D H et al 1995 Barriers to reproductive health maintenance among women with physical disabilities. Journal of Women's Health 4(5):505–518

Nosek M A, Howland C, Rintala D H et al 2001 National study of women with physical disabilities: final report. Sexuality and Disability 19(1):5–39

Nuefeld J A, Klingbell F, Bryen D N et al 2002 Adolescent sexuality and disability. Physical Medicine and Rehabilitation Clinics of North America 13(4):857–873

Robinson-Walsh D 1997 Disabled—not unable! Baby Magazine April:16–19

Sawin K J, Buran C F, Brei T J et al 2002 Sexuality issues in adolescents with a chronic neurological condition. Journal of Perinatal Education 11(1):22–34

Servais L, Jacques D, Leach R et al 2002 Contraception of women with intellectual disability: prevalence and determinants. Journal of Intellectual Disability Research 46(part 2):108–119

Shackle M 1994 I thought I was the only one: a report of a conference 'Disabled People, Pregnancy and Early Parenthood.' Part of the Maternity Alliance Disability Working Group Pack. Maternity Alliance, London

Shakespeare T 1996 Power and prejudice: issues of gender, sexuality and disability. In: Barton L (ed) Disability and society: emerging issues and insights. Longman, New York, p 91–214

Sharpe K, Earle S 2002 Feminism, disability and abortion: irreconcilable differences? Disability and Society 17(2):137–145

Sherrard J 2001 National guideline on the management of trichomonas vaginalis. British Association for Sexual Health and HIV. Online. Available: http://www.bashh.org 23 June 2006

Shipway L 2004 Domestic violence: a handbook for health care professionals. Abingdon, Routledge

Sobsey D 1994 Sexual abuse of individuals with intellectual disability. In: Craft A (ed) Practical issues in sexuality and learning disabilities. Routledge, London, p 93–115

Swain J, French S, Cameron C 2003 Controversial issues in a disabling society. Open University, Buckingham

Szarewski A 2006 Contraceptive dilemmas. 2nd edn. Altman, St Albans

Taleporos G, McCabe MP 2003 Relationships, sexuality and adjustment among people with physical disability. Sexual and Relationship Therapy 18(1):25–43

Tepper M, Whipple B, Richard E et al 2001 Women with complete spinal cord injury: a phenomenological study of sexual experiences. Journal of Sexual and Marital Therapy 27(4): 615–623

Vasey S 1996 The experience of care. In: Hales G (ed) Beyond disability towards an enabling society. Sage with The Open University, London, p 82–87

Welner S L 1997 Gynaecologic care and sexuality issues for women with disabilities: proceedings of the international seminar on women and disability. Sexuality and Disability 15(1):33–40

Welner S L 2004 Genital infections—diagnostic and therapeutic challenges. In: Welner S L, Haseltine F (eds) Welner's guide to the care of women with disabilities. Lippincott Williams & Wilkins, Philadelphia, p 131–144

Welner S L, Temple B 2004 General health concerns and the physical examination. In: Welner S L, Haseltine F (eds) Welner's guide to the care of women with disabilities. Lippincott Williams & Wilkins, Philadelphia, p 95–108

Whipple B, Komisaruk B R 1997 Sexuality and women with complete spinal cord injury. Spinal Cord 35:136–138

Whitman B Y, Accardo P J 1990 When a parent is mentally retarded. Paul Brooks, Baltimore

## Further reading

European Disability Forum 1999 Manifesto by Disabled Women in Europe. UK Disability Forum Women's Committee. Online. Available: http://www.edfwomen.org.uk/manifesto.htm 10 Sept 2005

# 3 Maternity services and women's experiences

*Jackie Rotheram, Stella McKay-Moffat*

## INTRODUCTION

The past two decades have witnessed a dramatic change in maternity care. Despite these changes however, disabled women are still being marginalised in that their specific and individual needs are not being met in our traditional healthcare settings. From my experience as a specialist midwife in disability, more disabled women are seen in our healthcare settings in the UK. Despite this, statistical data for this client group are not readily available as birth register records do not routinely include details of maternal disabilities. The women are seen as vulnerable adults, as a minority within a minority and therefore experience of need is limited. Furthermore, society in general assumes that disabled women neither want nor are able to have children, and if they do have children are unable to care for their well-being. In this latter situation many care professionals concentrate on the needs of the child at the expense of nurturing parenting skills.

It is estimated that there are in the region of 1.2–4 million disabled parents in the UK but exact numbers are unknown because of difficulties with calculations (Disabled Parents Network 2006). People with physical and sensory impairments appear to be the most prevalent. Of this number there are many who face barriers both in their maternity care and their parenting role. Expectations are not met, and overall experiences have not always been positive. This is often the same for their carers; midwives in particular find themselves unprepared, lacking in disability awareness and knowledge of disability issues.

This chapter focuses on the needs of women with physical or sensory impairments. Within these criteria, no boundaries are set for age or type of impairment, however women with mental health needs will not be considered as they are not within the remit of this book. Using experiences from my personal and professional life and information from contacts, I have included three composite case scenarios at the end of the chapter to illustrate service provision. None of these 'cases' actually refers to an individual case therefore there are no issues of breach of confidentiality. One of these 'cases' describes a couple with learning disability; the specific needs of women with learning disabilities are discussed in Chapter 5.

The aim of this chapter is to explore the maternity needs of disabled women with physical and sensory impairments as perceived by disabled women themselves. It will also address the specific maternity care priorities and needs of this client group. Women's own experience of pregnancy and parenting will help identify gaps in service provision and make services better targeted to need. It will enable health carers to focus on the needs of disabled women to ensure a maternity service that is woman centred and evidence based.

Specific chapter objectives listed below will help service providers to:

- overcome prejudice and barriers by offering equal choices with services;
- help women to make an informed choice about their care;
- identify issues and areas of concern for the women and themselves;

- use adaptive and creative approaches to meet individual needs;
- inform and empower disabled women by giving accessible and accurate information;
- consider the need to provide appropriate equipment.

## BACKGROUND AND LITERATURE REVIEW

A systematic, computer-assisted search of the literature showed that there is little research into the maternity needs of disabled women. Some qualitative evidence exists and reports of case studies, but much of the literature is primarily anecdotal in nature. My experience in this area has also identified a lack of relevant literature available for disabled women and their health carers. There is some evidence in the area of learning disabilities, but here the literature tends to focus mainly on the needs of the child and not always the needs of the parent. Furthermore, other writers confirm that there are relatively few published studies on the maternity and parenting experience of disabled women (for example Thomas & Curtis 1997). Campion (1990) and later Shackle (1994) both reported disabled women's experiences of negative attitudes in relation to their sexuality and parenthood. The latter information was the report of results from a conference organised by the Maternity Alliance giving details of disabled women's experiences of the maternity services. Findings from this conference generated the UK midwives' professional body: the Royal College of Midwives (RCM) to publish a position paper (1996) to give midwives guidelines for their practice which was updated in 2000.

Despite these guidelines however, Shackleton & Goddard (1997) claimed that disabled women who choose to become parents still experience discrimination, disempowerment and insensitivity from health professionals. They discussed the need to explore emerging themes identified by disabled women themselves in order to make recommendations for change. However, it must be acknowledged that the experiences reported by the women may have occurred long before the first RCM position paper was published. Furthermore, some women are reluctant to focus on the impairment alone preferring to adopt the social model of disability.

Personal contact with disability specialists and support groups also confirms that research in this area is needed. In view of this therefore, there is clearly a necessity to determine the needs of this minority group to meet individual requirements. Without this, obstetricians, midwives and other health carers will be faced with providing care and support often in situations where they may have little or no experience (Carty 1998) and with little evidence to guide practice. Indeed, as disability and maternity are two words rarely seen together in the same sentence according to Campion (1997), it is not surprising that many health carers are unsure how best to provide maternity care to this minority group.

Culley & Genders (1999) confirm this need for more information as highlighted in a research project designed to examine the role of learning disability nurses in supporting people with learning disabilities who become parents. They argue that training is essential to providing a person-centred service where disabled people are valued and respected and where attitudes are positive and appropriate.

Disabled women have been identified as a group that the present maternity services are failing. The RCM (2000) believe that midwives have a key role to play in meeting the needs of disabled women and supports the woman-centred principles set out in the UK government's document *Changing Childbirth* (DoH 1993) that physical access and the attitudes of professionals do not prevent access to services.

Inadequate services are no longer acceptable and some legislative progress has been made to help rectify the issues. The most significant legislation of the decade in the UK is the Human Rights Act 1998 which came into force in October 2000 (Dimond 2000). It is extremely likely that this Act has ensured that more concern is directed to the rights of the individual. Similarly the UK Disability Discrimination Act (DDA) (1995) draws attention to the duty of care for service providers in the respective parameters of access, communication and disability awareness training, embracing these concepts to improve the quality of healthcare provided. The DDA states that it is unlawful to provide a lower standard of service to disabled people and focuses on three areas of concern:

- Access to goods and services.
- Physical barriers.
- Care by professionals. Attitude and behaviour of others.

Maternity services can place barriers for disabled women which Dimond (2003, 2004) points out is illegal as it is discriminating against them. Left unaddressed these barriers often give rise to prejudice and ignorance of individual needs. Problems may arise if these needs are not met. The DDA states that reasonable adjustments are to be made to ensure that services are not impossible or unreasonably difficult for disabled people to access and use. Part 3, Section 21 identifies three key areas for action:

- Disability awareness training—the most significant barrier cited by disabled people was that of inappropriate staff attitudes and behaviour.
- Communication and information, to include policy and procedures.
- Access/removing barriers.

The legislation in the form of the DDA, and more recently the new maternity services standard published as part of the National Service Framework for Children Young People and Maternity Services (NSF) (DoH 2004) sets out the principles of care that midwives should offer to all women and that of course includes those with a disability. The latter document continues to revolve around promoting women centred care and advocates informed choices as did *Changing Childbirth* (DoH 1993). Access to up-to-date and relevant information, in particular preconception advice, care and support; working in partnership; appropriate care pathways; and alliances and networks, are all highlighted.

Standard 11 of the NSF addresses the requirements for women during pregnancy and maintaining contact before and after the birth process. Maternity services are to be proactive in engaging all women early in their pregnancy, particularly women from disadvantaged groups and communities. The principles of the government which initiated the Sure Start system, whereby midwives and other health professionals work with disadvantaged groups of pregnant women and new mothers and babies, should be extended across other services i.e. working with parents and children. This should be started early, be responsive to women's needs and

be flexible at the point of delivery. There must be provision of services for everyone ensuring they are community driven and professionally coordinated across agencies, and outcome focused. Sure Start midwives engage with disadvantaged groups and midwifery-led centres are being developed in deprived areas to ensure care is locally based and accessible.

Maternity care providers and Primary Care Trusts should plan the provision of maternity services based on an up-to-date assessment of the needs of the local population e.g. identifying specific vulnerable groups. Involving service user groups to explore the reasons why women from these groups find it difficult to access and maintain contact with maternity services will improve the access to, and effectiveness of, maternity services for minority groups. This means that providers must ensure that local maternity services are inclusive for women with learning and physical disabilities taking into account their communication, equipment and support needs.

Services need to be innovative and flexible in meeting the needs of women with communication difficulties and other disabilities, and informed by best practice from settings and regions caring for disabled women across the country. To aid this it is suggested that a directory of local and national agencies is developed that can provide expert advice and support for professionals working with women from disadvantaged and minority groups and communities. There should be inter-agency arrangements, including protocols for information sharing. Additionally, to promote the health and well-being of the mother and her baby, it is highlighted that there is the need for a lead professional who will help to ensure that women from disadvantaged groups have adequate support from other agencies.

It is clear from the literature and my own experiences in practice, that the most common themes for disabled women are lack of relevant information, barriers to access to services, and negative attitudes from professional carers. Disabled women want to be treated like all other women but not at the expense of the disability being overreacted to or ignored. There is a tendency for the needs of disabled women to become more medicalised as professional carers often view pregnancy as problematic. As a consequence the experience of childbirth becomes one of 'high risk'. This usual traditional view is not the case for every disabled woman. Being realistic however, one must be aware that problems may arise, but this is also the case for non-disabled women. Disabled women themselves live within their strengths while recognising their limitations: knowing what they need and what they do not. Carers should, therefore, respect their individuality, seeing them as women first, disabled second.

These issues cannot be viewed in isolation but need to be embraced within the context of the wider determinants of health and the link between economic, social and environmental conditions as these also have implications for health. Furthermore, providing maternity services for disabled women represents a challenge to many health professionals who often find themselves under resourced and not adequately prepared for the role.

The rationale for this chapter emerged not only from these factors but from my own personal experiences of disability, childbirth and parenting (I am a disabled parent myself) and my professional role as a specialist midwife/disability advisor working in a maternity care setting in one of the largest specialist centres for women in Europe. This specialist role has enabled me to offer care and support to disabled women with physical, sensory, learning and mental health issues.

Investigating the needs of disabled women helps to identify gaps in service provision to enable health providers to be better able to target the needs of this client group and to provide a maternity service which is woman centred and evidence based. It is the responsibility of all carers to prepare themselves to meet this challenge. With this in mind I conducted a small-scale qualitative study using semi-structured interviews with 12 disabled women with a physical or sensory impairment. This highlighted the perceived needs of this client group, giving further experiential evidence of requirements. These experiences highlight some of the negative attitudes that exist, and the gaps in service provision to meet individual needs. Making reasonable adjustments will enable health care services to offer maternity care that is woman centred, evidence based, meeting the needs of disabled women.

## DISABILITY AWARENESS

One of the components of the UK Disability Discrimination Act (1995) is 'Disability Awareness': the process of informing and empowering individuals in disability etiquette. The biggest barrier cited by disabled people is that of negative attitudes and behaviours.

The view of many disabled people is that professional carers are not disability aware. There is a lack of understanding by many GPs, obstetricians, midwives, and other carers as to their needs. Women are not asked directly, there is no mention of the impairment and the implications thereof, and there is an obvious lack of specialist knowledge. The duty of care is the responsibility of all carers in order to be informed, enabled and empowered to provide an inclusive philosophy of care.

## BARRIERS

Thomas and Curtis (1997) support the claims made in *Changing Childbirth* (DoH 1993) in that professional practice and other features of maternity services can place barriers for disabled women. Left unaddressed these barriers often give rise to prejudice and ignorance of individual needs. The current literature identifies three predominant barriers faced by disabled women: attitude and behaviour, access to services, and care by professionals. The experiences of disabled women highlighted by Shackle (1994) summarises the negative attitudes that exist, poor access to services and the lack of relevant literature available for disabled pregnant women and their health carers; as one disabled parent commented to me: 'it should not be down to informal conversations with other parents and the luck of the draw with professionals as to whether relevant information is given'.

Following a recent opportunistic survey, Wates (2003) claimed that the level of support given is often dependant on the individual relationship between a disabled woman and her professional carer, and that certain professional groups are more supportive than others, although variations between groups do exist. In the report, 'It shouldn't be down to luck', Wates (2003) describes what over

150 disabled parents said about access to information and support. Although midwives and maternity services were not specified directly, this study highlighted that even to the present day disabled women who choose to become parents are still experiencing discrimination, disempowerment and insensitivity from health professionals.

My professional experience of midwifery, parenting and disability reflects and confirms these findings in that negative attitudes abound, and the need is for more midwives and other carers to provide individualised care centred on each woman to make a difference. The level of services received by disabled women is often influenced by the underlying beliefs and attitudes of service providers. Attitudes towards disabled people are often negative. This is highlighted in the UK Disability Discrimination Act 1995 as the most influential and most common barrier to this client group.

This negativity is associated with the many myths around disabled pregnancy and parenting. For example, assumptions are made that women with a physical impairment do not want, or are unable to pursue the role of parenting. Similarly, it is often thought that disabled women cannot adequately care for and meet the needs of their child. Typically these views focus on issues of the individual coping and the associated 'problems'. Therefore they concentrate on the impairment and pay little attention to the social perspective. There is also popular belief that people with learning difficulties have more children and that their children will be neglected because of inadequate parenting skills (Shackleton & Goddard 1997).

Although these issues may be real in some cases, this is not the norm for the majority and is not the perspective from which healthcare policies should begin. Positive attitudes can only be developed as people have regular contact with disabled women and mutual respect in their diversity. Change is therefore necessary in order to provide equity in maternity care provision for disabled women. It is the responsibility of all carers to explore their own attitudes, to investigate the needs of this minority group, and be willing to be prepared to meet the challenge.

Ask yourself, why is it that so many disabled women struggle in these areas, having to justify their reasons to become parents, to convince health carers that they are women first and want to fulfil the role of motherhood? Do *you* give disabled parents the credibility and respect they deserve? Many have planned and considered the implications of disabled parenting very carefully. It is often the belief that disabled people are irresponsible, that the pregnancy is a mistake or that they will be unable to cope with the needs and demands of parenting. This results in women having concerns about pressure to become good mothers due to professionals' unhelpful support.

Disabled women need to be accepted and supported in their choice to become parents and to be cared for and informed like all other women. Evidence suggests that information aimed at parents and families tends to omit the issue of disability, whereas information for disabled people rarely covers parenting (Wates 2003).

## THE RESULTS OF THE STUDY: WOMEN'S EXPERIENCES (SEE APPENDIX FOR QUESTIONS)

### Expectations and fears

Women's expectations of their maternity experience often depended on the type of their impairment, and the support and information they received during their pregnancy. Many disabled women feel confident in this experience, others have many fears. When these fears are left unaddressed the maternity experience for both user and carer will not meet expectations.

Some of the most common fears for disabled parents are highlighted as follows:

- Concern about well-being throughout pregnancy and delivery.
- Vulnerability—may not have been a patient before. Nervous seeing doctors, fear of the unknown. Not able to care for baby, coping as a disabled mum.
- Implications of delivery: the need for caesarean section and choice of anaesthetic. Knowing about the procedure from the experience of others or maybe their own can be fearful causing upset. Being admitted the night before can be problematic for some, for others it can feel more reassuring and secure.

- Not being able to have a normal labour, pain relief, and recovery time postnatal. Implications of delivery, possibility of epidural/tear.
- Loss of independence, having to ask for help to shower, to mobilise, requiring use of specific equipment, bed, cot, Zimmer frame, help with childcare: handling, lifting, changing, feeding, bathing.
- Exacerbation of impairment following pregnancy and delivery—effects unknown.
- Depression due to fatigue and maybe doubting own parenting experience; some mothers can become depressed due to the change in emotions, the added responsibility, impairment itself or just being a new mother.

## Information

Information enhances knowledge: to have knowledge is to have control and autonomy. The information needs of disabled parents are variable according to the type of impairment but on the whole they are the same as that of non-disabled women in respect of pregnancy and birth. Disabled parents, however, may also need appropriate, relevant and up-to-date information specific to the impairment and in a format which is accessible. The Disability Discrimination Act 1995 highlights accessible information as one of its themes in providing equity in goods and services.

From the results of my study the following information requirements were identified.

- Availability of specific preconception services for those who require specialist advice before becoming pregnant because of pre-existing medical or familial conditions.
- Specific information to parents and family requesting referral for genetic counselling following the diagnosis of a genetic disorder in a previous child.
- Early provision of preconception information and then more emphasis on early pregnancy information to meet the needs of second-time parents.
- Information on the effects of disability on pregnancy and vice versa: For some there was *no* specific information, for others not enough information was given.
- There was much information on pregnancy and very little on disability—nothing on being pregnant and disabled.

- More specific information related to the disability to fill in gaps in knowledge.
- More information on medication, its effects on pregnancy and risk to baby: 'risk to baby only explored by one support group'.
- Information needed 'on what to do in an emergency'.
- More practical hands-on information—what to do, how to do it and what to expect.
- Lay knowledge of medical terms to be used for easy-to-understand everyday language.
- Information on all methods of contraception not just sterilisation.
- Explanation to be given when care is medicalised.
- Parent education to be offered at weekends— Sundays for women with families and to accommodate working partners, building a relationship of trust.
- Classes to be more focused on disability issues or at least to have disability more integral to session: Parent education to also cover general issues: 'what it's like to be a parent'.
- More reassurance to have the confidence to ask questions.
- Effects of pain relief in labour, effect on baby and what to expect.
- Maternity hospital to work in partnership with Primary Care—effective communication one with the other, exchanging relevant information and instruction.
- Network to sources of information, newsletters, and phone lines.
- Closer liaison with support groups and other specialists to share information.
- Accessible information in different formats and media, large font, Braille, audiotape, disc, video (with subtitles, British Sign Language).
- Information on conditions associated with pregnancy e.g. symphysis pubis diastases (SPD), depression, and postnatal depression.
- More explanation of caesarean section, preoperative care, postnatal, what to do, what not to do when at home, long-term implications.

Disabled parents access information from many sources, primarily from midwives who are seen as the main carers. Other professionals also give specific information (see responsibilities of midwives) and many are given information from family members who share their own experiences. Disabled parents have individual needs which are impairment specific. Many will make their own enquiries exploring equipment resources and other service provisions.

## Best and worst moments of maternity experience

The experiences of many disabled parents are variable, depending on their own personal experience. My research revealed some of the best and worst moments for disabled women.

The following quotes from disabled parents show how experiences can vary.

### Best moments
- 'Whole experience was good'
- 'When pregnancy confirmed was my best moment knowing that I had done what some women couldn't do'
- 'When my baby's first picture was taken in theatre, I was afraid I would miss it'
- 'When I found out on the scan that my baby was OK'
- 'The first hour when I was left alone in the recovery area in theatre, just me and my baby'
- 'The care I received from my midwife after delivery, it was brilliant'

From my experience disabled women also report that:

- 'Yes, needs asked by consultant, midwife, maternity care assistant and others'
- 'Shared care good e.g. Sure Start and team midwives, other professionals seen in pregnancy, specialist consultant, fetal centre'
- 'Choice for delivery given by midwife who discussed issues'
- 'Staff on wards were informed of care needs from the plan of care'
- 'Supported by consultant, having all appointments at hospital'
- 'Closely monitored, pleased with this, needs not ignored, taken seriously'
- 'Care needs during labour always good'
- 'Scared of delivery/nervous, helped by tour, also seeing theatre'
- 'Partner always encouraged to get involved'

- 'Staff supportive, pleasant, good fun'
- 'Happy with outcome of delivery/position restrictions'
- 'Information given on folic acid, heparin, pain relief and other medication, this explored in detail'
- 'Good video in antenatal clinic. All kinds of leaflets, books, someone to ask questions'

### Worst moments
- 'When the pain relief stopped working'
- 'My fear of delivery'
- 'When my impairment got worse, I couldn't move'
- 'There was not enough info on symphysis pubis diastases, my needs were unmet'
- 'I was ignorant of the equipment that was available to use, I struggled on my own'
- 'Not being able to bath baby because of my impairment'
- 'Long labour, I was left too long before any intervention: I was exhausted, it exacerbated my myalgic encephalomyelitis (M.E.)'
- 'When I was told the sex of the baby' (psychological issue)

Other negative experiences of disabled parents are quoted below:

- 'Midwife not aware of my impairment. Impairment and needs only explored by Disability Advisor.'
- 'Hospital should take a more proactive role e.g. a referral to see specialist for care and support before discharge home'
- 'Did not want caesarean section—not prepared enough for this'
- 'Not enough nursing care after caesarean section—needed extra support'
- 'Caesarean section planned because of my impairment, I was sad not having first sight of baby because had a general anaesthetic'
- 'Little help given with self care'
- 'Long postnatal stay—too long'
- 'Own room key factor to recovery'
- 'Had complications postnatal, not prepared for this'
- 'Pain relief discussed on ward postnatally, too late should be discussed earlier'
- 'Not enough care at home'

## Tests and investigations

The assumption is made that disabled women require more tests and investigations than others. The majority of disabled women are happy with all tests performed but the experiences of women are varied in this instance in that they report:

- Good care clinically, impairment was not ignored.
- Many scans performed, drugs, and the effects on baby, fear of ectopic, size, sex of baby.
- Usual bloods taken and urine samples as other women, no extra tests.
- Glucose tolerance and other tests in fetal centre reassuring.
- Reassured that pregnancy was monitored closely.
- Enough information on tests and investigations seen in leaflets, books available, also midwife availability to explain.
- Age influenced decision to have blood test. There is an assumption that more tests are done because of age; when test refused, attitudes of professionals can be negative.

## Attitudes

To develop positive attitudes towards disabled parents, all carers need to explore their own attitudes in order to offer respect and not impose their own values and beliefs.

Disabled people on the whole face negative attitudes, however in my experience comments have been positive when the impairment is acknowledged and needs identified and supported.

To follow are comments from disabled parents in their maternity experience:

- 'I was not treated differently or made to feel different'
- 'My experience was good'
- 'Overall positive'
- 'No unacceptable terminology or words used'
- 'Not patronised or patronising attitude seen, however pockets of negative attitudes observed'
- 'Treated like other mums, made to feel special'
- 'No problems really'
- 'Some negative attitudes by a community midwife, she was unable to care for specific needs'
- 'Lack of knowledge by midwife seen'

- 'Negative attitudes seen but not intentional more inappropriate behaviour'
- 'Good it was to be spoken to direct and not to my mum or partner'
- 'Assumptions were made because of being a wheelchair user'
- 'Positive support from younger midwives—those newly trained were creative and up to date. The older the midwife the more negative the attitude' (more interested in paperwork)
- 'Midwife very busy, not enough time to get to know individual needs, too many tasks, not enough time for individual needs'
- 'Very busy, so many other mums to care for, attitude abrupt'
- 'Made to feel uncomfortable, my partner was told to use downstairs toilet' (partner has sensory impairment)
- 'Midwife from black cultures, very good'

## MATERNITY SERVICES

## Inclusive philosophy of care

An inclusive philosophy of care is the key to success for all parents as they prepare for pregnancy, birth, and parenthood. From my own midwifery experience, disabled parents seek acceptance from their carers; there is a desire to be accepted and supported like non-disabled women. The way parents are treated by health professionals can influence their maternity care and early days of parenting.

When starting to consider the provision of an inclusive philosophy of care the terminology used to identify those with a disability is the first aspect. There are many words associated with disability and the terminology is changing all the time as society looks for alternative words. Whatever term is used, it will never be tolerable to all disabled people. The correct way is to ask the individual directly and for them to decide on the term most acceptable. One must consider that impairment gives the label but society gives the definition.

In the past, words associated with disability were spastic, handicapped, cripple, invalid, deaf and dumb, and wheelchair bound. These are not terms that would make one proud. Terminology is personal to the individual and should be respected as such. Some definitions, terms and labels are vague, for example 'partially sighted': is a person 'more blind' or 'less blind'? 'Wheelchair bound' implies being tied to the chair. A few will use the condition to describe and define an individual, for example 'epileptic', others are called victims of polio. But the word 'victim', it could be argued, implies punishment and subservience. Referring to people as deaf and dumb may not be acceptable. Deaf people have their own community, language and grammar (see Chapter 7). Using the term 'the blind' refers to a homogenous group, whilst the word cripple refers to a fixed state.

In my experience young women, particularly during pregnancy, do not use the word or even want to be known as 'disabled'. It has a negative view, one of weakness, with 'problems', using aids or adapted equipment, having 'special needs' and requiring extra help which implies having to rely on someone else. These notions are all negative in a maternity setting. Being referred to a 'specialist midwife' is more acceptable than referral to the 'disability advisor'. It is all in the word, but to a disabled person it can make all the difference between being accepted and included or rejected and separated.

Disabled parents want their needs to be met alongside those of other women. However, the experience of antenatal, labour and postnatal care for many can cause anxiety as they consider the barriers they may face. To overcome barriers to providing an inclusive philosophy of care, we must start by asking disabled parents themselves what their needs are. This is explored during the needs assessment interview where women are consulted and involved. For many women this does not happen and their own specific care needs are not addressed i.e. direct questions specifically related to the impairment are *not* asked. Assumptions are made, equipment is provided that is not required, there are unhelpful care needs and too many professionals are involved.

## Choice

Choice is a crucial issue for disabled people not least for women during their maternity care. Disabled people often have choices made for them, dictated by society in order to conform to the 'norm' and be accepted. It is the assumption that 'we know best'

therefore information is not given in full, hence women are not able to make informed choices for their own care and that of their baby. *Changing Childbirth* (DoH 1993) advocated that choice be given to all women to empower, educate and instil confidence in their ability to become confident, competent parents. There needs to be a dialogue between disabled parents and their carers where individual strengths and weaknesses are discussed and needs identified by the parents themselves. It is also important for disabled women to be able to make their own choices without influence from their own parents (especially mothers), family members, professionals and other carers. Making choices for oneself instils confidence.

Choice of hospital to attend for maternity care may be essential but for many there is very little choice as many maternity units are now becoming large tertiary hospitals. Therefore some disabled parents may choose to travel to specialist units with specialist midwives and specialist services. A few are guided by the experience of others, yet this is not always the best way to choose where to have a baby but it is the choice of some. From my experience disabled parents have made their own enquiries and made their own decision where they want to go. A few, however, are not sure and look to health professionals to make the decision and choice for them. It is our duty of care to inform and instruct, to support and guide. Whatever choices disabled parents make we need to respect and acknowledge their right.

All women have the right to choose the lead professional in their maternity care: consultant obstetrician, midwife or GP. This can be confusing as many are not sure whilst others make specific requests to their GP to refer to a particular obstetrician. The cultural beliefs of women from some ethnic minority groups dictate that they will only be seen by a woman. Disabled women should be given the same choices as other women regardless of their impairment but if they are viewed as 'at risk' because of their disability they are more likely to be referred to a consultant obstetrician. This 'medicalises' the pregnancy immediately.

Additionally choosing to have a home or hospital birth or a water birth must be considered for its suitability, safety and good practice. Many professionals make the assumption that disabled women will give birth by caesarean section, being the best outcome for the impairment. It should not be an automatic decision and it cannot be the decision of another. It must be the choice of the individual following discussion with the respective consultant and/or midwife.

To assist disabled parents in their decision-making process the specialist midwife or disability advisor can support women to reinforce their choices. There is an urgency therefore to redress the balance, giving disabled women autonomy and choice in their maternity care to empower, educate and instil confidence in their ability to become confident parents. There needs to be a dialogue where individual strengths and weaknesses are discussed and needs identified by the client herself and not from the assumptions of her health carer.

## Flexibility

Maternity care for disabled parents needs to be flexible, creative and specific to need. Flexibility in care provision needs to be discussed and explored with both user and carer alike, primarily client led but depending on the urgency of need and the availability of resources. Disabled parents are familiar with their own impairment but may be unfamiliar within the context of maternity. Care is individually tailored towards the type of impairment and need; flexibility is key to control and choice. Disabled women often feel more reassured having all their antenatal care in hospital seeing a doctor and a midwife. Others on the other hand prefer shared care with primarily the midwife as the lead carer and only seen by the medical team if there are any concerns. Nevertheless, care for women, for example with medical disorders, twin pregnancies, and who substance misuse will be consultant led. The well-being of mother and baby will dictate the degree of flexibility of the care.

There is often a feeling of control in flexibility of care and timing of hospital appointments. However, because of the impairment some may require care in the community with home visits by midwives. This is particularly necessary for women whose impairment is exacerbated because of the pregnancy. Poor mobility can also be a problem making hospital visits difficult whilst others prefer home visiting to avoid the organisational barriers. As with all mothers, those working depend on the flexibility in time and frequency of antenatal appointments around employment or child-care.

After the birth disabled parents may need a longer in-patient stay given flexibility of time spent on the postnatal ward. Many prefer to be discharged home as soon as possible where their own facilities and equipment lessen the disabling effects of their impairment. Others may have had a traumatic or long delivery or have young children at home and need a longer time to recover and rest. Continued flexibility in postnatal care with visits from the community midwifery team can be discussed directly with midwives giving care.

Standards 11, 9.4 and 9.5 of The National Service Framework (DoH 2004) suggest that community postnatal care has not extended sufficiently long enough for the identification of health problems, for example postnatal depression, that develop later than the traditional 10–14 days midwives visit or even the 6–8 weeks postnatal check. This is equally important, perhaps more so, for the disabled mother. Now the role of midwives is no longer restricted to providing care only up to 28 days following the birth (NMC 2004); there is the potential for continuation of midwifery care as long as necessary. Life with a new baby is challenging for all mothers but likely to be more so for the disabled mother, therefore the key to aid effective parenting is to be as flexible as mother and baby's needs dictate.

## Child-care with a disability

Caring for a new baby as a disabled parent can be a challenge. Disabled parents are aware of their limitations and will apply their own coping strategies to overcome them. Time and consideration will be given to types of equipment to buy such as prams, cots, car seats, baby bath. Some will have different ways of performing certain tasks, for example feeding, bathing, changing, lifting and carrying depending on the type of impairment. Others will be creative in the types of clothing to buy, for example a mother with rheumatoid arthritis may choose to use clothing with hook and loop (Velcro) fastening rather than buttons and ribbons.

Parents know their own strengths and weaknesses and what areas of child-care may be hard. When in hospital on postnatal wards disabled parents may need help to lift baby from the cot, with handling, bathing, changing, dressing and then help to put baby back into the cot. Additionally, how to adjust these aspects of child-care when baby's weight increases. New parents, whether disabled or not, are nervous at first and will seek support from their carers to increase their confidence. To suggest that disabled parents cannot care for their baby without added resources and support could be a stumbling block and erode their confidence as new parents. Too much unhelpful care can also be seen as interfering and undermining. The key to successful parenting is onward, forward, upward and higher, learning on the way, adapting to changes and needs as they occur. Life with a new baby can be challenging. It is important therefore that all parents find good support networks and practical help. Support can come from primary care teams, GPs, midwives, health visitors, and specialist health and social services.

## Responsibilities of midwives

Midwives have a responsibility and duty of care to be available to reassure, support and advise all parents (NMC 2004), not least disabled people. Just 'being there' providing a 'safe place' can be comforting to new parents. The parenting role is a time of much change and increased responsibility for all parents. Disabled parents may be overly anxious being aware of the expectations made on them and having to justify themselves to others and making allowances for their impairment. Many give the impression that they are 'super mums' not being allowed or afraid to ask questions, or dare to make a mistake for fear of being seen as a bad parent, or worse still not being able to cope. However, the effect of pregnancy and delivery on a person's impairment often causes a struggle particularly for women with myalgic encephalomyelitis (ME), multiple sclerosis (MS), and rheumatoid arthritis. Referrals to their respective specialist may be necessary. From my experience some use alternative therapies to aid recovery.

The practical responsibilities of midwives are the same for the disabled parent as they are for any other parent under their care, but they may need to be innovative and adaptable in the way that advice and service is offered. Additionally, knowing what questions to ask and to be sensitive to needs, and to be ready to share in problem solving to find the best solution to overcome difficulties is vital. This also includes embracing the needs of partners and the extended family that may have fear of being unable to cope and the added responsibility. Key skills of perception and communication are necessary to be attentive to the silent fears and moods, and the relationship and interaction with others. To be able to instil confidence and allay any overt or covert fears requires skills of encouragement and insightful advice.

Liaison with other professionals, support groups and disabled parent networks not only enables the expertise of others to be channelled into helping mothers, but helps to reinforce the reality of parenting with a disability for midwives. This in turn will aid the enhancement of services to parents. As the 28-day limit has been removed from midwives' time of attendance (NMC 2004) the midwife is able to reinforce support from the health visitor for a much longer period of time. Additionally she can be involved in the 6-week postnatal examination with or without mothers' GPs. This will enable midwives to fulfil their public health and health promotion role, for example by offering information about contraception and family planning, preconception care and issues around women's health if needed.

To enable midwives to fulfil their role, a training and development programme would be of significant benefit. This could include issues promoting disability awareness during all induction courses for new staff and as mandatory training and professional development days for existing staff. It would utilise a strategic training programme that could be based on the 'Positive about diversity and equality' NHS training materials and the DDA. There is also the potential to develop an e-learning package. Outside trainers and speakers, and the inclusion of disabled service users would enhance learning.

## Physical access to services

Physical accessibility of premises should be a priority to enable equity of access for all. This concept does not just assume physical access alone. Many people are of the assumption that when lifts and ramps are available then physical access is addressed. However, this notion extends to equity in access to all aspects of healthcare. It also revolves around actually having facilities that are appropriate to enable care to be undertaken. To aid clarity here, access is divided into specific sections.

### General access issues

General access issues (Box 3.1) relates to the ability to actually reach the buildings where services are provided and move about the inside of that building with the maximum of ease. It is important that reception to a clinic or hospital feels welcoming to all those using the services. For people using a wheelchair or short in stature a low reception desk that enables direct eye contact with the receptionist (Fig. 3.1) will make a greeting more personal and facilitate communication. To assist people finding their way around a hospital or clinic environment, visual signs should have both large text to make them more readily visible, and symbols/pictures to indicate a location for people with language diffi-culty (Figs. 3.2a, 3.2b, 3.2c). From my experience people become confused, even lost, when signage is not clear, for example when asked to attend other departments like ultrasound.

Lift call buttons that are at a height readily reached by someone using a wheelchair or short in stature, with tactile numbers and/or Braille, as well as an audible indication of floor number and door operation, will aid independence in moving from one floor to another in a building.

### Waiting areas

Thought needs to be given to waiting areas within a clinic as well as other parts of a building to ensure that they do not disadvantage disabled people, draw unnecessary attention to their disability, or result in their discomfort (see Box 3.2). Advanced preparation following effective communication from other health professionals will make a woman feel more welcome. If midwives and support staff are aware that a disabled woman is due to attend clinic and what her initial needs may be then they can be prepared to ensure that they know how to communicate with her e.g. taking her name at reception and calling her for her appointment (see Box 3.2). Additionally relevant equipment/facilities can be made available (see below and Box 3.3).

### Ward environments

All ward environments must be considered for in-patients and for visitors who may also be disabled. Many wards have intercom access for security purposes which can create a barrier for many deaf people, making that ward or department inaccessible. Deaf organisations suggest that intercoms should include a light to alert the visitor when the doors are opened. A video entry system can be more accessible and give more effective security (Fig. 3.3) and a light that illuminates to indicate that a door bell had been activated or a door is unlocked is helpful for deaf people (Fig. 3.4). An audible buzz will alert people with visual impairment that the door is open.

It may be better for some mothers to be in a large side ward or separate room with spacious en suite facilities and a wheel-in shower for wheelchair users if possible. Most hospitals have height-adjustable beds, but a height-adjustable cot (Fig. 3.5) on the ward, or when a baby is in need of special care,

---

**Box 3.1  General access to maternity services**

- Disabled parking that is accessible, clearly signposted, at an appropriate height for drivers to see and near to the entrance, with some disabled parking to be rear exit bays.
- Encourage the use of taxicabs that are able to accept wheelchairs.
- Accessible hospital wards and departments with permanent or temporary ramp, dropped kerbs, automatic doors, wide doors, non-slip and tactile flooring at entrances.
- Simple, short and clear signage in large font with a good background contrast and visual or pictorial symbols especially for clinics and wards.
- A voice-over on lifts and tactile buttons at a height accessible for wheelchair users or people short in stature.
- Provide escort to other wards and departments especially in an emergency. It may be difficult for people with a physical impairment to access long corridors therefore a wheelchair may be useful.
- Wheelchairs that are regularly maintained should be available at entrances for disabled people to use.
- Flexible visiting for partners and set times for others.
- Inform users of equipment and communication aids in an accessible information leaflet.

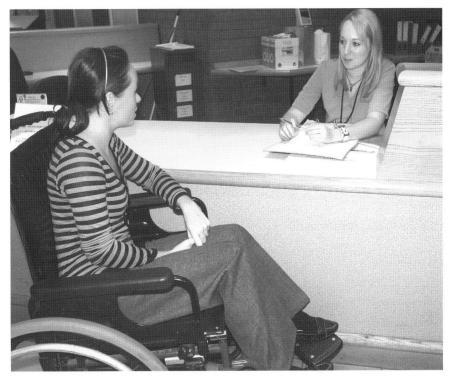

*Figure 3.1*   A low reception desk is more welcoming for someone using a wheelchair or of short stature, and enables eye contact with the receptionist to enhance communication. Photograph by Martin Baxter, with kind permission from Liverpool Women's Hospital.

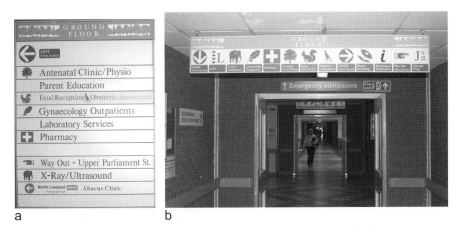

a                              b

*Figure 3.2*   **a), b)** A location can be found by following directions signs with large, clear letters and an individual picture. Photographs by Martin Baxter, with kind permission from Liverpool Women's Hospital.

(*Continues*)

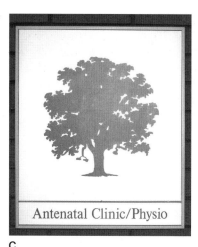

C

*Figure 3.2—Cont'd* **c**) A large individual picture indicates the location has been reached. Photograph by Martin Baxter, with kind permission from Liverpool Women's Hospital.

---

### Box 3.2  Waiting area set up

Waiting areas should be set up to:
- alert disabled people by using electronic displays or ticket/number systems enabling deaf parents and others to know their name has been called to avoid people missing their turn;
- ensure a receptionist or clerk informs midwives that a woman is deaf and will need to be approached personally when it becomes her turn;
- provide flexible seating—some soft and firm chairs with and without arm rests, variable in height, large seating for women who have a large frame. Seating at appointment desks;
- offer enough space for wheelchair users to pull up alongside a seated companion;
- enable readily accessible toilets with plenty of room to manoeuvre and with clear signposting towards the facilities;
- provide a lower reception desk enabling wheelchair users to communicate at eye level with the receptionist;
- provide separate cubicles to ensure confidentiality.

---

### Box 3.3  Equipment/facilities that may be useful during antenatal visits

- Wheelchair to tour hospital wards—information may be required regarding long-term wheelchair loan services.
- A 'Way Finder' map if available—this can be tactile and pictorial to meet individual needs or may be in an audio form for women with sensory impairments.
- Guide dogs and dogs for deaf people are acceptable in health settings.
- Height-adjustable examination couch which will aid both user and carer—enables more independence and maintains greater dignity when getting onto the bed.
- A large clinic room with large doors for easy wheelchair access.
- Availability of a hoist if needed.
- Accessible toilet and baby changing area.
- Televisions with subtitles in the waiting area.
- Loan of crutches (this is provided by the physiotherapist).
- Adequate lighting in corridors.
- Availability of minicom/textphone, or information on where to access one.
- A named midwife who can communicate by text, particularly in an emergency.

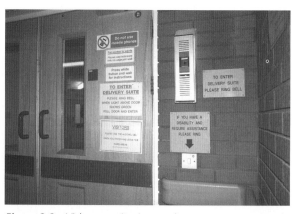

*Figure 3.3*  Video monitoring at the entrance to a ward or department enables staff to see who is awaiting entry, and if help is needed. Photograph by Martin Baxter, with kind permission from Liverpool Women's Hospital.

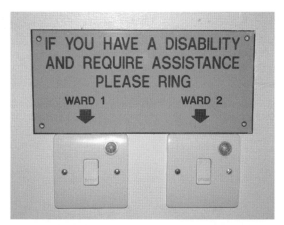

**Figure 3.4** A low-level door bell at the entrance to a ward or department is easily reached by someone using a wheelchair. The light illuminates and a buzzer sounds to indicate that the bell has rung and when the door has been unlocked. Photograph by Martin Baxter, with kind permission from Liverpool Women's Hospital.

a height-adjustable incubator (Figs. 3.6a, 3.6b) (see Chapter 9 for supplier), will make it easier for a mother to care for her baby with less need of help.

For women who are deaf a single room would cut down on background noise and make communica-

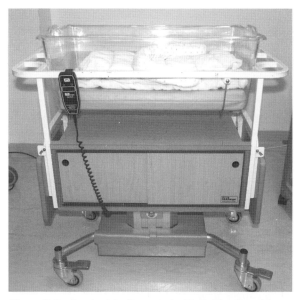

**Figure 3.5** An electrically operated height-adjustable cot. Photograph by Martin Baxter, with kind permission from Liverpool Women's Hospital.

tion more effective. The bed should face the door so that a woman can see if someone comes into the room. On the ward a deaf mother will benefit from being in a bed with a clear view of the midwives' work desk to make it easier to see what is going on and to signal if help is needed. However, if a mother is using a baby alarm that vibrates under her pillow when baby cries a single room is better as the alarm will react to the cries of other babies.

For mothers who have a visual impairment the environment of the room can be changed around so that the layout of the room or ward area becomes more familiar. If she is completely without sight, lighting is not an issue although the needs of her partner may have to be considered. If on the other hand she is partially sighted then lighting levels need to be considered and additional lights may need to be provided. Some people find a magnifying glass useful. If a mother uses a guide dog it should be allowed in the room with her but of course dog walking/care must be catered for by her partner or family member.

Women with a physical impairment may request that a partner or carer be allowed to stay on the ward overnight to support and care for their needs. If this situation arises the sleeping needs of a woman's carer must also be addressed. But for the 'high-risk' mother, for example following caesarean section, rather than being alone a bed in a four- or six-bed area may be more appropriate.

### Equipment

Equipment needs vary according to a person's impairment. Many disabled parents will have aids and adaptations in the home, for example a bath buddy, raised toilet seats, handrails, stair lift, wheelchair and deaf aids. Some will have had an occupational therapist assessment to identify additional needs. During their maternity care midwives and other carers need to focus primarily on what equipment disabled parents may require when accessing services (see Boxes 3.3, 3.4, 3.5). Many parents are unaware of what is available or what to ask for. Having leaflets itemising available equipment or suppliers of equipment will benefit all women. The Disabled Parents Network (see Chapter 9) offers a comprehensive list of equipment suppliers that can be downloaded from the internet. Some women may prefer to bring in their own equipment

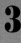 

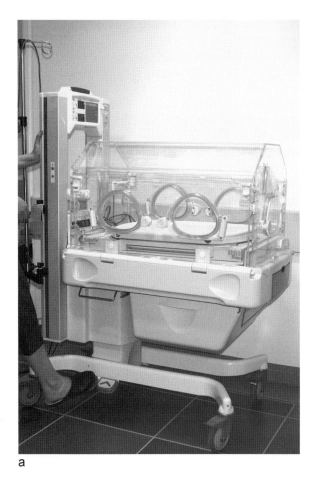

a

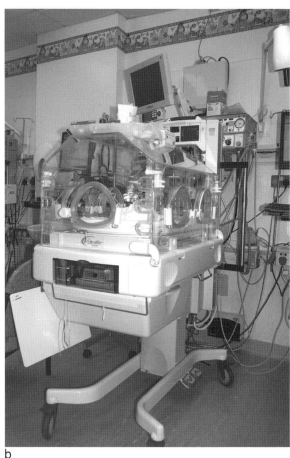

b

*Figure 3.6* **a)** A height-adjustable Giraffe® incubator (see Chapter 9) on charge and ready to be set up. The drawer is accessible from both sides and slides across to give a knee space for someone sitting. **b)** The height-adjustable Giraffe® incubator set up ready for use in the neonatal unit. Photographs by Martin Baxter, with kind permission from Liverpool Women's Hospital.

for a hospital stay that they know works for them. An added benefit here may be with infection control e.g. when a raised toilet seat is needed.

When planning for women's attendance at clinics or for hospital admission, forward planning is essential and an important part of the role of midwives. One vital piece of equipment that has the potential to maintain a woman's dignity by aiding her to more easily get into position for examination, is a height-adjustable couch (Fig. 3.7) (see Chapter 9 for supplier). These are electronically operated with

---

**Box 3.4  Specific equipment that may be useful in the delivery suite**

- Accessible en suite toilet/shower.
- Adjustable-height bed.
- Large bed if person has body mass index (BMI) above 25.
- Access to hoist if needed.
- Stools.
- Appropriate chairs relevant to need.
- Fans to cool environment.
- Extra lighting in rooms if woman or partner has a visual impairment.
- Clock in room—this is important for many.
- Labour information sheet for deaf people.

## Box 3.5 Equipment/facilities that may be useful during a hospital stay

- Large single en suite room to accommodate and manoeuvre a wheelchair.
- Overnight bed/settee or similar if partner/carer is to stay.
- Height and back rest adjustable; electronic bed if required (beds can be hired).
- Accessible toilet and shower grab rails, non-slip floors, low shower seat. Parents are encouraged to bring in their own equipment, and this will provide familiarity for the parent, and aid infection control.
- Room with a bath may be preferred.
- Alert button for safety and to summon help in an emergency.
- Height-adjustable cot and incubator in the neonatal unit.
- Magnifying glass.
- Availability of textphone/minicom. If not, parents are encouraged to bring in their own. A very few may request access to a fax machine as mobile telephone use is not allowed in hospitals.
- Televisions with subtitles if available.
- Baby alarm mattress—these specialist monitors vibrate under the mother's pillow when the baby cries. This may be difficult to use in an open-plan ward as it will pick up other babies' cries. Arrangements will need careful planning.

great ease by a foot pedal i.e. lowered for the woman but raised to ensure comfort and safety for the professional performing the examination.

## THE GENERAL WAY FORWARD

The key to success is for the multidisciplinary team to work in partnership in terms of communication, education and removing physical barriers. To further improve service provision midwives need to continue asking individual disabled parents and groups what their priority of needs are and thereby give disabled parents a voice. Work needs to be ongoing in relation to removing any offensive or upsetting barriers and providing equity in service provision and care.

The principles are:

- To eliminate discrimination by being advocates of good practice.
- To offer equity regardless of ability.
- To develop an action plan and estimate costs to prioritise the implementation plan required across the hospital Trust.

Issues seen as priorities for disabled parents can be summarised as:

- Writing and publishing a current up-to-date newsletter containing relevant information for today's parents. The journal 'Disability Pregnancy and Parenthood International' (DPPi) can be seen as an example of such a resource.
- Telephone support—Disabled Parents Network (DPN) has a contact register.
- Availability of specific support groups relative to impairment and need.
- Multidisciplinary advice and practical help.
- Access to relevant organisations and networks.
- Literature that is accessible in other formats and media.
- Parenting classes to include topics on infancy as needs of children change.
- Peer support, contact with other mothers and fathers and to continue links with professional carers and other voluntary groups.
- National Childbirth Trust equipment/links i.e. where to purchase second-hand equipment and clothing.
- Evaluate and further develop services through audit and research.
- Inviting users to share their knowledge and experiences by participating as speakers at conferences, teaching seminars and publishing articles.

## THE WAY FORWARD FOR MATERNITY SERVICE PROVISION

- Identify the target population and consult all stakeholders.
- Review current practice and refocus specific services.
- Develop the existing structure with a new role(s) of an agreed key worker(s) e.g. specialist midwife disability advisor, and develop a competency framework.

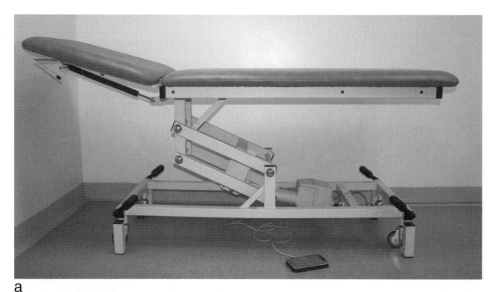

*Figure 3.7* A height-adjustable couch (see Chapter 9) at high level for carrying out an examination **a)**, and low level for ease of client transfer **b)**. Photograph by Martin Baxter, with kind permission from Liverpool Women's Hospital.

- Create an effective multidisciplinary referral mechanism.
- Design a joint working framework with common pathways of care and joint working in the decision-making process.
- Location of integrated services—this may be more difficult due to policies around staffing, health and the need for more flexibility.
- A key worker to be involved in facilitating training strategies for all staff.
- Ongoing audit and the monitoring and evaluation of services.

## THE WAY FORWARD FOR MATERNITY CARE

- Enhance midwives' and other professionals' knowledge and understanding and facilitate disability awareness to change attitudes.
- Develop midwives' and other professionals' communication and listening skills to enable disabled parents to be heard.
- Meet individual mother's needs by assessment and planning.
- Provide creative, flexible and innovative care.

- Develop networks by forming health alliances.
- Involvement in research to further develop service provision.

### CONCLUSION—KEY POINTS

- The provision of client-centred maternity care is the right of all women, not least disabled women.
- Disabled women are often marginalised because of their disability, and are viewed as a minority group unable to cope with the role of parenting. To redress this imbalance and to provide equality within the maternity service disabled women need to have an active role in their maternity care, to be given back the control and be full participants in their own health care.
- Women need to explore the options available to them and be supported in the decision-making process. Similarly health professionals having a significant role in meeting the needs of disabled women will be required to focus on how to make services more accessible and appropriate to need. The emphasis is to develop excellence in the provision of care.
- A health service that meets the needs of disabled women, will meet the needs of *all* women well.

## CASE SCENARIOS

### Scenario 1—Parents with hearing impairment

Joy is deaf due to a genetic condition. She has a little hearing in her right ear but not enough to communicate effectively. She has speech and uses Sign Supported English to communicate and she lip-reads. Her partner David is also hearing impaired or hard of hearing. His hearing started to deteriorate from the age of 10 years but because of this age of onset he has good speech.

Joy was excited about being pregnant but she was also a little anxious because of her deafness.

David was also anxious about being a father because of concerns about how he would cope and he was also worried that their baby might be deaf.

When Joy was 12 weeks pregnant she attended hospital for her first booking appointment. She informed the midwife that she was deaf. A needs assessment identified Joy and David's communication requirements. She did not want the hospital to provide interpreters as she wanted her mother to interpret for her because, as she said, 'she trusted her'. The DDA states that it is the responsibility of service providers to make available sign language interpreters for deaf people. Some, however, prefer to use family members and friends to interpret. If this is their choice it must be documented in the notes and this was carried out in Joy and David's case. It then needs to be explained that for quality assurance purposes interpreters must be registered and trained to NVQ level 3 and are accountable for all information given.

At most antenatal appointments Joy's mother was present to interpret but when she was not available information was written on paper for Joy to read. There was one occasion when an appointment had to be cancelled and rearranged for a later date when her mother was available to interpret. Fortunately, on this occasion the information was not urgent. In an emergency Joy was happy for a midwife to use basic interpreting to communicate as well as using pen and paper.

Following the needs assessment, specific resources and equipment were identified. A baby alarm mattress (a specialist monitor that vibrates under the mother's pillow when baby cries) was required for Joy to know when her baby cried at night. At home they both had all the deaf aids they required. It was suggested that they bring their own baby alarm into hospital to use during Joy's stay and any other equipment they may want to use, for example, a textphone. All parents are encouraged to bring their own aids and equipment from home. This avoids having to wait for specific equipment to become available and then having to learn how to use it. It also gives parents confidence and a feeling of being in control.

Joy's labour went well. Her mother and David were present at delivery and her mother was able to interpret for them both. David was then able to concentrate and support his partner. They had seen the delivery room before delivery and were reassured that the bed was positioned in a good light and there were no long shadows from windows. Importantly, there was also a clock in the room situated on the wall opposite, and not behind the bed, for Joy to know the time and to be able to record timing and duration of her contractions. This was something she could do without asking for help. They were both able to communicate effectively. During a contraction Joy had her eyes closed but after each contraction she relaxed and David was able to communicate with her, passing her instructions from the midwife.

To be able to see the delivery room before labour will prepare disabled parents and remove some anxiety and fear. If changes are necessary, for example moving the bed near a window or under a light, then these can be managed before admission. This forward planning can avoid gaps, overlaps and surprises but it must be noted that meeting needs and making reasonable adjustments to remove barriers must not compromise health and safety.

Joy wanted to breast-feed her baby as soon after delivery as possible. This was done on the labour suite and to encourage mother–baby interaction skin-to-skin contact was encouraged. At this time David went outside to text on his mobile phone to make the important calls. He did not require the use of the hospital minicom (textphone). To meet the needs of deaf parents specific equipment can be made available, for example a minicom, loud-ring telephone (available from British Telecom) or the facility to text on a mobile phone. Having a named midwife with a designated mobile phone number, televisions with teletext and subtitles, use of fax machines or communication by email is very valuable. There are many ways midwives and other carers can be innovative and creative to meet needs. Cost should not be an issue as all equipment can also be used by non-disabled people.

Mother and baby were transferred to the post-natal ward soon after delivery. David was concerned that Joy might not be able to hear the baby cry, and also not be able to communicate effectively and feel isolated. Allowing a partner or relative to say overnight will reassure and support both mother and midwife. To support Joy, especially at night, and to interpret for staff David was able to stay overnight. This request was easily managed

by giving Joy a single room during her hospital stay, and with the help of a bed settee that was made available for him. The single room served an additional purpose in that using a baby alarm mattress in an open-plan ward may be difficult as it will pick up and vibrate when other babies cry. Many deaf parents request a single room for this reason. Joy was happy about the single room as she was able to communicate better without background noises or distractions in her room from other people. She asked for the bed to be moved to face the door as she wanted to see people as they entered her room because she could not hear a knock on the door.

Access to the ward was not an issue for Joy as she was an in-patient. David wanted to visit during the day, in the evening and outside of visiting hours. However he encountered new barriers as access to all areas is by intercom which caused delays. Many hospital wards and departments have intercom access for security which can create barriers for many deaf people. If intercoms are used they should include a light to alert the visitor when doors are opened. A video entry system can be more accessible and give more effective security. As David was allowed to stay in the hospital overnight he required ease of access. To remove this barrier a security pass was provided which gave him access to the place where Joy was a patient. This was seen as a reasonable adjustment to overcome this barrier. David was able to collect this pass at the main hospital entrance and return it there if he went outside of the hospital premises. This met both his needs and the needs of staff.

On the postnatal ward Joy met many people. Some were unaware that she was deaf and there were some awkward moments but on the whole ward staff were very caring and supportive. Joy took the opportunity to inform them how to be more deaf aware and seek ways to remove barriers by discussing some of the key issues identified above.

To alleviate parents' concerns about congenital deafness hearing tests can be carried out before mother and baby leave hospital. Therefore, while on the ward Joy's baby was given a hearing test. Although no concerns were identified, because of the parents' history an appointment was made for a further hearing test at a later date. As an additional service to make life less stressful, an appointment was made for Joy and David to register their baby before discharge home. Mother and baby both went home on the fourth day postnatal as they were both well. No specific support was required although primary care and support was given as usual following liaison with the community midwifery team.

## Scenario 2—A mother with a physical disability

Susan, aged 28, visited hospital in January 2006 to book with her second pregnancy at 13 weeks. She had severe spinal problems following a road traffic accident in 2003. Her GP had managed her care initially until symptoms worsened in 2005 when she was referred to an orthopaedic surgeon for further assessment and management. She was experiencing discomfort in the left side of her pelvis and had softening of both knees; she was quoted as saying 'my femur is not aligned straight'. She was in constant pain, experiencing more 'bad days' than 'good days'. Her mobility was deteriorating; she walked with a limp and required the use of crutches. She was diagnosed with a chronic back condition and had investigations, tests and physiotherapy.

Based on this information arrangements were made for the midwife to see Susan at home where a needs assessment was performed and a plan of care for pregnancy, labour and postnatal period was discussed. Her limitations were explored and entered on the plan. Her fears and concerns were many. She had a rapid delivery with her first child and was particularly concerned that the same would happen again. Susan was afraid that the pregnancy and the weight gain would exacerbate her condition. She had a fear of epidurals and was concerned about coping with child-care with her impairment.

In order to provide individualised care it is essential to involve disabled women in their own healthcare planning. Disabled people can give their own account of the impairment and the needs they see themselves requiring. Health carers need to respect individual choices, opinions and views whilst not making assumptions about how a disabled person may or may not cope with parenting. They need to be given the same opportunity of choice as non-disabled women and be actively encouraged to participate in their own maternity care. Visiting at home will empower women and give them confidence being in their familiar environment with their own aids and adaptations.

An appointment was made for Susan to see the anaesthetist in order to discuss her concerns and to be informed of other choices of analgesia available to her. A Social Services referral was explored as Susan recognised that she would need extra help and support when discharged from the maternity services. She believed this support would be required long-term for her own self care and her parenting role. Additional referrals were made to the health visitor requesting a pre-birth visit for support and to the occupational therapist (OT) for a needs assessment for aids and equipment in the home. All disabled people are entitled to an OT assessment and this can be made by a GP referral to services.

Working with Social Services is a task that is often time-consuming and in this case, where adult services are required, the process can take even longer. When midwives consider child protection issues it can make them feel very vulnerable, especially when having to attend a case conference called by the Social Services. Adequate support from her supervisor of midwives may be required especially if a decision is made to remove a baby.

As her pregnancy progressed Susan's back condition affected her activities of living and she was becoming increasingly distressed and anxious about the delivery. To address her physical impairment she was referred to a physiotherapist. A support belt was given and she was also encouraged to try aqua natal and some light exercise. A manual handling assessment was completed and arrangements made with the post-natal ward for a height-adjustable cot (Fig. 3.5) and a back rest adjustable bed to be made available. To help further, Susan was referred to an aromatherapy midwife for relaxation which helped her to become calmer.

Towards the end of the pregnancy Susan was seen by her consultant obstetrician to discuss delivery. Susan was interested in the birthing pool as she thought it would help her relax and aid delivery. The plan of care discussed with Susan was put in her hospital notes and a copy was given to her to put in her hand-held notes. Further copies were sent to the delivery suite, postnatal ward, community midwife and health visitor thus ensuring effective communication of Susan's needs.

As her back condition deteriorated and she was no longer coping, it was decided to induce labour at 39 weeks. A water birth was now no longer possible. In the end she had a quick labour of 1 hour 35 minutes with diamorphine and kapake to relieve pain. She had a beautiful baby boy and chose to artificially feed. Susan was discharged from hospital on the third day postnatal with much family support and the support of the primary care.

Disabled women should be treated and cared for the same as all women. They should be actively involved in their care, offered choices for their pregnancy and birth and enabled to make informed decisions on those choices. Midwives may not always feel confident to offer all choices and need to be empowered to do so. They need knowledge about local services for disabled parents. They need to feel confident to be able to signpost to relevant organisations and manufacturers of specific equipment, such as prams, baby slings and carrier, with an appreciation of how much these aids actually cost.

## Scenario 3—Parents with learning disability

Brenda and Joe both have learning difficulties. Brenda was pregnant with her second child; their first child who was four years of age was adopted at birth. Brenda was delighted to be pregnant but very anxious as she remembered her first experience of losing her child and was very frightened that the same would happen again.

Brenda initially thought she might have been pregnant because she recognised the first signs of pregnancy from the last time. She visited her GP who referred her to the maternity hospital for her care. Although very nervous the couple were very keen and wanted all the support available to them to help them become good parents. It is often assumed that this client group are unable to fulfil the role of parenting and that they are very vulnerable. However, according to Tarleton et al (2006) when appropriate support is given, people

with a learning disability can care for their children and be 'good enough' parents.

At the hospital booking visit a midwife suggested that they might want to meet with the Specialist Midwife in Disability to identify their needs and to network with other services to offer support. At that first meeting a history of the learning disability was given. Brenda had attended 'special' school as a child as she has specific educational needs. Joe attended mainstream school but had many difficulties that required support. They both communicated well and there were no barriers to communication provided the words used were short and in 'everyday' English. They did not understand medical words, abbreviations or jargon. Brenda asked sensible questions and had matured since her last pregnancy. She had attended child-care classes and was very confident about safety issues and care of the newborn. Her memory and concentration were limited when too much new information was given. She was able to comply when asked to repeat and recap information and this was further reinforced using visual aids and demonstrations. They had just moved to a new flat and were able to manage their own finances although on occasions Brenda did tend to overspend.

Midwives will need to identify the best way to communicate with people with learning disability and not to assume that new information is immediately understood. It is always best to ask a person to give feedback on the information they have been given to check understanding. People with learning disability may require information in accessible formats using diagrams, symbols and tactile aids. It is important that a midwife does not assume that non-compliance to instruction is lack of cooperation. It may simply mean that there is a lack of understanding. It is recognised that many people with learning disability also have a sensory and/or physical impairment. Providing one-to-one parent education, ideally in the mother's home, can meet individual needs through flexibility, it enhances teaching and supports parenting skills (Tarleton et al 2006). However, it is also good for parents to join mixed groups when they can meet and learn from others.

When the needs assessment was performed it was evident that networking with other services was necessary. A plan of care was written identifying the support networks that were required for Brenda and Joe in their parenting role. These included:

- Learning Disability Team to give specific support throughout pregnancy and early parenting.
- After Care Workers from the Learning Care Team to give extra help and support with child-care and activities of daily living.
- Health visitor to make contact in the antenatal period and an early birth visit.
- The community midwife to visit at home for an extended period. This is possible now the role of the midwife is no longer restricted to providing care only up to 28 days following the birth (NMC 2004) therefore the continuation of midwifery care can be as long as necessary.
- Support from the extended family.

This multi-agency approach worked well with midwives ensuring advocacy for the parents and 'joined up' care and support.

Performing the needs assessment interview will enable a midwife to identify the strengths and requirements of an individual. Providing the language and words that are used are understood, questions can be asked about physical, emotional, educational and financial needs. It is not acceptable to make assumptions about a person's disability or to assume that because someone has a learning disability they cannot be a good parent. A midwife can help a person learn new skills by making new information easy to understand. Visual aids such as videos, pictures of the developing fetus and anatomical models can be used to provide individualised parent education. A tour of the maternity ward is always useful for parents to see the environment in which they will receive care. It may also be appropriate to involve the extended family in all of these situations and opportunities.

Midwives need not work in isolation as dedicated learning disability services can be engaged in service provision but additionally to offer support to health professionals to enable them to provide a good quality service. To avoid discrimination it is important to apply the same standards of parenting support to people with a learning disability as to non-disabled women.

After Brenda's first pregnancy and the subsequent child protection issues, Social Services were already involved in her second pregnancy.

A parenting assessment was required during this pregnancy to assess both parents' ability to parent and support a child physically and emotionally. Brenda informed me that both she and Joe had just successfully completed a health and safety award. They wanted to show everyone that they were now more mature and sensible as they wanted this baby so much. In addition to this Brenda's carer, whom she saw three times each week, helped her with shopping and money matters. A health professional meeting was convened and chaired by a social worker. All carers and Brenda and Joe were present. Brenda and Joe were pleased to listen to the positive comments that were given. As there was enough evidence to suggest that, with appropriate support and care for Brenda and Joe, the baby could go home and a case conference was not required.

Maternity care can go beyond the boundaries of physical well-being and education to encompass wider and broader issues as identified here. It is important therefore that a midwife is empowered herself and has knowledge of how to access and work in partnership with other services to provide an inclusive philosophy of care. When considering child protection issues and working with Social Services midwives need to be aware of their individual responsibilities under Schedule 17 and Schedule 47 of the child protection law.

Brenda was nervous as she approached her estimated date of delivery but she also was excited. Joe and her carer were her birth partners. After a very short labour Brenda gave birth to a beautiful little girl who she called Emily. She wanted to breast-feed which she did, a little nervously, while still on the delivery suite. She was transferred to the postnatal ward where she particularly wanted to be with other mothers in order to talk, watch and learn. Her postnatal experience in hospital was good. She was supported to breast-feed and a bath demonstration was given to both parents. A bottle-feed demonstration was not given on the ward in order to promote breast-feeding, but the principles involved in feed preparation were highlighted. Brenda coped very well and was discharged from hospital on the seventh day postnatal. Unfortunately Emily had an infection which extended her stay. All services were informed of Brenda's discharge date in order that support was readily available and a record had been made on her discharge letter that if there were any concerns then the appropriate services were to be informed. With the right help and support from services working together across boundaries, parents with learning disabilities can be given the opportunity to care for their child.

## References

Campion M J 1990 The baby challenge: a handbook on pregnancy for women with physical disability. Routledge, London

Campion M J 1997 Disabled women and maternity services. Modern Midwife 7(3):23–25

Carty E 1998 Disability and childbirth meeting the challenges. Canadian Medical Association August 25th 159:4

Culley L, Genders N 1999 Parenting by people with learning disabilities: the educational needs of community nurses. Nurse Education Today 19(6):502–508

Department of Health (DoH) 1993 Changing Childbirth. Report of the Expert Maternity Group. HMSO, London

Department of Health (DoH) 2004 National Service Framework for Children, Young People and Maternity Services. Standard 11. Online. Available: http://www.dh.gov.uk/publications 12 April 2006

Dimond B 2000 The Human Rights Act 1998: implications for practice. British Journal of Midwifery 8(10):616–618

Dimond B 2003 Step 52: disability discrimination. British Journal of Midwifery 11(4):216

Dimond B 2004 Disability discrimination. British Journal of Midwifery 12(9):560

Disability Discrimination Act 1995 HMSO, London. Online. Available: http://www.drc-gb.org 1 March 2006

Disabled Parents Network 2006 Aims and values. Online. Available: http://www.disabledparentsnetwork.org.uk/about /aims.htm 12 April 2006

Human Rights Act 1998 HMSO, London. Online. Available: http://www.opsi.gov.uk 1 March 2006

NMC 2004 Midwives rules and standards. Nursing and Midwifery Council, London

Royal College of Midwives (RCM) 1996 Position Paper No. 11 May. RCM, London.

Royal College of Midwives (RCM) 2000 Position Paper No. 11a February. RCM, London. Online. Available: http://rcm.org.uk 1 March 2006

Shackle M 1994 I thought I was the only one. A report of a conference 'Disabled People Pregnancy and Early Parenthood'. Part of the Maternity Alliance Working Group Pack. Maternity Alliance, London

Shackleton P, Goddard L 1997 Pregnancy and disability. Birth Issues Dec-Jan 6(4):5–10

Tarleton B, Ward L, Howarth J 2006 Finding the right support: a review of issues and positive practice in supporting parents with learning difficulties and their children. The Baring Foundation. Online. Available: http://www.baringfoundation.org.uk

Thomas C, Curtis P 1997 Having a baby: some disabled women's reproductive experiences. Midwifery 13:202–209

Wates M 2003 It shouldn't be down to luck. In: Disabled parents network handbook project. Rowntree, London

## APPENDIX

## Evaluation questionnaire

Was there any evidence of negative attitudes/behaviours from carers?

Were you made to feel awkward or different?

What gaps (if any) were identified in provision of maternity care?

Were your specific needs met?

Were you given the opportunity to ask questions?

Was the information received satisfactory?

What type of carers did you meet? Who did you want to meet?

Is there a need for a specialist midwife for disabled women?

How was your impairment identified? Do you feel identification would raise awareness to need?

Was there a need you identified not addressed by your carers?

How flexible was the maternity service in meeting your need? How can maternity care be more flexible?

How can care be offered in a more creative way?

Who offered you the most support during your maternity care?

Was an opportunity given to explain the effect of medication?

Was breast-feeding promoted and specific support offered related to your impairment?

Was termination of pregnancy mentioned/offered?

Were risks to health explored?

Apart from being a parent what was your best experience?

What was your worst experience?

Were your expectations met? If no, then why not?

What unhelpful and unwanted care was received? (Fussing, carer 'taking over', confidence undermined.)

Offended by phrases, words used? (Labels, terminology, assumptions.)

Advice on specific aids in the home? (Availability, manufacturer, cost.)

Have you any suggestions on how to improve quality of maternity care offered to disabled women?

# 4 The role of the midwife in maternity service provision

*Stella McKay-Moffat, Jackie Rotheram*

## INTRODUCTION

Increasingly women with disabilities are making use of the maternity services (Royal College of Midwives (RCM) 2000) although the extent of that utilisation is unknown and is probably impossible and unnecessary to quantify. Nevertheless, anecdotal evidence exists that women with disabilities are undertaking parenthood. This is probably reflected in the slowly developing interest from professionals that is evident from the higher profile of the issues in professional journals. In order to respond to the increasing diversity of women with disabilities accessing maternity services, midwives and others providing those services during the childbirth continuum should have greater depth and breadth of knowledge, understanding and skill. This will then ensure the most appropriate services for this, still small, group of women whose requirements may need to be met in alternative ways. The interaction between effective, appropriate communication and the development of a trusting relationship, and midwives' interpersonal skills and their ability to be mothers' advocates can be seen to have an impact on the quality of care that women receive.

Maternity services should be both physically and psychologically accessible. Physical access has to do, for example, with entrance to buildings and the use of facilities whilst in that building; reception desks that are low enough for someone using a wheelchair or of short stature to readily interact with the person at the desk, and mechanisms to help communication and finding the way round the building (see Chapter 3 for more details). Psychological access has to do with the interaction with those providing the service, which means all

staff whether professional or support workers. The values, attitudes and beliefs of those people will be reflected in the type of welcome and approachability they present and the respect they offer to the service user. Nothing less than that which is given to other users is acceptable.

Overviews of some of the issues that need to be considered during antenatal, labour and postnatal care are included in this chapter. However, Chapter 8, contains a greater depth of information related to women with specifically identified conditions, including preconception issues, and needs to be read in conjunction with this chapter.

## COMMUNICATION AND INTERPERSONAL SKILLS

One key to successful maternity services is effective communication. That communication may be between clients and midwives, midwives and their peers, and midwives and other personnel. Fraser (1999) found that women's prime concern was good communication from their maternity service providers but they also wanted a special relationship with *their* midwife. To develop that relationship when working with mothers, a person-centred approach is important. But it could be argued that where a mother has a disability it is more than important; it is *essential* to aid the development of a partnership between equals, as people with disability may perceive themselves as subordinate to health professionals if previous experiences have put them in that role. Perceptions of equality will aid a two-way communication process (Ralston 1998), and can be helped by the mutual agreement that all parties use first names. Increasingly in all elements of social interaction the automatic use of first names is burgeoning. However it must never be assumed that use of someone's first name is acceptable.

Communicating effectively can have a life-long benefit to all concerned. As Ralston (1998) puts it '...how the midwife communicates [may promote] a therapeutic relationship ...or create barriers' (p 8). However, Goodman's (1994) report of the maternity experiences of women with disabilities indicated their considerable dissatisfaction with communication with health professionals, although midwives were not singled out. Nevertheless, midwives not only need to develop their communication skills but that development should be at an advanced level.

To participate in advanced communication midwives need to be self-aware and perceptive. Valuable communication requires appropriate speaking i.e. using words that are understood or explaining new words; suitable questioning techniques; and active listening skills i.e. not just hearing the words but understanding the meaning behind them. Butler & Jackson (1998) particularly highlighted midwives' need for effective listening skills but warned that these are influenced by their own experiences, attitudes, feelings and assumptions. Lack of experience associating with people with disability may mean that midwives feel anxious about communication, although they may feel comfortable interacting with people with disability. A sense of comfort interacting with people with a disability indicates a positive attitude towards them (Gething 1994) and there is evidence that this correlates with confidence in communication (McKay-Moffat 2003). However, uncertainty and negative attitudes may present as not knowing what to say or how to ask questions particularly related to actual or perceived sensitive issues, for example about the disability and how it affects daily life, and discussion about antenatal screening for fetal abnormality (McKay-Moffat 2003).

If mothers are unable to voice their feelings or needs, clues may come from the non-verbal signals that they display, therefore midwives need to be alert to recognise those indicators. In a busy practice situation with pressure of work and time constraints, perceptions of non-verbal signals may be inhibited. Perhaps the answer lies in using the 'chatty' conversation style identified by Stapleton et al (2002) that serves to enhance a mutually trusting relationship, thus increasing the likelihood of an openness of expression of thoughts and feelings.

Non-verbal communication from midwives or other carers, for example body language, eye contact and tone of voice, can be very powerful suggestions of both negative and positive perspectives including attitudes and availability of time. Women with disability may be especially sensitive to those signals depending on their perceptions of self and life experiences. People with a disability are often stared at, avoided or receive derogatory remarks from members of the public which may leave life-long sensitivity to non-verbal clues from those with whom they interact. Experience of contact with health professionals may also have left them with a sense of intimidation, vulnerability and inferiority. Therefore midwives must reflect on their own attitudes, opinions and preconceived ideas, and be vigilant to their own non-verbal signals that may betray them. Tone of voice and choice of words may reveal underlying acceptance or prejudices to which women are likely to be sensitive, especially those with learning disability. Verbal intonations will give a woman who is blind the clues others obtain from visual signals, whereas visual signals do not offer the person who is blind that background detail. Non-verbal communication may enhance the perceptions of people unable to hear and offer clues to what is actually meant.

Information giving and receiving are a vital part of the role of midwives. Given information needs to be clear, unambiguous and meeting a recipient's requirements. Women with disabilities will want the same information related to pregnancy and childbirth as other women but they may also require additional information. Having appropriate, relevant information leaves women in a better position to take control over their childbirth experiences and to make the choices that suit them. Despite being a large part of the daily work of midwives, the giving of information may not be achieved as effectively as practitioners may think (Blackford et al 2000, Stapleton et al 2002). Yet if women receive the information they need, satisfaction with their maternity service is greatly increased (McKay-Moffat 2003). What midwives must do is avoid the 'patter' of information giving, which means that what they say revolves around a set spiel that is given to everyone with little regard for individual preferences and desires. Further, the way information is delivered must be considered as the positive or negative aspects of an issue can indirectly guide the response and the choices made, or lead to misunderstanding (Stapleton et al 2002).

Despite using the word 'discussion' much of what Stapleton et al (2002) noted during antenatal visits was little in the way of opinion or thoughts elicited from women. If 'discussion' is inadequate with a mother with a disability, information and opinion gathering will be lacking, resulting in failure to identify her specific individual or alternative needs. The use of effective questioning techniques, in particular the use of open questions where relevant, will enhance midwives' ability to elicit what is required and facilitate two-way discussion. However, this type of genuine discussion takes time, therefore adequate preparation must be made to ensure availability of time for each appointment.

## Mothers with sensory impairment

Communicating with a mother who is deaf can prove challenging and stressful for all concerned without the right know-how or correct help. Pen and paper can be useful as can text using a computer or via a mobile telephone. If a woman lip-reads, knowledge and understanding of what to do and what not to do is vital, for example the speaker's face should be well lit, the mother looking at the speaker and speech should be at a steady pace without over-emphasis of the words (Iqbal 2004). Basic skills in British Sign Language (BSL) can be very valuable for midwives, as can a readily available finger spelling chart. Although it is time-consuming spelling out every word, it can be useful for the often new terminology that will be used. Literature to take away and read later is vital to ensure clarity of understanding and reinforce the information given.

The use of an appropriate interpreter is often the most efficient way of ensuring effective communication but caution needs to be employed to avoid talking to interpreters rather than mothers. Bramwell et al (2000) recommended independent freelance translators and dismissed the use of family members, especially children. They argued that using family members would mean that women

loose their privacy; that family emotional involvement may lead to misinterpretation of information; and that accusations of child abuse could even be levied. A regular female interpreter chosen by a woman is likely to be the ideal. However, access at short notice or in an emergency could be problematic (Iqbal 2004). The private, intimate time of giving birth may be the time when mothers want no one other than a close significant other person present. Therefore planning and preparation for communication between a mother and her midwife who is going to provide labour care during pregnancy would be of great advantage to all concerned. However, realistically this may not always be possible.

Verbal communication with mothers who are blind or partially sighted is usually not a problem but additional or supporting information needs to be in a format that is useable. This may be in the form of literature in large print or Braille, or audio tapes. To be innovative in this area there is nothing to stop midwives recording the content of commonly used leaflets or information packs for women to take away. As the women will not be able to read their hand-held records it is also important that midwives actually read to mothers what has been written. This means that each mother can ensure accuracy and clarity of information, and that confidentiality will not be breached because she had to ask family or friends what was in her notes.

Midwives need to be proactive in ensuring that aids to communication for women who find communication difficult are available, for example a loop system, minicom (textphone), hearing aid amplifiers, flashing lights, and literature in Braille or large print. Some Trusts, however, due to the financial implications, may find this difficult or impossible to fund. This leaves it up to individual midwives to use their skills of flexibility and adaptability, and resources from outside agencies to fill the gap in facilities. If this is the case then the respective organisations need to be reminded of their duty of care under the Disability Discrimination Act (1995).

## Mothers with learning disability

The ability of mothers with learning disability to communicate will vary depending on their level of disability. In general people with learning disability have a reduced capability of understanding new or complex information and abstract concepts, and they may not be able to read letters or complete documentation (DoH 1999). Straightforward language should be used when both seeking and offering information. If understanding of time and dates is difficult focusing a question related to a specific event may elicit more accurate information, for example when trying to determine the date of a last menstrual period.

Taking a social, medical and obstetric history may be difficult therefore liaison and information sharing between service providers, for example GPs, health visitors and social workers will enhance the quality and accuracy of necessary information. However, that information sharing should be a two-way process therefore it is important that midwives share information about a woman's progress during pregnancy and childbirth, but still remain within the boundaries of confidentiality (NMC 2004a). So this means seeking permission from each woman to share necessary information about her to other relevant service providers or carers. If permission is refused, her rights are respected the same as everyone else.

People with learning disabilities may not have difficulty communicating their ideas and preferences (DoH 1999) so it is important that they know about and understand that they do have choices the same as everyone else. However, extra time may be needed to enable that choice to be informed. Visual aids will enhance learning and if written material is appropriate it should be in a language that is readily understood. Information may need to be repeated and alternative ways of giving that information may need to be explored to ensure or reinforce learning. Terminology and bodily functions are often difficult for those *without* learning difficulties to understand, and for women with learning problems models (see Figs. 6.1, 6.2) and pictures can be of great use. Skill acquisition may be slow and additional time will be needed to not only explain how to perform a procedure, for example basic baby care, but to give opportunities to practice.

## Interpersonal skills

In order to try to counteract any previous negative experiences of healthcare and to focus help and support for mothers, midwives need good interper-

sonal skills. Their conduct needs to be one that radiates approachability and it needs to be obvious that they are non-judgemental and offer unconditional regard. Research by Tinkler & Quinney (1998) demonstrated that when women were treated as individuals in a supporting, enabling partnership as opposed to one where midwives were dominating or interfering, mothers gained the most benefit and satisfying experience. Application of those same principles should be implemented in care provision for mothers with a disability who may feel vulnerable, particularly if they have received negative attitudes from family, friends or professionals towards their decision to become a parent.

Women with a disability may strive against all manner of difficulties to achieve conception and a child. Like Neville-Jan (2004) some avoid analgesia to enhance their ability to conceive, thus enduring what could be considered as unacceptable pain. Others may alter or omit medication that may be harmful to the fetus challenging their own health and well-being. Therefore a sincere, sensitive and caring approach to a mother's possible emotional and personal feelings is a must.

## Records and care planning

The most effective way(s) of communication with mothers should be recorded in their notes as appropriate to ensure speedy instigation of that method by all concerned who work with them. This will not only enhance all parties' knowledge and understanding by ensuring that the exchange of information between mothers and helpers is readily available, but will help to prevent a disempowering relationship.

Record keeping, care planning and liaison with other members of a multi-professional team require effective communication skills. Adequate records about a mother's disability, how it affects her daily living and what treatment if any she needs will lessen the need for repeated history taking that can cause her considerable distress. But it is not just about making the records, it is important that those records are read by a person taking over care. Plans of care should be made in conjunction with mothers and other experts as appropriate, for example occupational therapists or specialist consultants. However, the pressure of work may make it difficult or impossible for all those concerned to get together. So it is important that the midwife acts as the coordinator, taking the lead by liaising with all those concerned to provide a holistic plan of service. A plan of care is formulated by first undertaking a thorough assessment of the mother's needs and wishes (see below).

## MIDWIVES AS ADVOCATES

Midwives believe they are women's advocates and the directives in the Code of professional conduct (NMC 2004a) and 'Midwives rules and standards' (NMC 2004b) demonstrate that this is a key part of the role of midwives. Indeed, women expect midwives to be their advocate (Fraser 1999). However, as Warrier (2003) explains, in today's ethos of practice where risk management is all embracing, this is a challenging element of the role. Where a mother with a disability is concerned, that challenge may be even greater because she may be perceived as 'at risk' because of her disability. Midwives providing care may find the role demanding and testing of their ability particularly if they are confronting 'the system' on mothers' behalf. Yet meeting that challenge is potentially very rewarding for both mothers and midwives.

Advocacy goes hand in hand with trust. Midwives need to trust women: their knowledge of self and their capabilities. Woman need to trust midwives because that relationship can affect women for the rest of their lives (Gould 2004) but of course that trust needs to be earned. A philosophy of openness and honesty will facilitate the development of that trust. Midwives need to trust themselves: their knowledge, skills and ability to support women through the whole birth process. A philosophy of mutual trust and respect will enhance a working partnership that will benefit all parties. A trusting relationship will enhance women's satisfaction with their care and lessen the chance of them holding back i.e. not asking for information or help, or not sharing information (Fraser 1999).

To act as an advocate midwives need to be proactive in championing the needs of women. From her research with parents with a disability Wates (1997) identified four main characteristics of a good professional allay as one that:

- provides encouragement;
- supports parents' way of doing things;
- is helpful in finding solutions to practical challenges;
- sees parenthood as a right of passage into society.

Midwives, whilst being the experts in normal midwifery and with an extensive depth and breadth of knowledge and skills, are unlikely to have all the information and ability to meet the needs of all women with a disability. This means that liaison with other disciplines from the health, and a social or voluntary sector, is vital. This will not only enhance the level of expertise that is available to women, but will enable midwives to develop their helping skills. Both aspects will initially benefit mothers concerned, but knowledge and skills gained by midwives will be available for mothers in the future.

Midwives' advocacy role for mothers may have to be extended to function with colleagues and women's families. Not all professionals appear to have positive attitudes towards mothers with disabilities, and family members may also be sceptical about their undertaking to have a child. Situations may arise where a woman makes a choice about a specific issue that professionals and the family feel is inappropriate, for example refusal of antenatal screening for fetal abnormality or a decision on place or mode of birth. This may result in unacceptable pressure being put on a woman to conform and, particularly where professional advice is rejected, it may result in an insensitive or even antagonistic approach. If midwives have discussed the issue(s) adequately and given women all the information available; if they have been honest about their concerns; if there truly is an open relationship where mutual trust is evident; then even if midwives disagree with decisions women make, those decisions should be respected. Midwives are then being supportive: that is genuine advocacy.

## CHOICE AND CONTROL

In 1993 the philosophy of the government's *Changing Childbirth* report (DoH 1993) promoted the rights of women to have care that centred on their needs and was based on their choice and control over their childbirth processes. However, 5 years later Baroness Jay, the then Minister for Health (DoH 1998), acknowledged that women-centred care for minority or marginalised groups requires special effort. Policies and procedures that lack flexibility, and NHS Trusts' financial constraints make some innovative practices slow to be implemented, therefore the needs and choices of some women remain unmet. However, midwives spearhead midwifery practice and they can be a powerful force to bring about change if effort is made. Much of that change may have little in the way of financial implications because it revolves around patterns of care and the attitudes of midwives and other professionals.

The more recent government document, the National Service Framework for Children, Young People and Maternity Services (NSF) (DoH 2004), continues to promote the rights of women to have choice and control over what happens to them during pregnancy and childbirth. But this document makes much greater emphasis on including women from disadvantaged or vulnerable groups (of which women with a disability are frequently a part) and focusing on their individual needs.

Conventional choices for mothers with a disability may be inappropriate, therefore midwives may need to make a special effort to empower women with a disability to make choices appropriate for their needs. Midwives need to adopt an attitude of flexibility and adaptability as these will be the key elements in meeting those choices. This may mean that midwives utilise local resources or contact self-help or voluntary organisations (RCM 2000) or statutory bodies to enhance the level of practical and financial support for mothers. They may need to be proactive in ensuring that there is a list of readily accessible contact details of local and national organisations, or people who could prove very useful to the mother to help fulfil requirements.

By empowering mothers to make the choices that best meet their wishes and requirements midwives are enabling them to take control over their maternity services and childbirth experience. Participation in decision-making could ensure that women know they are being treated as the expert in their care (Tinkler & Quinney 1998). Midwives also need to recognise that women with a disability are the expert in their own situation, therefore they are in the best position to make the decisions that affect them and the care they receive.

## CONCERNS WITH NORMALITY

Women with a disability are likely to be concerned about the 'risk' related to pregnancy (Thomas 1997) both for themselves and their baby, but they may not always verbalise that concern. Pregnant women generally want to know that their pregnancy is progressing normally, paralleling those of other women but they may also want to be seen as different and unique (Earle 2000). Earle attributes midwives' expertise and authority in normal childbirth to their ability to confirm normality for women providing the key reassuring element of care provision. Conversely, Earle explains that good communication with women, knowing them individually and using their name promotes a sense of being individual and special. On the other hand, if a mother with a disability sees herself as achieving womanhood and developing her perception of self as a mother (Grue & Trafjord Lærum 2002, Thomas 1997), she may not want to be seen as different or special. Wates (1997) declares 'Asserting one's "normality" is linked ultimately with asserting the right to retain control over one's life' (p 14).

Women may not want to be praised or seen as special any more than they want to be blamed or receive sympathy. With two possible contrasting perceptions of being a mother with a disability, midwives need to use their own insight and sensitivity to elicit how a woman feels about her pregnancy and future motherhood. This will then guide appropriate responses and the ability to offer a maternity service that is focused on mothers as individuals.

All women, but particularly women with a genetically linked disability, need accurate information about prenatal screening. However, midwives and obstetricians may not always be fully conversant about screening guidelines (Wray & Maresh 2000) and the probability of genetic abnormality occurring. Sometimes this is because of the lack of concrete evidence to underpin information. This may then result in women lacking understanding about their babies' risks of abnormality and even the possibility of inaccurate screening test results (Bramwell & Carter 2001). Rowe et al (2002) postulate that additional communication skills training may improve information giving. This is particularly necessary when needing to explain to mothers that there is no information available.

## CONTINUITY OF CARER

Women should have the choice of lead professional for their maternity care although in reality that choice may not be readily offered or taken up. Continuity of carer has been a much discussed issue in maternity services mainly since the *Changing Childbirth* report (DoH 1993). Although women often appear to benefit from continuity of midwife carer, evidence in the literature is not always conclusive. Nevertheless, it is recognised as a marker of good practice in the NSF document (DoH 2004). Indeed, a mother with a disability is likely to benefit considerably from seeing the same midwife and by the development of a close positive relationship. Regular visits by one midwife or a very small team of midwives will aid the development of a trusting rapport particularly if a woman feels vulnerable or finds it difficult to interact with new people. Where communication is challenging, for example with a mother who is deaf or has learning difficulties, midwives will have time to develop their skills to improve their chances of communicating effectively (see Chapter 7 for how this can be done).

A sense of relaxation and confidence during interaction with another person aids greater depth of discussion about feelings and wishes, and can have a positive impact on perceptions of experiences. Therefore issues that require solutions will be more transparent and sensitive topics more easily addressed without embarrassment or ill feeling. Having the depth of knowledge and understanding of a mother's individual disability and her ways of managing daily living will enhance midwives' ability to advise on practical things like coping with body changes in pregnancy, positions for giving birth, and baby care.

A partnership of care where mothers know their own expertise is respected will strengthen the decision-making process and give confidence to all parties concerned. That decision-making process will be aided by readily available channels of communication and consistency of information. This in turn will boost mothers' self-confidence and feelings of security with their own and midwives' judgement and ultimate decisions.

## NEEDS ASSESSMENT

All women regardless of ability should have a detailed need assessment performed. This analysis will form the basis of a plan of care for the antenatal, labour and postnatal period. The purpose of this plan will be to inform midwives and other carers of an individual's general needs and care requirements (see Box 4.1). Ideally this process should be undertaken in a mother's own home as this is a non-threatening environment, and will allow the physical, emotional, psychological, educational, spiritual and financial dimensions of health to be explored. Mothers should be encouraged to give a history of their impairment and any consequent limitations. They should consider, discuss and focus on the details of their own specific needs (see Box 4.2) and be supported to seek ways to overcome any obstacles in an innovative, flexible and creative way.

Midwives' enhanced knowledge and skills, and the employment of lateral thinking and logical planning have the potential to successfully help mothers solve any difficulties. Ingenious or alternative ways of doing things may help mothers maintain their independence and control over their childbirth experience.

## ANTENATAL CARE

The pattern of antenatal visits has changed in recent years and fewer are now recommended by the

---

**Box 4.1 General requirements identified in the needs assessment process**

- Support and advice required.
- Emotional and psychological needs.
- Access issues.
- Specific equipment needs.
- Communication needs.
- Requirements for specific relevant literature.
- The format of information.

**Box 4.2 Specific requirements identified by the needs assessment process**

- Priority of need during pregnancy, birth of baby and postnatal period.
- Length of time needed for appointments.
- Type and timing of support required.
- Information required during pregnancy.
- Effect of pregnancy on disability and vice versa, for example safety/risks of any medication and fetal well-being.
- Place of care e.g. hospital, home or clinic visits.
- Lead professional e.g. midwife or obstetrician or shared care—continuity of midwife throughout is of great advantage.
- Place and type of birth planned.
- Communication needs for deaf parents.
- Types of equipment and other aids.

National Institute of Clinical Excellence (NICE) (2003) for the healthy pregnant woman. Mothers with a disability may be in good health therefore the suggested schedule of appointments requires no alteration. However, they may have medical concerns that indicate they should be seen more often. They may have anxieties or worries that mean they would benefit from more frequent appointments, therefore a rigid pattern should be avoided and substituted by one that is flexible and reflects individual requirements.

The initial visit or 'booking' interview is of vital importance in any pregnancy because of the vast exchange of information that is undertaken. This visit may need to be undertaken over more than one appointment to allow adequate time for all necessary information to be gathered or given. This could be of particular relevance for women with learning difficulties. In this situation midwives would need to prioritise the content of their discussion in order to provide and gain information that requires immediate action. Suitable literature should then be provided to aid understanding and reinforce what has been said.

The location of the booking interview and subsequent antenatal appointments is a matter for discussion with individual mothers. Some women will prefer home visits because of mobility difficulties or because they feel in control in their own home. In many ways a home visit is ideal because

midwives will see a woman's adapted way of living. This will then offer midwives potential inspiration for suggestions for alternative solutions to practical problems related to pregnancy, labour and childcare. However, caution must be exercised as perceptions of how manageable a task is may be negatively or positively biased. This is because the functional ability and performance of our bodies gives what Rogers et al (2004) call 'movement reference' or 'kinesthetic memory' (p 170). Everyone's understanding of how their own body moves and adapts to different circumstances reflects perception of how easy or difficult a task is to perform. Bias has the potential to inhibit understanding of what, if any, help or support a person with a disability may require.

Time of day for antenatal appointments may need to be considered. If a condition and/or the pregnancy make a woman tired, for example someone with cerebral palsy or multiple sclerosis (MS), she may not be able to attend early morning visits, or mid-afternoon appointments if she needs an afternoon rest. Antenatal appointments may take considerably longer than normal therefore midwives must ensure that they are not pressed for time. However, excessive time should be avoided as this could be tiring for mothers and concentration for both mothers and midwives may not be retained.

Appointments with experts may need to be arranged, for example consultant physicians for advice on medical and medicinal aspects of mothers' conditions, or occupational therapists, physiotherapists or specialist midwives (if one is available) to offer their skills to mothers and midwives. It may be up to midwives to take the lead and instigate these appointments. It could be of great advantage if midwives attended with mothers to liaise with those specialists and to enable a multi-professional discussion with individual mothers about their plans of care. However, with the pressure of work this may not always be realistic. One way round this will be to encourage mothers to take their midwifery notes with them and for them to ask specialists to record pertinent information in the records.

## Pregnancy issues

### Health promotion advice

An important part of the role of midwives is health promotion for all women in their care. Women with disability will receive the same information and advice as all women but there are some issues that may require addressing with a greater focus. One of the key aspects that all women can control during pregnancy with the potential to impact on their own and their babies' health and well-being is diet and nutrition, and the consumption of a well-balanced diet. For some women diet may need to be modified during pregnancy to increase fibre content as pregnancy has a tendency to increase the incidence of constipation because of the relaxation effects of progesterone on peristalsis. Women with a poor nerve supply to the bowel, for example due to a spinal cord condition or MS, may find that modification of diet alone is ineffective therefore midwives may need to recommend a mild laxative, e.g. Lactulose.

Women with mobility difficulties need to avoid excess weight gain during pregnancy to avoid compromising their mobility further. The advice of a dietician may be useful for some women so midwives need to make an appropriate referral. Dietary advice related to the prevention of anaemia is also important as anaemia would add to the tiredness that women develop with some conditions, e.g. cerebral palsy, fibromyalgia and MS. Prophylactic iron may be beneficial in some cases, but will be needed if blood tests indicate iron deficiency anaemia. Some anaemia is due to folic acid deficiency rather than iron, therefore it is important that blood films are scrutinised to differentiate between the two causes ensuring appropriate treatment.

One prophylactic supplement that is advised for all women during the first three months of pregnancy, to lower the risk of fetal neural tube conditions, is folic acid (NICE 2003). For women with spina bifida or who are taking certain medication for epilepsy the routing dose of 400 mcg is commonly raised to 4 mg.

Another prophylactic dietary addition that midwives may recommend is cranberry juice. Irvin's (2005) comprehensive literature review led her to conclude that cranberry juice is an effective remedy to lower the incidence of urinary tract infection (UTI) and is safe in pregnancy. However, Mario (2004) disputed the benefit saying that 4 litres would need to be consumed daily to significantly alter the pH of urine to be effective in lowering bacteria levels. It would appear then that there is some lack of clarity about the benefits of the juice. If women wish to drink it and they find it beneficial there appears to be no contraindication during pregnancy.

Discussion about general health and well-being includes consideration about adequate rest and exercise. Tiredness is a widespread effect of pregnancy and commonly a side effect of some conditions, for example MS, cerebral palsy and muscular dystrophy. Mothers may need encouragement to take additional rest and seek the help of family and friends to take on some of the daily tasks. Exercise is also important to maintain good circulation and muscle tone, and to alleviate compression on pressure areas which will be increased due to the weight of the pregnancy.

Advice on specific exercises or massage from a physiotherapist may be needed to lessen muscle contractures and to aid muscle relaxation if spasms are a problem. Leg movement is of particular importance in the prevention of deep vein thrombosis as the risk generally increases during pregnancy for all women. This is potentially compounded for women with little or no lower leg mobility but this is not only from immobility. Venous congestion due to the smooth muscle relaxation of blood vessels as a result of progesterone, and compression by the growing uterus are the other factors involved. Passive exercise may be the answer as well as changes of position and body lifting movements using the upper arms. Prophylactic anticoagulants may rarely be considered.

Physiotherapy may also help if backache or pain develops or existing back problems are exacerbated, for example in women with fibromyalgia and achondroplasia. Altered gait and balance, the additional weight and the effects of progesterone on the soft tissue of joints, i.e. ligaments and cartilage, may also be implicated. Muscle strengthening exercise may be beneficial. Some people find alternative therapies, for example aromatherapy, can reduce stress and relieve physical impairment.

### Routine screening tests

Routine screening tests are offered as usual but midwives need to be alert to the significance of some tests that may be pertinent for women with some conditions. It can be seen from the section above, the importance of a full blood count for the detection of iron or folic acid deficiency anaemia.

Women with chronic UTI or infection in pressure sores are more prone to anaemia. This blood test will also give an indication of chronic infection from the white cell count and the white cell differentiation.

Women with poor innervation to their bladder e.g. due to spinal cord conditions or MS or with a catheter, are more at risk of UTI. Therefore regular laboratory testing of urine to detect asymptomatic or low-grade infection will be necessary, rather than when infection is suspected because of illness. This then enables rapid treatment to minimise the risk of illness and will lessen the chances of acute or chronic nephritis that has the potential for short- and long-term health consequences.

Vaginal infections are not uncommon during pregnancy because of the altered pH of vaginal secretions and the changes in vaginal flora. Vaginal infections appear more common in women with spinal cord injury (Jackson & Wadley 1999) when not pregnant. Women with continence problems may also be more susceptible. Midwives need to ask women pertinent questions, and suggest a visual examination or possibly take a vaginal swab to enable effective diagnosis and subsequent treatment. Additionally, routine examination of pressure sore areas for women using wheelchairs may be offered to identify any skin lesions and infection, enabling appropriate advice and treatment. Chronic infection needs to be eliminated as far as possible to increase maternal and fetal well-being. Anaemia as a result of chronic infection is not the only consequence. As Baschat & Weiner (2004) and Jackson & Wadley (1999) point out chronic UTI and infection in pressure sores may lead to intrauterine growth retardation.

Ultrasound screening and certain blood tests are routinely offered to all women to aid detection of anomalies during pregnancy (NICE 2003). Mothers with a disability may be happy to avail themselves of those services. On the other hand they may equally prefer not to take up that offer. The choice is for individual women to make. For some mothers with certain conditions e.g. spina bifida and achondroplasia, this may be of prime importance to detect the condition in their fetus. However, it must never be assumed that all mothers will wish to know if their baby is affected, and they may have concerns about pressurisation to end their pregnancy.

Midwives may be apprehensive about being considered to devalue people with a disability and feel reluctant to discuss screening for fetal abnormalities.

### Physical examination

Abdominal examination and palpation of the uterus is a routine part of the role of midwives. There are factors that may need to be taken into consideration when examining women with a disability. Some women may have developed muscular contraction or may have muscle spasms, for example women with cerebral palsy or MS. It is important to make slow changes of position when helping women to prepare for examination to avoid the sudden onset of muscular spasms and pain or joint pain, for example in someone with arthritis. Care should also be exercised when moving women with achondroplasia as sudden movement may cause neck or spine damage.

Vaginal examination during pregnancy, for example to take a high vaginal swab when infection is suspected, may present some challenges if a woman is unable to abduct her legs. An alternative position such as the left lateral may make the examination possible but requires midwives to have a little more dexterity performing the procedure. Excess stimulation of the cervix must be avoided as this can cause a sudden muscle spasm or in a more serious situation it may lead to autonomic dysreflexia in women with spinal cord conditions (see Chapter 8 for a description and the consequences of the response). Caution must also be taken when examining a woman with spina bifida as latex allergy is more common than in the general population (May 2005, Welner & Temple 2004).

If there are medical conditions some women may need to be referred to a doctor, perhaps a physician, to have lung and cardiac function monitored. Pregnancy creates additional work for heart and lungs and if either are already compromised a woman's health may suffer. As pregnancy advances and the uterine fundal height rises lung capacity falls. For women with spinal cord damage or those with a small chest cavity, e.g. women with achondroplasia (Trotter et al 2005), there is an increased risk of chest infection. If a chest X-ray is needed this is best done after the first trimester but early enough during pregnancy for a shield to be used over a mother's abdomen whilst it is being performed. If a woman has any concurrent cardiac condition an electrocardiograph is commonly taken. Results of both tests will enable necessary action during pregnancy or relevant preparations to be made for labour and birth.

Monitoring of blood pressure is again a routine procedure during pregnancy. It is worth noting here that Gordon (2004) warns of the increased risk of pre-eclampsia in women who have been taking steroids, for example these may be taken by women with MS, and they are more at risk of developing diabetes. A loading dose of steroids is likely to be needed at the onset of labour and if there is a sudden period of illness at any time during pregnancy, labour or postnatal period.

## Parent education

Parent education plays a major part of the service that midwives offer (NMC 2004b). Preparation for parenting during pregnancy is challenging for all prospective mothers but even more so for mothers with disability as they may feel at risk and insecure. Inadequate preparation for parenthood can be a source of stress (Blackford et al 2000). Mothers with disability will have the same learning requirements as other mothers, for example about diet and nutrition, labour, pain relief and infant care, but different teaching and learning methods may need to be used.

Midwives often consider parent education as meaning participation in formal classroom-type group sessions. However, individual opportunistic teaching and learning occasions often present themselves during the childbirth process and make up the majority of instances of learning. Sometimes midwives appear to grasp those opportunities and utilise them fully, while at other times chances are missed. This is possibly due to inexperience as junior midwives are more likely to lack confidence in their parent education skills than those with more years in the profession (McKay-Moffat 2003). In relation to mothers with disability, there may also be a lack of confidence in knowledge particularly related to practical advice for 'parenting with impairment'.

Mothers may want one-to-one sessions in their own home or hospital but should be able to attend group sessions if they wish. If a mother chooses a group session midwives need to ensure that adequate preparation is made. The RCM (2000) states that parent education should be 'flexible, creative and accessible' (p 3). Physical access must be possible and teaching techniques will need to be appropriate for mothers' learning needs. If midwives themselves are not running the particular sessions they must liaise with the relevant colleague(s) to ensure they are aware that a mother with specific requirements will be attending, and what those requirements are. Failure to do this has the potential to make the whole experience negative and even psychologically destructive by undermining a mother's confidence in herself and the maternity services.

Mothers or midwives can liaise with outside agencies offering specific aids and equipment. This will enable selection and trial of chosen equipment to ensure that it meets requirements. Having a 'dry run' using a life size and weight baby doll may prove useful for developing adaptive care techniques, for example lifting or moving the baby, or when having to use one hand. A supportive 'can-do attitude' (Rogers et al 2004, p 169) could aid positive thinking and women's self-confidence in baby care.

Part of the service for preparation for parenthood includes exercises, relaxation and breathing techniques. For mothers with mobility issues these may be a crucial factor in maintaining or even improving function and perhaps aiding a normal birth. Usual classes are unlikely to meet mothers' requirements and they may find the prospect of participating in a formal class with non-disabled women unacceptable. Specific one-to-one sessions with an obstetric physiotherapist would be the ideal although a mother's willingness to participate might depend on previous experiences. Rogers et al (2004) point out that physiotherapy may have negative implications particularly related to women's *inabilities*. Here then, midwives can promote the benefits of strengthening and training muscles to respond to specific actions. This has the potential to enhance a mother's ability to cope with increasing weight and altered centre of gravity during pregnancy; positions for childbirth; and subsequent handling and lifting skills for baby care.

Ideally an initial group session should be planned, where mother, midwife and physiotherapist work together to discuss an exercise regime.

This will ensure that the knowledge and expertise of each is combined to formulate the most appropriate strategy. Additionally, the selection of mobility aids or specific equipment could be undertaken, possibly helped by the services of an occupational therapist. Before aids or equipment are selected it is not only a mother's physical needs that have to be considered but her family and other helpers, and social and environment factors, for example housing, income and life-style. This is where a holistic assessment is of prime importance.

One element of parent education is the opportunity for a visit to the delivery suite in the maternity unit. The majority of prospective parents find this visit both informative and anxiety relieving. Becoming familiar with a strange environment before it will actually be needed can have a positive influence by lowering stress and enhancing confidence on admission during labour. Mothers with a disability could find this exceptionally beneficial if their midwives were with them. Additional time could be planned to enable mothers and their birth partners the chance to become very familiar with the room and equipment. Midwives take for granted what all the equipment is for but an explanation of function may be helpful, and for mothers with learning difficulties or mothers with little or no sight, a chance to actually handle the equipment could be useful.

Mothers with mobility difficulties would benefit from the opportunity to practice moving on and off the labour bed or in and out of the birthing pool. The feasibility and comfort of different labour and birth positions could be tested for both mothers and midwives. This will enable any specific equipment to be obtained and tried, for example cushions and wedges, and ensure adequate preparation is made for labour which will aid confidence for both mothers and midwives when labour begins.

## INTRA-PARTUM CARE

Women should have a choice about place of birth (DoH 1993, 2004) but realistically that choice is not always made readily available. Perceptions of mothers with a disability as 'at risk' because of their disability may make that reality even more distant. However, mothers who are well may be at no greater

risk than any other mother with an uncomplicated pregnancy. For mothers whose home is adapted to make life as independent as possible, giving birth at home may enable them to maintain that independence and with it their dignity. Therefore home birth should not be dismissed. If this does in fact appear to be a sensible option and is a mother's choice, then all necessary discussions and preparations should be made as usual. In the event of a mother choosing home birth, but her midwife has concerns about safety, as with all mothers those concerns should be discussed honestly and openly. Support by a supervisor of midwives is sought in the usual case.

If a hospital birth is the preferred choice then ideally midwives who have provided care during pregnancy should be available to provide care during labour. As this may not always be possible the lead midwife in the antenatal period should liaise with and prepare the labour ward team of midwives in advance to discuss the use of a plan of care. Effective records and a birth plan will assist midwives during labour to meet mothers' additional or alternative needs. In the main their needs are going to be the same as every woman, for example information about what is happening and progress; availability and choices of analgesia; safe, effective care and support; as well as support for their birthing partners.

Labour is a time when most women have fears and worries. For mothers with learning difficulties lack of comprehension about what is happening or why there is so much pain may make them severely afraid. This could lead to behaviour that is out of character. Mothers with sensory impairment may also be unnecessarily afraid because of the strange environment and difficulties with communication. Early and effective preparation for labour during pregnancy would minimise fear but if this was not achieved then it is up to midwives providing care in labour to do their best to give explanations and offer a calming influence. This may not be easy if labour is advanced when women's attention span is particularly limited. Midwives are likely to need all of their interpersonal and advanced communication skills to make the experience as stress free as possible.

Mobility in labour is known to aid progress and for mothers with joint and muscle stiffness mobility may be essential for as long as possible to avoid making their mobility worse. Moving in and out of bed may need assistance, particularly if muscle tone is poor or in spasm, for example in women with MS and cerebral palsy. As many disabling conditions lead to tiredness it is important that midwives are sensitive to mothers' abilities and to ensure they obtain as much rest before and during labour as possible. Adequate analgesia must be offered and choice of type of analgesia will depend on mothers' specific circumstances and requirements. Entonox is suitable for all women although women with upper airway difficulties or physical impairment of arm(s), for example following a cerebro-vascular accident (stroke), hemiperisis or amputation, may find it difficult to use. Patience may be needed in teaching mothers with learning difficulties how to effectively use the equipment. Epidural, spinal and general anaesthetic may be suitable in some situations (see below). Mothers who rely on lip-reading or sign language may find pethidine unacceptable as the drowsy side effects inhibit communication.

## Possible issues to be prepared for

There are some issues that may need to be considered for women with disability. As during pregnancy, abdominal and vaginal examination may need additional care (see above). Vaginal examination, to monitor cervical changes and to ascertain the progress of labour, needs to be performed with particular consideration to avoid over-stimulation and pain. This is because muscle spasm or autonomic dysreflexia may suddenly develop (see above and Chapter 8). Muscle pain, stiffness and autonomic dysreflexia may also be stimulated by uterine contractions or a full bladder. Epidural analgesia will help to prevent these conditions from developing and frequent bladder emptying is advisable. Midwives also need to be aware of the possibility of latex allergy in women with spina bifida (May 2005, Welner & Temple 2004) therefore gloves made of an alternative material, usually readily available in the NHS, are used.

The onset of labour may not always be easily recognised if there is some inhibition or absence of nerve pathways, for example in women with MS or spinal cord damage e.g. spina bifida, spinal cord lesions, or from cord compression from spinal damage due to achondroplasia. Midwives

need to prepare women during pregnancy for this possibility and show them how to palpate the uterine fundus to recognise the contractions of labour and advise when to seek help. During labour midwives need to be vigilant to recognise the onset of the second stage of labour to ensure that birth does not go unattended. Conversely, progress in labour may be slow if uterine muscle tone is poor. An oxytocic infusion is successful in stimulating effective contractions (Baschat & Weiner 2004) and should be used for the third stage of labour.

Although epidural analgesia is likely to be beneficial for some women with disability, and it is often recommended generally for women undergoing caesarean section, it may not always be technically possible in some cases even with a skilled anaesthetist. Women with a tremor due to cerebral palsy, a damaged spinal column or limited space between the vertebrae because of trauma or achondroplasia, or those with scar tissue or chronic back conditions may not be able to have an epidural. However, if epidural can be sited then there are no contraindications. Grace Parker (2006) and Sevarino (2004) warn against spinal anaesthetic for women with achondroplasia. This is because the narrow spinal space makes the effects of the anaesthetic unpredictable whereas an epidural using a spinal catheter enables a limited and controlled dose. A spinal is also not recommended for women with MS (Sevarino 2004) as there is the potential for further impairment to an already compromised nervous system. Therefore it is important that women in these situations are advised to see an anaesthetist during pregnancy to discuss possible issues and explore other choices.

Whilst a normal vaginal birth is the aim of most women there are times when instrumental of operative delivery is needed. For women whose condition causes tiredness their energy levels may be diminished during labour, making expulsive efforts impossible, therefore they may require help using vacuum extraction or with forceps. Operative delivery may be planned during pregnancy if there is concern about pelvic size or shape but should never be considered routine just because a woman has a disability. However, women with achondroplasia frequently have a small contracted pelvis and are therefore more likely to need operative delivery. Experienced anaesthetists should always be present for induction of anaesthetic and during surgery for all women with a disability. Additional care may be needed for women with achondroplasia as jaw size and the structure of the neck may make intubation and induction of anaesthetic potentially difficult (Sevarino 2004). Women with the condition may develop upper airway obstruction so midwives need to be particularly vigilant for early signs of obstruction or apnoea in the immediate post-operative period. Extra care may also be needed when moving unconscious or semi-conscious women to avoid trauma to already compromised soft tissue, joints and nerves.

Experienced anaesthetists also need to be involved in the care of women with possible lung or cardiac compromise. Continuous cardiac and respiratory function monitoring will probably be standard and it may be necessary for women to be cared for in a maternity unit with readily accessible intensive care facilities. Midwives with expertise in special or intensive care would ensure knowledgeable and skilful care.

## POSTNATAL CARE

Initially the majority of postnatal care is in the hospital setting as few births occur in the home. But this is unlikely to be the ideal location for mothers with disability as their own homes will be adapted to their individual needs. Transfer home as soon as possible will be the best plan of care for most women. As the time that midwives can attend women in the postnatal period no longer has a time limit (NMC 2004b) the opportunity for a longer period of continuity of care from the same midwife or small team of midwives has improved. Mothers with a disability may benefit from a prolonged plan of visits which provides greater opportunities for midwives to liaise with other members of the multidisciplinary team. This has the potential to enhance assistance and provide mothers with a seamless service.

The postnatal period is the time when mothers with disability may need midwives to have practical suggestions for managing infant care in alternative ways. First, of course, midwives need to understand an individual mother's abilities and ways of tackling everyday tasks. Wates (1997)

argues that adhering to non-disabled behaviour without recognising the significance of impairment actually makes the situation abnormal for the individual, as '...every family's way of doing things is normal to them...' (p 56). However, midwives need to balance keeping their distance while remaining approachable. Therefore flexible professional involvement and interaction that is responsive to mothers is the key to avoiding an oppressive presence. Few people enjoy someone watching over them and assessing their actions. For mothers with disability this experience is likely to be even more stressful. They may have fears of failure and of being seen as unable to cope in case the baby is removed from their care by someone from the Social Services department.

Although there may be some grounds for that anxiety, a survey conducted by the Social Services Inspectorate of disabled parents in eight councils in England between November 1998 and July 1999 found that 60% of the respondents felt that social workers actually helped the families to stay together (Goodinge 2000). Parents did not find it easy to ask for help but when they did they were satisfied with the assistance received. Nevertheless, Goodinge (2000) felt that Social Services do not always focus holistically on families' needs or even have the ability to identify parents with a disability in order to offer help. With this in mind a key role that midwives may need to undertake, with mothers' consent, is to liaise with Social Services on their behalf. However, a note of caution must be given here as women may perceive visits from Social Service staff as intrusive and unwelcome (Prilleltensky 2003).

When assessing mothers several factors need to be taken into account. First, do they know the basics of infant care and parenting requirements? If this is a mother's first baby and she has received little or no parent education then midwives need to be ready to offer parent education on a one-to-one basis to ensure she has the required knowledge and skills. Second, does a mother have and know how to use any specialised equipment that could make her physical tasks achievable, less tiring and easier? Equipment has the added advantage of minimising injury, for example back strain. Finally, if a mother is unable or chooses not to participate physically in a task is she participating by interacting with her child and making the decisions about the helper's actions? This is a vital element ensuring a mother is her child's point of reference and for her to be in control of her child's long-term upbringing. Taking all of these elements into consideration will enable a complete picture of mother–baby interaction process to be formulated. This ensures that the correct support and guidance is offered, and only when needed.

Rogers et al (2004) advocate building up a 'visual history' of how a mother successfully copes with baby care with or without the aid of special equipment. However, this may not always be feasible taking into account a first-time mother's lack of experience. Additionally, the potential bias from understanding how easy or difficult another individual with the same disability finds a task, may lead to inappropriate or deficient help. Nevertheless, building up a visual history may aid midwives to form the 'can do' philosophy advocated by Rogers et al (2004).

Moving and handling may be challenging for mothers with an upper limb disability or a lack of upper arm strength. As an alternative some mothers may find using their teeth to lift their baby by the clothes another possibility. Rogers et al (2004) explain that if verbal commands are used regularly with a specific action a baby soon learns to follow such cues and 'help' with the task by lifting or even just keeping still. The use of a sling to carry baby over the chest may be useful. For mothers using a wheelchair a sling over the chest or on the lap can do much to solve the problem of moving baby in this situation.

## Infant feeding

The promotion of breast-feeding is an integral part of midwives' role. The contraindications to breast-feeding by mothers with disability are no different to other mothers. The main issue is likely to be the type of medication a mother is taking for her condition as some are unsuitable. During pregnancy some women will have omitted or changed medication to minimise the risks of fetal abnormality and they may need to restart that medication to alleviate pain or make the condition more tolerable.

Depending on a mother's upper limb dexterity and strength she may need to try different positions to ensure her breast is in a suitable position to facilitate her baby latching on. Midwives may need to help with this process initially until her baby has learnt to 'help itself'. Trial and adaptation may be needed using additional support from pillows or cushions. It is important that mothers are comfortable as tension and pain may inhibit lactation and the let down reflex. Perineal and wound pain need to be minimised, particularly for women with spinal cord damage, as autonomic dysreflexia (see Chapter 8) may be stimulated by undue pain.

If a mother chooses to use infant formula it is important that midwives ensure feeds are correctly prepared and stored. For women with upper limb impairment feed preparation may need to be undertaken by a helper. Now that the government recommend that freshly made feeds are no longer stored but used when made (DoH 2005) this may prove inconvenient if a mother's helper is not available at every feed time. The solution would be to use ready-prepared feed that is sterilised but that, of course, incurs greater expense. Feeding techniques i.e. positioning of the teat and bottle, may need to be practiced to find the best position that ensures safety.

## Family planning advice

Midwives commonly ask postnatal mothers about contraception and family planning. There is no ideal or set time to prompt discussion on the topic and for some women it is the last thing they wish to consider. Nevertheless, women should be asked if they wish to discuss the issue. Midwives need to be able to offer information and advice when necessary and that should be pertinent to an individual mother's wishes and situation. Not all methods are suitable for every woman and women with disability may have specific requirements (see Chapter 2). If a midwife feels unable to offer appropriate advice, referral to a local family planning clinic should be made.

Mothers should be given the times and locations of clinics and what services they provide, as not all clinics offer every service. If a woman has a specific time and location in mind her midwife could liaise with the clinic staff. This would ensure they have relevant information about a woman's situation and that they are adequately prepared for her appointment, for example regarding access and appropriate equipment for any necessary examinations. If work time permits, it may be possible for a midwife to go with a woman if she wishes. This could be of particular benefit for mothers with a learning disability who may be afraid or uncertain about attending. Additionally this would be a learning opportunity for midwives thus enhancing their own knowledge and ability to offer information and advice.

## ROLE OF THE MATERNITY SUPPORT WORKER

Midwives are not the only maternity care provider, particularly in maternity units where staffing by midwives is at a premium. The services of support workers are increasingly being used. Midwives must remember that in essence they are *delegating care* to support workers and therefore must assure themselves that the standard of care remains at or above minimum requirements, as it is clearly indicated in the 'Midwives rules and standards' (NMC 2004b) that they remain ultimately responsible for the care that women receive.

Maternity support workers generally work towards NVQ Level 3 and some will be undertaking a new Foundation Degree (qualifying with a diploma) in health. They have considerable input to postnatal and transitional care. A further dimension to this role can be developed by providing additional support to parents with a disability and working alongside the named midwife to coordinate care. They may ultimately have considerable levels of responsibility (see Box 4.3). This enhanced role will improve communication with other healthcare professionals and provide continuity of care for women with a disability, particularly in a maternity unit where there is a shortage of midwives.

As support workers increasingly become the team members providing a large proportion of 'hands-on' care they need the education to enable them to increase their disability awareness, and relevant knowledge and skills to be effective helpers. The curricula of NVQ and Foundation Degree courses need to reflect the learning requirements of these vital members of the midwifery team.

---

**Box 4.3  Possible responsibilities of a maternity support worker**

- Improve communication with ward staff regarding needs of women with physical, sensory and learning disabilities.
- Keep a file on the postnatal ward for plans of care for reference and instruction.
- Provide continuity of care for disabled women providing specific input and support if required.
- Inform ward manager of any changes in care needs e.g. issues following caesarean section, equipment needs, manual handling assessment.
- Hire specific equipment needs as identified from plan of care (height-adjustable cots, specific beds, height-adjustable incubators etc.).
- Enhance midwifery care given by offering practical help and quality time: they are often more available to listen.
- Meet with the lead midwife or specialist midwife in disability on a regular basis as needs arise giving feedback to other support workers.
- Attend disability awareness training programme to further enhance knowledge and skills.

---

## PARTNERS' NEEDS

Having a baby can be stressful on any relationship but for the couple where the mother has a disability, additional issues may cause extra strain on the relationship, although, conversely, the relationship may be strengthened. Therefore the needs of partners are important to consider; some fear the responsibility and huge role of parenting. Regardless of their ability, all partners want to be informed and supported. Whilst some play a more active role in maternity care, others do not. All, however, will benefit from consistent care and continuity of carer.

Partners who are deaf may need communication aids to be fully inclusive therefore midwives need to be aware of this and support accordingly. If however a partner is hearing he should not be expected to act as interpreter, particularly during labour when he may be anxious or stressed. Very few deaf parents request an interpreter in labour therefore another birth partner of their choice to act as an interpreter would meet this need.

Many believe that a partner faces fewer barriers if he has impairment, however his individual needs should also be addressed. Some partners view care from an objective view only i.e. task orientated, but it is important to consider the emotions of both mothers and fathers as the key to a positive experience. Women have stated that a partner has been 'brilliant', others are 'traumatised' by it all (Rotheram unpublished research).

Partners need to be invited to parent education classes to become involved. This will include a tour of delivery suite and postnatal wards to become familiar with the environment. Attention must be given to the needs of partners who are partially sighted or blind. The layout of rooms could be altered if necessary to make better use of natural or artificial light and to avoid shadows. This may also be necessary for partners who communicate by lip-reading.

Some partners may have access issues if they have a physical impairment or are wheelchair users themselves. It is necessary to overcome barriers of access, provide escorts if necessary, offer volunteers to support and assist and to have flexibility, for example use of an accessible toilet on the ward. It may be important therefore to discuss the partner's requirements in order to provide a positive experience.

Partners of women with a disability often request to stay in the hospital ward overnight to offer care, assistance and support and this involvement should be encouraged. They generally request little during their stay, but a single room should be provided with a bed or mattress to sleep on. There should be no discrimination between partners who are non-disabled or disabled.

## THE EXTENDED FAMILY AND HELPERS

It is not only partners of women with disability that may require support by midwives but so too may a woman's extended family and her helpers. This could be especially necessary if a woman's partner also has a disability. With a woman's consent the significant support people in her life can participate in any aspect of antenatal, labour and postnatal care. Attendance at parent education sessions could be useful for all concerned particularly when an issue needs an alternative solution. The people

providing a woman with help and support may have ideas that resolve any difficulties.

There is another area that midwives may be able to offer help and support in. Much of the literature reporting women's experiences indicates that women frequently experience negative attitudes towards their pregnancy and forthcoming parenthood. By being a mother's advocate during pregnancy and parenthood, midwives may be able to enhance helpers' understanding of a woman's capabilities and guide them on how, when or *if* to offer help. A mother's independence and decision-making may be enhanced and her autonomy promoted whilst ensuring helpers still feel their services are valuable.

---

### CONCLUSION—KEY POINTS

- Effective communication between mothers and midwives, midwives and their peers, and midwives and the multidisciplinary team will enhance the care mothers receive and enable a seamless service within an ethos of partnership.
- Positive attitudes towards mothers with a disability will promote mutual respect and increase mothers' satisfaction with service provision and midwives' job satisfaction.
- Midwives acting as advocates for mothers will help the development of a mutually trusting relationship in which women are in control of their pregnancy and birth experience.
- The fundamental factors to a successful maternity service are based on practitioners' knowledge, skill and confidence, and their ability to be creative, flexible, adaptable and innovative.

---

## References

Baschat A A, Weiner C P 2004 Chronic neurologic diseases and disabling conditions in pregnancy. In: Welner S L, Haseltine F (eds) Welner's guide to the care of women with disabilities. Lippincott Williams & Wilkins, Philadelphia, p 145–158

Blackford K A, Richardson H, Grieve S 2000 Prenatal education for mothers with disabilities. Journal of Advanced Nursing 32(4):898–904

Bramwell R, Harrington F, Harris J 2000 Deaf women: informed choice, policy and legislation. British Journal of Midwifery 8(9):545–548

Bramwell R, Carter D 2001 An exploration of midwives' and obstetricians' knowledge of genetic screening in pregnancy and their perception of appropriate counselling. Midwifery 17(2):133–141

Butler M S, Jackson L 1998 The value of listening skills to midwifery practice. British Journal of Midwifery 6(7):454–457

Department of Health (DoH) 1993 Changing Childbirth. Report of the Expert Maternity Group. HMSO, London

Department of Health (DoH) 1998 Equality is key to future of maternity care. Baroness Jay says: "Maternity services must be accessible to all women." 4th Feb. Department of Health, London

Department of Health (DoH) 1999 Once a day. Online. Available: http://www.dh.gov.uk 24 March 2006

Department of Health (DoH) 2004 Standard 11: Maternity Services, The National Service Framework for Children, Young People and Maternity Services. The Stationery Office, London

Department of Health (DoH) 2005 Bottle feeding: 2005 edition. Online. Available: http://dh.gov.uk 20 June 2006

Disability Discrimination act 1995 HMSO, London. Online. Available: http://www.drc-gb.org 1 March 2006

Earle S 2000 Pregnancy and the maintenance of self-identity: implications for antenatal care in the community. Health and Social Care in the Community 8(4):235–241

Fraser D M 1999 Women's perceptions of midwifery care: a longitudinal study to shape curriculum development. Birth 26(2):99–107

Gething L 1994 Interaction with disabled persons scale. Psychosocial perceptions on disability. Journal of Social and Behaviour and Personality, A Special Issue 9(5):23–42

Goodinge S 2000 A jigsaw of services: inspection of services to support disabled adults in their parenting role. Department of Health, London

Goodman M 1994 Mothers' pride and others' prejudice: a survey of disabled mothers' experiences of maternity. In: Maternity alliance disability working pack. Maternity Alliance, London

Gordon C 2004 Hormones, pregnancy and inflammatory arthritis. Arthritis Research Campaign. Online. Available: http://www.arac.org.uk 28 April 2006

Gould D 2004 Trust me, I am a midwife. British Journal of Midwifery 12(1):44

Grace Parker J H 2006 Achondroplasia. Emedicine from WebMD. Online. Available: http://www.emedicine.com 18 May 2006

Grue L, Trafjord Lærum K 2002 'Doing motherhood': some experiences of mothers with physical disabilities. Disability & Society 17(6):671–683

Iqbal S 2004 Pregnancy and birth: a guide for deaf women. RNID & the National Childbirth Trust, London

Irvin S K 2005 The cranberry: therapeutic properties. Clinical Excellence for Nurse Practitioners 9(1): 37–40

Jackson A B, Wadley V 1999 A multicenter study of women's self-reported reproductive health after spinal cord injury. Archives of Physical Medicine and Rehabilitation 80(11):1420–1428

McKay-Moffat S 2003 Midwifery care for women with disabilities. MPhil thesis. Liverpool John Moores University, Liverpool

Mario B 2004 Cranberry juice and UTIs: no evidence of benefit. Canadian Pharmaceutical Journal 137(2):41

May P L 2005 Latex allergy and spina bifida: a medical view. Association of Spina Bifida and Hydrocephalus (ASBAH). Online. Available: http://www.asbah.org 13 May 2006

Neville-Jan A 2004 Selling your soul to the devil: an autoethnography of pain, pleasure and the quest for a child. Disability & Society 19(2):113–127

NICE 2003 Antenatal care: Routine care for the healthy pregnant woman. National Institute of Clinical Excellence, London

NMC 2004a Code of professional conduct: standards for conduct, performance and ethics. Nursing and Midwifery Council, London

NMC 2004b Midwives rules and standards. Nursing and Midwifery Council, London

Prilleltensky O 2003 A ramp to motherhood: the experiences of mothers with physical disabilities. Sexuality and Disability 21(1):21–47

Ralston R 1998 Communication: create barriers or develop therapeutic relationships. British Journal of Midwifery 6(1):8–11

Rogers J G, Tuleja C V, Vensand K 2004 Through the looking glass. Baby care preparation: pregnancy and postpartum. In: Welner S L, Haseltine F (eds) Welner's guide to the care of women with disabilities. Lippincott Williams & Wilkins, Philadelphia, p 169–183

Rowe R E, Garcia J, Macfarlane A J, et al 2002 Improving communication between health professionals and women in maternity care: a structured review. Health Expectations 5(1):63–83

Royal College of Midwives (RCM) 2000 Position Paper No. 11a. Maternity care for women with disabilities. RCM, London. Online. Available: http://rcm.org.uk 1 March 2006

Sevarino F B 2004 Obstetric anaesthesia. In: Welner S L, Haseltine F (eds) Welner's guide to the care of women with disabilities. Lippincott Williams & Wilkins, Philadelphia, p 159–168

Stapleton H, Kirkham M, Thomas G, et al 2002 Language use in antenatal consultations. British Journal of Midwifery 10(5):273–277

Thomas C 1997 The baby and the bath water: disabled women and motherhood in social context. Sociology of Health & Illness: A Journal of Medical Sociology 19(5):622–643

Tinkler A, Quinney D 1998 Team midwifery: the influence of the midwife-woman relationship on

women's experiences and perceptions of maternity care. Journal of Advanced Nursing 28(1):30–35

Trotter T L, Hall J G, Schaefer G B, et al 2005 Health supervision for children with achondroplasia. Pediatrics 116(3):771–783

Warrier S 2003 Midwives: advocates or arbitrators? British Journal of Midwifery 11(9):532–533

Wates M 1997 Disabled parents: dispelling the myths. National Childbirth Trust & Radcliff, Cambridge.

Welner S L, Temple B 2004 General health concerns and the physical examination. In: Welner S L, Haseltine F (eds) Welner's guide to the care of women with disabilities. Lippincott Williams & Wilkins, Philadelphia, p 95–108

Wray J, Maresh M 2000 Midwives, obstetricians and prenatal screening. British Journal of Midwifery 8(1):31–35

# 5 Women with intellectual disabilities

## Linda Moss

## INTRODUCTION

The purpose of this chapter is to provide guidance to practising midwives when working with parents who are learning disabled. During the production of this chapter, the question was asked, what about mental illness? The fact is that there are many conditions that could be included in a weightier tome. Learning disability is a condition that causes people to be marginalised and devalued, often in favour of people who are mentally ill. For this very reason this chapter attempts to address the wide gap in the literature, where meaningful work carried out with people who are learning disabled is highlighted and used to direct midwives towards available resources and good working practices. Ironically, the adoption of such strategies will help midwives to work more effectively with people with other conditions if the skills are incorporated into everyday practice.

This chapter will explore the terminology used in various services. Often the terms 'learning disability' and 'mental health' are confused; this will be clarified within the text. Following the closure of the institutions and the backlash against the eugenics movement, people with learning disabilities have started to live ordinary lives. A discussion of rights issues for people with learning disabilities is included. This discussion will examine issues such as the way services have taken control of people's lives in the past and the lack of empowerment for people to enable them to have control over their own packages of care. Most of us take the components that make up our everyday lives for granted. These components make up the principles of choice, respect, inclusion, relationships and development; these are explored from the point of view of the person with learning disability. These principles are the fundamental issues in people's lives and serve to illustrate how people with learning disabilities have limitations imposed on their lives. Rights issues and the European Convention of Rights for Disabled People are discussed to highlight the fact that services should encourage advocacy for people to enable them to realise their rights. The *Valuing People* White Paper produced by this government is the first piece of legislation specifically for and about people with learning disabilities in 30 years. Issues within this White Paper are discussed, with the emphasis being on the areas relating specifically to families and the right of the person with learning disabilities to have a relationship and start a family.

Booth and Booth from Sheffield University and McGaw from Cornwall NHS have all written extensively about people with learning disabilities and parenthood. Their work is used to discuss assessment of parents in areas of child-care and the coping strategies employed by parents. The issues affecting parents from socio-economically deprived backgrounds are discussed in relation to the parallels that can be drawn with the way people from such backgrounds cope and the similar issues for parents with learning disabilities. The conclusion to this argument is discussed; in that support networks are highlighted as being paramount in the success of parents especially those with learning disabilities. It is the strength of such networks that govern whether a person with learning disability is successful or not in their endeavours to be a parent.

## HISTORICALLY SPEAKING

Institutions housed many people with learning disabilities over the years. Out of sight and out of mind was the norm for anyone who appeared to be different in any way. It can be said that disability is a social construction, that is to say that in a non-disabled world, there is an expectation for people to function in a certain way. Any deviation from this norm becomes problematic. In our non-disabled world, services, shops, entertainment, partnerships, procreation, all aspects of life, are geared towards the social norms. In the 1980s when the UK Community Care Act decreed that institutions should close on human rights grounds, people with learning disabilities more than ever started to live ordinary lives in ordinary houses in ordinary streets (O'Brien & O'Brien 1995).

The Declaration of Human Rights was adapted in 1979 by the United Nations to a Declaration of the Rights of the Mentally Handicapped. The aim of the declaration is to ensure that disabled people have the right to 'freedom of expression, liberty and security, respect for private life, marriage, education, and prohibition of discrimination' (Atherton 2003, p 56.).

Along with this territory came the wishes from the people themselves to lead ordinary lives, including marriage and producing families. Relationships are an important part of the socialisation process for all of us. We take for granted the benefits of such relationships of sharing and caring during both good times and not so good times. Just to be able to have someone there to talk to about everyday things is something many of us take for granted. If we were unable to form relationships we would more than likely be very lonely and isolated and suffer from low self-esteem and even depression (Carson & Docherty 2002).

The work of David Pitonyak (2006) illustrates this very point. According to Pitonyak (2006), relationships are paramount in all our lives. Relationships enable us to have a sense of self and worth. Where we have relationships we have a personal history as social functions are centred on our own histories and the intertwined histories of those we have relationships with. Shevin (1999) talks about loneliness as being the most disabling of conditions. People who have disabili-

ties tend to live in situations where they have to depend on others to help them to function in their everyday lives. The people who provide the help more often than not are paid to be in those people's lives. The nature of employment is that people tend to work in one place for a while but will eventually move on. The majority of people take it for granted that there are friends and family around them that they can share their lives with. Even the simple question of 'how was your day' is very important to show that we are cared for and others care for us. If there is no one around to ask that question the consequences can be severe. Loneliness means that there is no one there to ask how your day was. There is no one to share in recapping memories of shared events of last week, last year or even last decade. As well as sharing, a family can provide kindness, acceptance and above all love. We all need to feel loved and that we belong somewhere. This need is the same for all people especially people who have disabilities. It is no surprise then that as opportunities to form relationships increase for people with learning disabilities so too does the desire to create a family of their own. In the institutions many people grew up in an environment where males and females were separated. This meant that inevitably some people who were more able would form secretive relationships. Often residents would talk of being 'engaged' in a desperate attempt to have a normal life as portrayed to them in the media and by staff, often their only link with the outside world. We have indeed moved far from this situation in terms of community care and people living in ordinary houses. Life is still very limited for many as a balance is sought between allowing people independence and an ordinary life and the desire to protect vulnerable people from exploitation.

The present government brought out a White Paper entitled *Valuing People* (DoH 2001b) in order to address the needs of people with learning disabilities living in the community. In it the DoH states 'good services will help people with learning disabilities develop opportunities to form relationships, including ones of a physical and sexual nature' *Valuing People* DoH 2001b, p 81. This paper addresses the issues of parenthood and how people with learning disabilities need the same considerations as anyone else in a similar situation. There is also a necessity to consider the individual needs of each person, to ensure that their experience is as positive as possible for everyone involved.

## TERMINOLOGY

A fundamental issue to begin any discussion around people with learning disabilities is around the terminology and array of terms used within services and the community in order to meet people's needs. In an effort to clarify the situation these will be explored here.

There exists a wide range of conditions causing learning disability and a resulting wide range of abilities. Some people are so affected by their disability that self-care and verbal communication are severely impaired (Roffman 2000). At the other end of the scale is people affected in such a way that they can self-care and communicate verbally, but may have some social inadequacies within our non-disabled literature-dependent world. The current legislation refers to the term 'learning disability', to indicate such people and their needs (Race 2002). The education system on the other hand works to meet the needs of people from a wider span of difficulties and the term used here is learning difficulty. This term incorporates conditions such as learning disability, autism and dyslexia amongst others. The legal system uses yet another term, referring to people as 'mentally impaired'. This term includes mental illness. The people being considered within this chapter are learning disabled. This is a condition usually present at birth or caused by some insult to the central nervous system in the formative years. This might be as a result of drug use by the mother or some trauma whilst the child was in utero. It might be the result of an instrumental birth, the use of forceps for example, or prolonged delivery and caesarean section causing anoxia. It could be as a result of the infant or toddler having trauma or disease such as meningitis. Any insult to the central nervous system during these formative years usually causes an arrested state of development which means that the person's capacity to develop cognitively is limited. This does not mean that the person is limited in all ways, just that the ability to learn may be limited. Mental illness on the other hand can be caused at any stage of life, a pertinent example being postnatal depression. The student who is stressed with studying for final exams can become suicidal; the increase in drug use in our society is causing an increase in schizophrenia. These are all examples of mental illness. Such conditions are usually responsive to treatment, whereas learning disability is usually a permanent condition. That is not to say that a person is incapable and shouldn't be given every chance to lead a similar quality of life as others of a similar age and social position. Learning disabilities span a wide scope of abilities. This is where the difficulty lies when the question of sexuality arises. Some people may only need to be advised about masturbation and appropriate behaviour and privacy, whilst others may need to have an understanding of more complex issues such as relationships, contraception and safe sex (Fegan et al 1993).

## EMPOWERMENT

Power is mentioned briefly here to illustrate how awareness on the part of health professionals can serve to change the lives of people they provide a service to. Talcott Parsons is discussed extensively in Giddens (1995) as writing extensively about issues of power and the sick role adopted and given to people using the health service. The inverse care law usually applies, whereby a person who is seen as more powerful receives a better service, whereas the least powerful person, who is often most in need of services, does not always receive an adequate service. Therefore empowerment becomes a central issue when attempting to deliver a service to a person who has a learning disability. Holmes (1999/2000) details work of Guttmann as alluding to the fact that prejudice can cause people with learning disabilities to feel inferior and even to have low self-esteem. Holmes (1999/2000) argues that people should not be made to feel this from health professionals. Professionals therefore have a responsibility to understand the issues that may face people with disabilities and so act as a resource to promote physical care, emotional support and give advice.

The difficulty is professionals are only human and according to Miller & Sammons (1999), we have a tendency in psychological terms to form patterns in our minds that make the world predictable, comfortable and familiar. When we come across an event that does not fit our usual scheme of the world, we are likely to react. Anything that is unfamiliar or unexpected therefore, can be unsettling. Our reactions to difference then can range from admiration, inspiration or curiosity to fixation, apprehension, fear, disgust, shock and surprise and even sadness. This is often the type of reaction people experience when they come across somebody who is learning disabled. If that person decides to start a family, rather than being congratulated, questions will be asked: why? How will they manage? Will they pass the disability on to their own children? Rather than considering, how can we help? What assistance will they need? Or even, what a wonderful event (Hevey 1993).

The questions asked are usually based on our historical tendency to devalue people who are different in any way. Even the term 'learning disability' is the culmination of years of attempts to define a group of people who are seen as different, labelled and experience devaluation in all aspects of their lives (Boxall 2002). As a consequence, the terminology used to describe such people becomes, in turn, devalued and is used as a derogatory term in everyday language. Examples are 'mentally handicapped', 'mentally subnormal', and a whole range of terms used in official capacities over the years that have been reduced to terms of ridicule and abuse: 'spaz', 'mencap', 'subbie' being some of the milder terms for example. In our more enlightened times, people with learning disabilities are becoming more valued as citizens within our communities; along with this comes the overwhelming desire to lead an ordinary life, which for most people includes marriage and starting a family. With this comes the increase in numbers of people becoming pregnant (DoH 2001a). This is often the result of a relationship but unfortunately can still occasionally be the result of an abusive event. Whatever the circumstances the mother will need the same support and care as any other prospective mothers.

## SERVICE-LED DECISIONS VERSUS PERSON-CENTRED CARE

In the 1980s, the term, 'social role valorisation' was introduced by Wolf Wolfensberger within services for people with learning disabilities (Race 2002). This term was used to define a complex issue within these services. People with learning disabilities have, up until now, been the passive recipients of services, whether the service was appropriate, therapeutic or not, or even abusive in some cases. Wolfensberger and others looked at human rights issues and saw that people with learning disabilities needed to lead ordinary lives with whatever support they needed to enable them to do so (Atherton 2003). Thompson (2005) refers to 'the professional gift' model of care, where professionals have the qualifications, knowledge and status, which put them in a position of power when deciding the service a person will receive. People themselves have no control or say in the service they receive. Social role valorisation saw a change in thinking, in that the services should enable a person to lead a valued life with valued social roles, which most people enjoy. These roles include simple things like being a customer, a colleague, and more complex roles like family roles, partner, and parent (Atherton 2003). There is therefore a need to redress the balance of power within services. Rather than a service providing care to passive individuals, individuals needs to have a say in the service that they want and the care they receive (O'Hara & Martin 2003).

Thompson (2005) agrees that this is no easy task since a person with learning disabilities will need guidance, especially in the situation of impending parenthood. The fact remains that a person using a service needs to have some control over the way that service is given rather than the relationship being an issue of power imbalance. This will help to ensure that people with learning disability have equity with other citizens and that the service they receive is not just a 'professional gift' but an equal partnership that meets the needs and choices of each individual.

At one time the life of a person with learning disability did not include any responsibility. Indeed the person's life would not follow the usual pattern of the life cycle. Even people who were more able could be treated as though they were incapable of having any responsibility for their own lives. A person often would be hidden from view and kept indoors. The case of a woman admitted into care after being shut in the house by her mother for the majority of her life illustrates the shame attached to the birth of a child with learning disabilities in the past. It wasn't until the then elderly mother passed away that the young woman, in her forties now, was moved from the family home in a very unkempt state into an institution where she started to mix with other people. Another woman, was kept locked in her bedroom away from her brothers and never received any schooling. Eventually she was put into an institution never to be seen by her family again. The normal patterns of schooling often did not take place and as a result people didn't receive the socialisation of mixing and learning from peers that the rest of us take for granted. Consequently the opportunities afforded to everyone else did not happen for either of these women and thousands of others like them. They certainly had very little choice or control in their lives and no chance of forming healthy, loving, valued relationships with others. Consequently any role they did have was seen to be a burden or shameful by their families and those around them, and by today's standards is quite shocking.

Following on from social role valorisation is the development of ordinary living principles. These are issues that most people take for granted but are often missing from the lives of people with learning disabilities. Race (2002) discusses work by O'Brien who developed five principles: choice, participation in everyday life, respect from others, development of skills to lead a fuller life, and relationships, but not just with people paid to be in the person's life, like teachers, carers and bus drivers. Services need to be based on these five principles. The *Valuing People* document (DoH 2001a) reiterates these principles in making its central objective aims to promote 'rights, independence, choice and inclusion for people with learning disabilities' (DoH 2001a, p 106). In relation to maternity services, choice is an important issue in giving people enough information, so they can make informed choices from the start of the pregnancy and antenatal care through to the birth plan and an individual's preferences. Participation means to be able to participate in all aspects of life and not being excluded on the grounds of having a learning disability.

Individuals with learning disabilities are often looked at from the view of what they cannot do, rather than the positive aspects of what they can do or could do with support. Booth & Booth (1999) refer to factors that are exacerbated by well-meaning professionals, one of which is the presumption of incompetence. Parents who are learning disabled often feel discriminated against as professionals mistakenly make the assumption that any limitations caused by their learning disability will automatically make them unfit parents (Booth & Booth 1999).

Development is a thing we all take for granted usually, but if we were treated as perpetual children, as often people with learning disabilities are, then life may become very frustrating. A person needs to be allowed to develop through learning new skills and being treated as an adult. Being allowed to develop real relationships remains a bone of contention but many people with learning disabilities develop lasting and enduring friendships (Brackenbridge & McKenzie 2005). Brackenbridge and McKenzie refer to the positive aspects of friendship as raising self-esteem, preventing depression and improving quality of life. Who are we then to prevent individuals from developing friendships and even relationships that include expressing sexuality? These issues are all part of ordinary living that the rest of us take for granted. The person with a learning disability can become very isolated. If siblings leave the family home to go on to develop their own families or go to college or just to make their own way in life, the person with a learning disability is often left behind. This can cause a sense of loss. Pitonyak (2006) refers to this situation where the person may lose a close friend, someone who advocated for them and who helped them in many aspects of their life. Such support is now gone and is an extension to the usual sibling relationship and therefore, according to Pitonyak (2006), the loss felt may be even greater. Pitonyak (2006) suggests that we ask ourselves, 'if this person died today who would care?' Whilst this may seem an extreme question to ask, the answer has serious implications. The majority of people with learning disabilities rely on people being paid to be in their lives or close family for their relationships. Even where relationships are facilitated in the person's life, little regard is given to the sexual aspect of any relationship. Relationships are usually considered as platonic and information is often limited to stopping any kind of loving relationship. Information that is given needs to include sexuality and any issues that are useful to that individual should be included. In a world where we still have difficulty in teaching our own children about sexuality and the taboos that surround sex education, teaching people with learning disabilities about sexuality is still seen as a great risk rather than a necessity. It can be argued that if both children and people with learning difficulties are taught about sexuality when it is appropriate for them, a lot of problems related to sexuality can be eased.

## ADVOCACY AND EMPOWERMENT

Since the closure of institutions, many advocacy groups have developed throughout the country. Groups such as, 'People First' for example (Ward 1995), are usually run *by* people with learning disabilities *for* people with learning disabilities. They have gathered momentum and are contributing to major government initiatives including the White Paper *Valuing People* (DoH 2001a). This said there is still a long way to go before people with learning disabilities have a say in the care they receive from everyday services. Booth & Booth (1999) discuss a project funded by the Joseph Rowntree Foundation, entitled 'Parents Together'. The project explored aspects of support needed for parents with learning disabilities, such as advocacy. This was rather than concentrating on the child and its development or on actual parenting skills. The key areas within this project were 'lightening the load on parents, challenging discriminatory practice and improving their self esteem' (Booth & Booth 1999, p 472).

Arnold (2003) details a similar service in North Tyneside. The emphasis within this service is also on support for parents and offers a support group to parents as well as a personal development programme to help individuals to develop their self-esteem. The service also offers support in the form of an outreach service.

In order to empower an individual, professionals need to enable that person to have a voice. Often this can mean a great deal of patience to allow a person with learning disabilities their say. In a busy clinic this is not always easy, and guidelines have been drawn up to help services to meet the needs of people with learning disabilities. The key requirements as detailed in *Valuing People* (DOH 2001a) include the most important issue for the NHS to address, that of staff developing the necessary skills to consider the needs of people with learning disabilities.

Linda Ward (1995) quotes 'People first' as putting the emphasis on accessible information: 'People with learning disabilities find their community inaccessible to them in many formats, but none more powerful than inaccessible information' (Ward 1995, p 16). This meant that many documents were written for people who are literate and have a certain level of cognitive functioning. Accessible documents would include pictures or illustrations, would be written in non-jargon language and would even have large font print to enhance readability. According to Ward (1995) 'People first' went on to develop initiatives in this area and there are now many documents in accessible format, *Valuing People* being an example. It is worth considering, therefore, in maternity services, the format of information given to prospective parents and considering just how accessible it is. Such a strategy may indeed help many parents and not just those who have learning disabilities.

## PROFESSIONAL ISSUES

The 'Once a day' document: 'A primary care handbook for people with learning disabilities' (DOH 1999) was produced by the government to emphasise the need for meeting the health needs of people with learning disabilities. This document details that people with learning disabilities have a reduced ability to understand new or complex information, to learn new skills and to cope independently.

There is a need, when communicating with people with learning disabilities, to ensure effectiveness of the communication and specific principles need to be considered (see Box 5.1). They were developed as a communication strategy *by* people with learning disabilities *for* people with learning disabilities from the CHANGE organisation website.

## Box 5.1 Principles to enhance effective communication

- Speak clearly.
- Use short words and not jargon.
- Use short sentences.
- Avoid giving too much information at once.
- Break down the information.
- List important things.
- Write it down if needed.
- Draw simple pictures to help make information clearer.
- Give the person time to think about what has been said.
- Check understanding.

Clearly in the case of a woman with a learning disability, there is a definite need to take her views into account during her pregnancy. This may just mean allowing time and engaging in thoughtful communication, but such measures can make all the difference to what could be a frightening and difficult time for that woman. However Booth & Booth (1999) do stipulate that whilst advocacy helps to empower people and raise self-esteem, in services that do not support families with special needs enough, advocacy is needed but the overall goal needs to be a change in attitudes and a change in the system to take into account a positive view of parents with learning disabilities.

When working with parents with learning disabilities, one of the starting points may be conception. Consenting to a sexual relationship between two adults is as normal a part of life as breathing and eating. When the two adults involved happen to have a learning disability, many issues arise.

Craft & Brown (1994) give an account of personal relationships and sexuality with people who have learning disabilities. Here they reiterate the point that in the past people have been treated under the medical model, whereby a cure or treatment for the condition has been the aim of services. Otherwise the educational model dominated; here the right kind of training could be seen to put people's faults to rights. The onus is always on the person as having a fault to be solved rather than a person who needed to be accepted in the society they live in. It is only in recent years that as

mentioned previously, the rights model has been employed. The rights of choice, development, community presence, relationships and respect (Race 2002) all link in to illustrate how, if the individual with learning disability is going to lead a full life, equal to their non-disabled peers, then services and others need to adopt this philosophy and allow people age-appropriate activities. This change does not happen overnight or indeed for all people; it is a process of social change away from the social structures and practices of the past in relation to people with learning disabilities.

## ASSESSMENT OF NEEDS

According to McGaw & Sturmey (1993), a starting point in assessing the needs of parents who have learning disabilities is in identifying that a person has a learning disability in the first place. There are assessment tools available that are commonly used by clinical psychologists, to identify people with learning disabilities. Given the time constraints of a pregnancy, midwives need to be able to identify if a person has a learning disability in order to ensure that individual needs are met. McGaw & Sturmey (1993) argue that the identification of complex issues such as Intelligence Quotient or I.Q. is problematic. People may be functioning within the community with an I.Q. of 50 to 70 but may not be using services, whereas another person with an I.Q. between 70 and 85 may be receiving services. Services need to be provided on a needs basis rather than a labelling scheme such as I.Q.

Baum (1994) discusses the case of a young woman who had an I.Q. of below 40 and had become pregnant. It was found that by law a person with an I.Q. below 54 is deemed to be incapable of giving consent to sexual intercourse. In this case then, a criminal act had been committed; this is another aspect of learning disabilities that needs careful consideration.

Tymchuk & Andron (1994) discuss the fact that I.Q. is not a reliable indicator of a person's ability to parent. Inevitably people that often come to the notice of services are those who are in need of the services. Others who are coping well and do not use services do not tend to be detailed in the literature, simply because they are absent from the available picture (Tymchuk & Andron 1994). A person who has learning disabilities and does not usually use any services will not always therefore be identified when they do need extra services to meet their needs during a life event such as pregnancy.

If prospective parents are already known to learning disability services, then identification of the individual and their needs will be easier (Booth & Booth 1996). Schooling may be an indication of the prevalence of learning disability. If a person attended a special school or had special tuition, a classroom assistant for example, this may indicate that a person has a learning difficulty.

The fact remains that identifying a person is problematic in that the person becomes labelled and the expectations and inequalities associated with that label are usually, unwittingly, instigated on the part of care providers, in this case midwives. If a person is labelled in such a way, the reactions as mentioned earlier, of shock, disbelief, revulsion etc., may be felt. A certain level of self-awareness is needed therefore on the part of midwife practitioners. The need for unconditional positive regard is paramount. That is to say, that midwives need to develop an awareness of their own attitudes in order to develop strategies to deal with feelings about prospective mothers or parents who have special needs (Booth & Booth 1996). This is in order that such feelings do not colour any clinical decisions taken and that the skills of advocacy and non-judgementality can be exercised in the practise of meeting the person's human rights (Blackford et al 2000).

McGaw & Sturmey (1993) identified that mothers with learning disabilities do not tend to receive adequate antenatal care. This is alarming since a high proportion of such mothers may go on to need further medical care as a result of complications (McGaw & Sturmey1993). There is a difficulty in identifying parents who are learning disabled as well as parents from a poor socio-economic background. More often than not a person with learning disabilities is likely to be socially isolated but both sets of parents may live in socially deprived or poor environments (Booth & Booth 1996). This, according to Booth & Booth, often leads to children being removed from the family on grounds caused by deficiencies in services, support and even

professional practice, rather than any failure on the part of the parents.

Tymchuk & Andron (1994) discuss the myths surrounding people with learning disabilities as parents. Such folklore includes whether the learning disability will be passed on to the child. This has been proved to be the same chance as the rest of the population. Other myths include promiscuity on the part of either parent or even numerous pregnancies. Given the same opportunities for education and guidance around contraception and sexuality, this too has been shown to be unfounded. Neglect of children and inadequate parenting skills as well as lack of discipline for a child are also issues that affect the rest of the population and can all be addressed with education and guidance and appropriate support (DOH 2001b).

McGaw & Sturmey (1993) discuss the effects of the 1989 Children's Act. The Act advocates that in the case of children in need, a preventative model needs to be adopted. This means ensuring a range of services are available to support both children and parents to prevent an abusive or neglectful situation arising. Such a model is dependent on the skills of professionals involved and their ability to work collaboratively (McGaw & Sturmey 1993).

Booth & Booth in 1999 found that between 40 and 60% of children were removed from homes where the parents had learning disabilities. This illustrates the point that lack of support and inadequate training for professionals leads to inadequate services to meet people's needs. Booth & Booth (1999) also argue that many children are removed from their families on the grounds of a narrow interpretation of the term 'abuse'. In actual fact it would be more appropriate to consider such children as being in need. This leads on to the argument that low expectations of people labelled as learning disabled means they are often expected to fail. The ensuing trauma experienced by these families when their children are removed is detailed by Booth & Booth (1996) and would seem to be yet another issue overlooked by well-meaning professionals. The strength of feeling and bonding within families needs to be considered.

Parents with learning disabilities do not always have access to positive role models for parenting skills. If they have been in care or suffered from abusive relationships with their own parents then this should not be an automatic bar for that person to be a parent (McGaw & Sturmey 1993). The emphasis is often placed on what the parents' deficiencies are rather than what their positive skills are (Booth & Booth 1993).

## COLLABORATIVE WORKING

There is clearly a need for collaborative working. It is useful for people working in midwifery and obstetric services to have some knowledge of other professionals and their roles. This will ensure health needs of individuals can be fulfilled by a service that caters for those needs. Blackford et al (2000) discuss the need for services to develop on from the run of the mill, standardised services that have been prevalent since services began. In our increasingly diverse culture, an awareness of the need for individualised and culturally sensitive care is an ever-increasing necessity. The days of one-size-fits-all care are gone (Blackford et al 2000. Blackford et al (2000) refer to Rankin et al (p 899) as detailing the value of 'recognising the importance of flexibility, communication, shared decision making and self care'. This will in turn, ensure that individuals have their needs met and most importantly have their rights realised through advocacy, empowerment and support.

There are some services that are establishing beacon sites for good practice. One such project is the Special Parenting Project founded in 1998 by Dr Sue McGaw, a Consultant Clinical Psychologist in Cornwall (McGaw et al 2002). This service provides assessment of parenting skills, interventions, advocacy, professional training, and research and has produced publications and resources for professionals and people using the service. This organisation runs the 'Family Ties' project, which is funded by the Sure Start programme, identifies families that are hard to reach and/or are socially excluded. Their work is centred on assessment of family needs and early intervention through multi-agency working (see Box 5.2) to achieve greater success in their parenting (see Box 5.3). The *Valuing People* White Paper explores this issue and stipulates that: 'In many places, people with learning disabilities and their families continue to be passed between organisations and professionals

> **Box 5.2 Multi-agency list of people who may be able to support parents**
>
> - Midwifery.
> - Community Learning Disability team; within such teams there is often a nurse or separate team dedicated to developing expertise in working with parents who are learning disabled.
> - Clinical psychologist, who may work closely with parents on a number of issues including teaching parents skills.
> - Psychiatrist, who may be a specialist working with people with learning disabilities and may advise on issues such as treatment required for conditions during pregnancy, such as epilepsy for example.
> - Other professionals that may be involved include social workers.

> **Box 5.3 With the right multi-agency support parents will be enabled to:**
>
> - increase their parenting skills;
> - gain a greater understanding of child development;
> - improve their child's health and hygiene;
> - manage their child's behaviour;
> - increase parental responsiveness;
> - develop home and management skills;
> - build self-confidence;
> - access appropriate support and resources.

with insufficient clarity about where responsibility rests for ensuring effective service provision' (DOH 2001a, p 107).

## ASSESSMENT OF PARENTING SKILLS

Tymchuk & Andron (1994) detail the importance of comprehensive assessment for the skills of the parents as a key issue. Wharton (2005) has also detailed an assessment tool for use with parents who have learning disabilities, based on the Department of Health Framework for the Assessment of Children in Need and their Families (DoH 2000) to assess need (see Box 5.4).

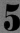 

> **Box 5.4  Issues considered in the parenting assessment tool**
>
> - Determination of areas of parental need.
> - The assessment will provide a basis to work on whilst establishing a relationship with parents.
> - Providing a basis for report writing, for reviews and child protection case conference requirements.
> - Identity of areas to increase client's self-esteem and willingness to cooperate.
> - Enable effective discussion with other professionals involved, ensuring the provision of the most appropriate support service.

Tymchuk & Andron (1994) discuss the features in the lives of parents who fare well in the role of parent or not. Such features tend to be a reflection of issues in the lives of the general population, usually associated with poor parenting skills. Interestingly, they are often considered as issues solely in the case of a parent who has learning disability. The characteristics of mothers who do well include those who have literacy skills affording the ability to read leaflets, prescriptions and other literature to help in the role of parent. This will also enable a person to read safety information and fill in forms which in turn will help with material benefits for the family. A person who copes well with stress and has no emotional or mental disorder and has a certain amount of motivation, possesses all factors that contribute to the success of this role. Financial considerations and having a partner who is also emotionally stable as well as having appropriate role models and supports, all contribute to a positive parenting role (Tymchuk & Andron 1994). The reverse is true, if the above are not in place then a person's parenting role will be jeopardised.

The work of Parents Together, as detailed in Booth & Booth (1999), found that the following issues of presumption of incompetence of a person in the parenting role by professionals; the conflicting responsibility to promote the rights of both parent and child on the part of professionals; and the tension between helping people to be empowered and issues of child protection, all had serious consequences for the parents with learning disabilities

and made this potentially happy time a time of trauma and hardship for all involved.

Booth & Booth (1999) also found that the focus was on the deficiency perspective, where deficiencies are focused on by professionals, rather than positive aspects and any skills the person may have. This serves to undermine the confidence of the prospective parents. It is often coupled with support that inhibits competence and professionals have a tendency to take over and not allow parents to make their own decisions for example. A person then becomes dependent on professionals for instruction and decisions and so their parenting skills are impaired. Deficiencies in support services are often masked by blame being apportioned to parents' learning disability and not the lack of resources. Lack of trust is also damaging in that parents may have had bad experiences of services in the past and so may not seek help when it is needed.

The Parents Together project (Booth & Booth 1999) works within the guiding principles of enabling parents by allowing them opportunities to succeed and so to exhibit their competence. Parents are also empowered by developing skills to improve their sense of control over their own situation. This in turn helps to enhance self-esteem and parents are assisted in improving their social networks. The Parents Together project aimed at reducing the pressures on parents, such as those detailed above, for example literacy, finance, environment, vulnerability and family breakdown. The project concentrated on these aspects rather than specifically on the development of parenting skills. Strategies to achieve this involved:

- Support groups to share experiences, learn from and support each other.
- Reduced isolation and loneliness.
- Combatting stress encountered.
- Encouragement of strengths and abilities to increase self-esteem.
- Outreach work for parents unable or unwilling to attend the group and to support parents in the community through:
  Crisis advocacy.
  Telephone helpline.
  Parent-to-parent links.
  A resource network.

Booth & Booth (1999) stated that this project worked well with parents who have learning disabilities whilst working in partnership with professionals. Given that most of their issues are the same for other socio-economically disadvantaged groups, they too could benefit from such a scheme.

Assessment of parents at the present time is carried out by the Community Learning Disability Nursing service. This occurs if a person or parents become known to the service. If a person is not known to the service, they may well slip through the net. Any involvement of midwives in the process or, at the very least, liaison between the professions will help to develop an adequate service for potential parents.

Consent is an issue that requires some consideration here. A person receiving care needs to consent to treatment and to have the capacity to consent to that treatment. This means that people need to have understanding of the intended treatment. Procedures need to be explained in non-jargonistic terms and understanding needs to be tested, by asking questions for example. It is not legal for a carer or relative to consent on behalf of another person. Therefore a person with learning disabilities needs to have the capacity to consent to any treatment. If this is not the case a doctor may act in the person's best interests. Capacity to consent to any treatment needs to he assessed on a regular basis (Wheeler 2003). People need to be allowed a fair chance to make their own decisions.

## GOOD ENOUGH PARENTING

Good enough parenting is a phrase coined by Booth & Booth (1998) to consider the question, what is good enough parenting? More often than not, this is not an issue and no one questions the competence of parents as they take their newborn child home. Support is given from community midwives and health visitors and even general practitioners. Further help is usually sought when something is needed or goes wrong. As a consequence, we have a service in the UK whose whole nature is to seek out problems and solve them. As the services are geared in this way the result is the testing of the person with learning disabilities to see if they are good enough parents, the outcome if not is often

the removal of the child. O'Hara & Martin (2003) found out that out of 79 live births to parents with learning disabilities, 16 children or 20% were taken into care as a result of the parent being learning disabled. Such a situation may be avoided if sufficient support networks were in place. Consideration also needs to be given to the usual informal support networks of parents, in-laws, friends, and relatives, all of whom ordinarily are drawn into the child-care arena at some point, even if it is in a purely advisory capacity. Often such networks are overlooked or absent in the case of a parent with learning disabilities.

A starting point for support is the assessment of parents. There appears to be a paucity of provision in this particular area. This is probably because women with learning disabilities were not considered to be fit parents in the past. This often resulted in enforced contraception or even sterilisation. Services are therefore patchy across the country and development of frameworks and tools to work with is a slow evolutionary process. Some tools are being developed and a review of the literature shows that it is usually learning disabilities services that are developing and using such tools (Baum 1994, Booth & Booth 1999, McGaw & Sturmey 1993, Wharton 2005). Admittedly, other services such as midwifery do have many other aspects of care and conditions to take into account. The development of knowledge about the tools available and how to use them can only serve to enhance the role of professionals and the experience and rights of parents (Booth & Booth 1998).

Wharton (2005) provides a model of assessment including areas to be considered when working with parents who have learning disabilities. The areas are reproduced here as a list to illustrate the need to consider issues more widely than purely specific child-care.

- Acknowledgement of problem and cooperation on the part of the parent.
- Practical skills.
- Preparation for baby.
- Housekeeping skills.
- How safe is your house?
- Establishing routines.
- Understanding the child protection process.
- Stability.
- Diet.
- Personal hygiene.

■ Healthcare issues.
■ Budgeting.
■ Interaction between mother/father and baby or child.
■ Emotional attachment.
■ Communication with other people/professionals.
■ Decision-making.
■ Timetabling—appointments for self/child.
■ Play stimulation.
■ Awareness of child development.
■ Behavioural management and consistency.
■ Coping with stress.
■ Developing networks.
(Wharton 2005, p 13.)

The multidisciplinary team could take these areas into account and develop support for the family in any areas of need. Preparation for these issues could be considered long before a baby is due, when lack of knowledge in these areas could result in crisis for the family.

An innovation by The Special Parenting Services in Cornwall is the development of skills cards for use by professionals when supporting parents with learning disabilities. These cards cover essential child-care activities, such as healthy eating, keeping healthy and warm, keeping safe and issues around love including providing an environment to enable child development.

In another account of pregnancy in a woman with learning disabilities, the assessment resulted in the development of best practice guidelines for the multidisciplinary team working with that particular woman. Issues arising included the need for mutual support within the team, and clear communication with all personnel on practical management issues and the specific roles of each professional. This allowed for privacy for the particular woman, the identification of the need for her to be told she was pregnant and what the implications of this were i.e. that there was a baby inside her, and the stages up to and including the birth and the birth itself. In this particular case, the need to allow grieving for the baby when it was taken for adoption was considered. The woman's physical needs and the needs of the other people in the house she lived in were also taken into account (Baum 1994).

Many other resources exist, and following initial assessment there needs to be a comprehensive programme developed to help both mothers and fathers to gain the skills they will need to operate as a family. Booth & Booth (1996) detail an account where a father was at a loss when mother and baby returned home simply because the mother had been taught skills such as nappy changing and bottle making but nobody had included the father. Fathers can be incorporated into such sessions but may sometimes need encouragement to do so. In the case of a father who may have a learning disability, extra encouragement may be needed.

## COMPLIANCE

Compliance may be an issue depending on how parents view their role, but working collaboratively with members from other teams can help to build up trust and confidence for parents. An emphasis on helping people to succeed can also help with compliance in parent education courses.

Baum (1994) gives an overall account of a programme set up to help a woman who has severe learning disabilities to cope with pregnancy and subsequent birth. This account details how thoughtful staff were when considering issues such as the woman's growing body as the fetus developed. Often it is an assumption that women have the knowledge of where a baby is developing and how this will happen and what will happen when giving birth. Even now the level of sex education and parent education in special schools is limited. There are a number of reasons for this, not least being the assumptions that people with learning disabilities will not go on to have children. Baum (1994) and her team used diagrams and calendars to show this woman how her body was developing and why. A similar system could be adapted for other women as their growing abdomen is measured and charted and linked to the growth of their child.

The concept of pain during childbirth needs to be taken into account. Familiarising a person with the environment could also take into account helping her to become accustomed to the masks used for Entonox for example. Women need to be prepared for the pain they will experience. This preparation also needs to include fathers to limit any alarm they may feel as their loved one goes into labour. Strategies employed to help mothers such as breathing techniques need to also take into account partners. Visual aids such as pictures and videos can help both parents to prepare for the event.

Baum (1994) adopted strategies such as using candles to demonstrate short and long breaths by blowing the flame. Tissues are another way of demonstrating breathing techniques and even perfume can be employed to encourage long and short breaths. Baum also included exercises to help the woman become accustomed to bending and opening their legs. All the techniques employed helped by preparing her long before the birth of her baby.

In another situation there was a case of a woman who had proved to be promiscuous. Although there is nothing unusual in promiscuity, this particular woman may have needed help to improve her situation. She may have been searching for the relationship that would satisfy her need to have loving, long-term companionship. Instead she was perpetuating her problems by becoming pregnant time and again. Here this woman needed advice and guidance from services around sex education and in order to make choices around contraception.

She was living alone with her six children, four of whom have learning disabilities themselves and attend special school. Her home is in council housing, not in the best of economical areas, and it is targeted by local youths pelting the house with eggs. Because of the intimidation and the house becoming infested with fleas from her children's pets she could be made to move. This is not too unreal a scenario. She clearly would have had difficulties coping if services were not able to help. Professionals therefore owed it to her to coordinate care and cross boundaries by working together to meet her needs. There was a real risk that because of moving around in order to escape her predicament, she may well have slipped through the supporting net. Therefore it is vital that services cooperate and work together in order to help her situation.

## COGNITIVE SKILLS AND COMMUNICATION ISSUES

The cognitive functioning of parents also needs to be taken into account. A person with a learning disability has a reduced ability to understand new or complex information, a difficulty in learning new skills, and may be unable to cope independently (DoH 1999, p 11). The *Once a Day* document (DoH 1999, p 1) is aimed specifically at health professionals and its purpose is to 'Promote good practice in enabling people with learning disabilities to access and receive good quality services from primary health care teams', and offers some indicators of good practice to guide professionals (see Box 5.5).

Actions suggested in the *Once a Day* document had been included in Baum's (1994) example of practice in that having a flexible and supportive approach and taking time to build up trust and confidence can all help with compliance with professionals and attendance at appointments. Developing familiarity of environments such as clinics and antenatal wards is also suggested in the *Once a Day* document (DoH 1999). Most people realise a fear of the unknown makes situations much worse to handle. Time taken to familiarise a person with the environment can pay dividends in ensuring compliance and resulting improvements in healthcare.

Learning disability by its definition is a neurological disorder which is why it affects a person's cognitive processes. Therefore, skills such as memory, perception, communication, understanding and problem-solving may be impaired (Roffman 2000). Roffman (2000) details the effects of such difficulties on a person as 'confusion with time and space, communication problems and related language disorders difficulties with social skills and perceptual impairments' (p 12). Roffman (2000) further

> **Box 5.5  Good practice guide for professionals to enable people to access services**
>
> - Asking questions in straightforward language.
> - Giving people extra time if needed.
> - Supporting plain language with visual information where possible.
> - Asking open questions, for example 'how are you feeling?' This will elicit more of a response than 'Are you OK?'
> - Change the question or information around to check the person's understanding and ask the person to explain what they have understood.
> - Understanding of time is usually difficult, so the document suggests linking time to familiar events such as 'was it before your birthday?'

discusses the difficulties experienced with taking in information as like trying to watch TV where the satellite signal is disrupted or listening to a radio that has interference with the signal. Consequently people do not always take in all the information they need. Strategies need to be employed to overcome these difficulties. There are many issues relating to perception that may affect a person with learning disabilities and these are usually the cause of misunderstandings. Some people manage to make adjustments to their lives to compensate for these difficulties with information processing. Understanding of possible difficulties on the part of professionals can also help people a great deal.

Roffman (2000) also details social skills that others take for granted but may cause difficulties for a person with learning disabilities. Eye contact is seen as an everyday skill that most people take for granted and so poor eye contact can be misconstrued as disinterest. Someone is then judged in a negative light as a result. Lack of self-awareness of the thoughts and feelings, even personal space of others, can lead to misunderstandings. Judgement of appropriate behaviour in a given social situation is also a skill that is taken for granted. Most of us have learnt the norms of level of voice, protocols for a given situation, for example queuing, and expected politeness. Many of these skills may prove difficult for a person who has learning disabilities. Again understanding of such processes can help professionals to find ways of working with individuals.

Shevin (1999) refers to the 'fluency principle'. Here he sees fluency within a language as being an advantage that people gain from being able to use the dominant language of a given society in a way that demonstrates competence. Shevin (1999) argues that it is in an issue of power as we give each other respect according to our use of the dominant language. This is highlighted in the case of a person with a learning disability and their use of services. If that person happens to be slow speaking or misunderstands then they can be seen as incompetent and unable to do whatever is expected of them.

Because language is constructed with many complex components, a person may have difficulty with any one of them. We tend to function at the level of language using punctuation, grammar and meaning as issues that are not considered until we come across a difficulty such as another dialect,

a person using another language or a person who has difficulties. When we look deeper at language and the issues of phonetics, syntax and vocabulary, and discourse, the complexities of the language we use everyday become a little clearer. No wonder then if a person has difficulties at the developmental stage of their life, that they may have difficulty with processing the spoken word.

Shevin (1999) also argues that we should strive to make connections with people and then negotiations, trust, cooperation, respect and even affection will follow. Interpersonal skills are paramount when working with people who have learning disabilities. This includes the ability to use listening skills, and to listen to individuals with respect. This is especially challenging in the climate of current day services with busy schedules and clinics. The emphasis needs to move away from the targets and task orientation of today's services and onto the individual and *making* time to listen. In the busy scheme of things it is all too easy to presume incompetence. It is only through respectful listening that we will start to make our jobs more satisfying as we start to work with people rather than relying on the power relations that allow us to fulfil our roles and targets rather than help individuals.

In the event of a mother or father having difficulties with verbal communication there are a number of other methods available. 'Augmentative' and 'alternative communication' are terms applied to methods of communication other than speech. Methods employed in this way are designed as supplementary to verbal and written communication. According to a paper written by the CALL Centre and Scottish Executive Education Department (2004), there are mainly two types of augmentative communication.

First, there are the methods requiring no technical equipment at all and the paper refers to these as methods that can be employed even in the sparsest of situations: camping as an extreme example. In other words, this type of signal can be used in a situation where no access to electricity or technical equipment is possible. Systems in this category would include sign language and the use of gestures. It can be argued that gestures can be used to enhance verbal conversation which in turn can be quite effective to emphasise a point or to request something. Signs that are used in daily life, for example, could be a telephone, drink or something to eat. All these activities can be indicated quite clearly in this way. When more in-depth communication is needed, the use of gestures could prove to be inadequate and rather limited, for example when trying to find information for assessment purposes.

Sign language can be used to provide much more information and is discussed in more detail elsewhere in this book (see Chapter 7). British Sign Language (BSL) is a system that has been developed by the deaf community and as a result is a complex language that includes the components of the spoken language. Consequently this still does not include the simplified visual cues that are more accessible to people with learning disabilities. The system derived from BSL and used extensively in schools to stimulate the development of language for people with learning disabilities who have communication difficulties is called Makaton.

The Makaton system is limited to around 350 signs. The signs are used in conjunction with the spoken word to encourage the development of spoken language. This allows people to develop a system of communication that can also enhance their spoken word. It is used by many people with learning disabilities and those who live and work with them, but is not used as extensively as BSL. Makaton has been found to help people to develop skills of communication such as eye contact, listening, interaction and the use of vocalised language and in turn the use of expressive language. Some people therefore whose spoken language is indistinct, in the case of uncoordinated musculature for example, may use the Makaton system to enhance their spoken word. (For more information see Chapter 7 and the Makaton website at www. makaton.org.)

There are many other methods of communication available. Simple boards with appropriate pictures to indicate a specific feeling or thing have proved to be very useful. Such systems include artificial voice boxes and sophisticated light boxes, all designed to give a person more control over their own life and the world they live in. The more complex systems hold messages and by pressing a key a number of messages can be accessed. (For more information see www.inclusive.co.uk.) Portable computers are sometimes used as software packages to increase or allow communication. They can also be used as teaching aids which is a useful point to consider when developing parenting classes, especially for people who have difficulty in understanding or retaining information in the conventional ways.

## Dyspraxia

Another condition worth mentioning, since it illustrates how associated conditions can affect people with learning disabilities, is dyspraxia. Imagine then a young lady who is able to express herself verbally and is largely able to care for herself. Her condition starts to deteriorate and she becomes clumsy and forgetful. She becomes careless in her college work and does not follow instructions. She used to enjoy games but now avoids them and her written work has deteriorated to the point that her handwriting is illegible.

Dyspraxia is a specific condition that can affect coordination and understanding of the spoken and written word. It is defined by the dyspraxia foundation as being 'an impairment or immaturity of the organisation of movement'. This means a person has a range of symptoms including lack of coordination, difficulties with perception and is often unable to remember and/or follow instructions. This can result in an individual becoming anxious and easily distracted. There are clearly implications for issues with a prospective mother and useful advice is available about this condition from the foundation's website at www.dyspraxiafoundation. org.uk. Advice includes the use of calendars and diaries to organise daily life, record instructions and use mind maps or charts to plan tasks. Relaxation techniques may help people cope with anxiety. These tips may be useful to bear in mind since this condition can affect any of the population and not just those who are learning disabled.

## PLANNING AND TEACHING SKILLS DURING PREGNANCY

If professionals work as a multidisciplinary team from the start, individuals or key workers can be identified as the main contact person within their own team. All professionals can then be involved in the assessment process with regular meetings to plan care and goals for the individual. The initial assessment could include specific areas of child-care and pregnancy so that strategies to teach a mother and her partner can be incorporated early on, giving the best possible chance for a person's role as a parent to develop.

When considering teaching skills to individuals with learning disabilities, there are strategies that can be employed whether the teaching is taking place on an individual basis or within a group of other mothers. A positive approach is needed to encourage the development of confidence and self-esteem. If achievements are made then these need to be praised and encouraged. If mistakes are made these need to be handled in a positive way with enthusiasm rather than chastisement or impatience. Task analysis is a strategy that can be employed when teaching a particular skill (Carr & Collins 1998). Task analysis allows the skill to be broken down into steps that can be tailored according to individual needs. The first step would be to consider breaking the task down into its component steps i.e. the macro steps. The task of bathing a baby will be used here to demonstrate this technique (see Box 5.6). Each of the steps may be taught in turn until a person has mastered that step and before moving on to the next step. The beauty of this system is that each step can be broken down further if needed into micro steps. So for example the steps of collecting bathing equipment could become more detailed (see Box 5.7). Each step would be repeated in a teaching session until the person has mastered that step.

Verbal presentation of information needs to be clear and free of jargon. Visual aids should be used whenever possible to help clarify a point and enhance understanding. Consideration needs to be given to building a person's confidence and self-esteem. Positive reinforcement is useful to reward success and a verbal 'well done' can count a great deal especially in helping individuals to feel confident and develop their skills.

There are of course many other methods of teaching skills to people. When working with people with learning disabilities it is worth remembering to include them in the planning process. Setting goals is a worthwhile exercise throughout the pregnancy. Providing positive reinforcement is a well-used technique that can improve the chance of the

---

**Box 5.6  The macro steps in preparing and carrying out a baby bath**

1. Collect bathing equipment.
2. Run water into bath.
3. Test temperature of water.
4. Undress baby.
5. Clean nappy area.
6. Wrap baby in towel.
7. Put shampoo on baby's head.
8. Rinse head.
9. Unwrap baby.
10. Hold baby securely underarm.
11. Put baby in bath still holding securely.
12. Use other hand to soap baby.
13. Rinse baby.
14. Wrap baby in towel and dry.
15. Dress baby.
16. Clear away.

---

**Box 5.7  The micro steps in preparing to bath a baby**

- Collect soap.
- Collect shampoo.
- Collect towel.
- Collect fresh nappy.
- Collect fresh clothes.
- Collect cotton wool balls.

---

goals being met. Reinforcers such as verbal praise, a simple 'well done' can easily build a person's confidence especially if given when the desired behaviour happens and will strengthen that behaviour (Carr & Collins 1998).

## PERSON-CENTRED PLANNING

A person-centred plan may be a good starting point in planning the care during pregnancy, especially if a person does not already have one. As part of the *Valuing People* White Paper all people with learning disabilities should have a person centred plan in place (DOH 2001a). Person centred planning is a lengthy process that will involve putting someone at the centre of the planning process and so empower them and give them control over their lives and the care they need and receive. Person centred planning begins when people decide to listen carefully and in ways that can strengthen the voice of people who have been or are at risk of being silenced (O'Brien & O'Brien 1995).

The focus of a person-centred plan is what an individual wants both now and in the future. The process is carried out in partnership with staff, the person themselves and family and friends. The fundamental principles of person centred planning are sharing power and making opportunities for community inclusion. Person centred planning is a detailed process that requires staff training and an investment of time in order to listen and positively hear what that person wants in their life. It is mentioned here since it is such a central theme to *Valuing People* but also because some of the underpinning principles are useful when working with a person who is learning disabled.

Sanderson et al (1997) set out these principles as follows:

1. Each person is at the centre. As mentioned earlier, power is an important issue and needs to be considered to develop ways of ensuring the power is shared in the healthcare relationship. People need to be consulted, and individuals choose who to involve in the process. A person-centred plan should begin with the process of getting to know the person. Plans cannot be formulated until enough information is gathered with and about the person in order to give an informed picture.

2. Family members and friends are partners in planning. The development of a good support network is important to ensure the success of a parent or parents, therefore it is good practice to develop networks from the start. Families may be able to provide important information to help in a person's care, as may other professionals and people who work with the parents.

3. The plan reflects what is important to an individual, their capacities and what support they require. Focus on capacities means a positive focus from the start. The identification of supports is an important aspect of pregnancy and people with learning disabilities, as mentioned

in the work by McGaw with parents in Cornwall. Shared understandings and rethinking the role of professionals involves guiding people and allowing them to make their own decisions. Too often services dwell on what people can't do and the negative aspects of the person's life rather than the positive.

4. The plan results in actions that have a bias towards inclusion. This means including parents as much as possible in the normal range of services available to new and potential parents. This also means making information accessible, easy to read and jargon free.

5. The plan needs to include ongoing listening and learning to and about a person, and taking further action as necessary.

Most of all Sanderson et al (1997) emphasise that working and learning together and being creative will aid problem-solving and bring about change in peoples' lives. That is to say, through the processes of listening, empowering and planning, the whole process of pregnancy and childbirth can be a positive experience for mothers with learning disabilities. The following case is used to emphasise this point.

A woman living in a house with her partner of 10 years may have been coping without help from services for many years. She has a good support network from her family; she attended an ordinary school but had some difficulties. She now manages to keep the house and motivate her partner. They have a good social life, attending the local social club for functions on a regular basis. Recently, at the age of 34, they decided that as they are not getting any younger they wanted to try for a baby. A person-centred plan would help in a situation like this since the family and the couple could work with the professionals to detail what is necessary in their lives and what is needed to help them cope in the future. The plan would usually be facilitated by the community learning disability nurse.

This is an example of how the process could be used with a woman who is more able. Clearly a plan would be equally useful in the case of a woman who is less able and more dependent on services. The emphasis being on putting individuals at the centre of the plan and making the effort to find out what is needed in their life rather than the care package as dictated by professionals.

Other tools used in the field of people with learning disabilities that have proved useful are 'paths' and 'maps'. A path focuses on the dream for a person—in this case it can be the event of giving birth. Working back from this, the team and an individual work together to devise a path incorporating the actions needed to reach the desired event. A map on the other hand, includes the history of an individual in an attempt to gain greater understanding and then focuses on who they are and their gifts. Both these processes can be used in meetings to focus the proceedings and to assist the process of advocacy for people using the service. If all the people working with the parents collaborate through a person-centred plan, the person can be empowered through the right support and guidance and positive relationships can be developed between parents and baby.

---

### CONCLUSION—KEY POINTS

■ The issue of people with learning disabilities deciding or becoming parents is controversial. This controversy is situated in deep-seated attitudes stemming from the eugenics movement in the early 1900s.

■ As institutions closed down in more enlightened, humane times, people started to live ordinary lives. Along with ordinary lives came ordinary needs and the need to be a parent is strong in people from all walks of life.

■ As professionals we cannot afford to continue with services that are one-size-fits-all. The need to consider the needs of individuals is paramount in the diverse climate of our society.

■ Whilst people with learning disabilities are in the minority, many are having their children taken away from them as a matter of course. If services are able to collaborate and develop proactive strategies, this can enable more parents to enjoy a family of their own, rather than it being a sad and tragic event.

---

■ A shift in attitude, to valuing people and seeing ways to enable them to cope is much needed. The strategies and skills developed will in fact help many people in their endeavour to lead fulfilling lives and become parents, and not only those who are learning disabled. Developing self-awareness and an understanding of available strategies and services is therefore a starting point.

## References

Arnold C 2003 Parenting skills. Learning Disability Practice April 6(3):10

Atherton H 2003 A history of learning disabilities, Chapter 3 Section 1. In: Gates B (ed) Learning disabilities, towards inclusion. Churchill Livingstone, London, p 41–60

Baum S 1994 Interventions with a pregnant woman with severe learning disabilities. In: Craft A (ed) Sexuality and learning disability. Routledge, London, p 217–236

Blackford KA, Richardson H, Grieve S 2000 Prenatal education for mothers with learning disabilities. Journal of Advanced Nursing 32(4):898–904

Booth T, Booth W 1996 Learning the hard way: practice issues in supporting parents with learning disabilities. Representing Children 9(2):99–107

Booth T, Booth W 1998 Growing up with parents who have a learning disability, Routledge, London

Booth T, Booth W 1999 Parents together; action research and advocacy support for parents with learning difficulties. Health and Social Care in the Community 7(6):464–474. Additional information online. Available: http://www.supported-parenting.com/projects/deadvocacy.html

Booth W, Booth T 1993 Accentuating the positive: a personal profile of a parent with learning difficulties. Disability, Handicap & Society 18(4):377–392

Boxall K 2002 Individual and social models of disability and the experiences of people with learning disabilities. In: Race D G (ed) Learning disabilities — a social approach. Routledge, London, p 209–226

Brackenbridge R, McKenzie K 2005 The friendships of people with a learning disability. Learning Disability Practice 8(5):12–17

CALL Centre & Scottish Executive Educational Department 2004 What is AAC? Introduction to augmentation and alternative communication. Online. Available: http://www.communicationmatters.org.uk 29 April 2007

Carr J, Collins S 1998 Working towards independence: a practical guide to teaching people with learning disabilities. Jessica Kingsley Publishers, London

Carson I, Docherty D 2002 Friendships, relationships and issues of sexuality. In: Race D G (ed) Learning disabilities — a social approach. Routledge, London, p 139–153

CHANGE organisation. An organisation run by people with learning difficulty. Online. Available: http://www.changepeople.co.uk 28 June 2005

Craft A, Brown H 1994 Personal relationships and sexuality: the staff role. In: Craft A (ed) Practical issues in sexuality and learning disabilities. Routledge, London

Department of Health (DoH) 1999 Once a day. A primary care handbook for people with learning disabilities; HSC 1999/103; LA C(99):17

Department of Health (DoH) 2000 Framework for the assessment of children in need and their families. Department of Health, London

Department of Health (DoH) 2001a Valuing People. A new strategy for learning disability in the 21st century. Online. Available: http://www.dh.gov.uk 13 June 2006

Department of Health (DoH) 2001b Seeking consent; working with people with learning disabilities. HMSO, London. Online. Available: http://www.dh.gov.uk/consent

Fegan L, Rauch A, McCarthy W 1993 Sexuality and people with intellectual disability, 2nd edition. Maclennan & Petty, Sydney

Giddens A 1995 Politics, sociology and social theory. Polity Press with Blackwell Publishers, Cambridge

Hevey D 1993 The tragedy principle, strategies for change in the representation of disabled people. In: Swain J, Finkelstein V, French S, Oliver M (eds) Disabling barriers—enabling environments. Open University with Sage Publishers, London, p 116–121

Holmes L 1999/2000 Nurses attitudes to disability. Paediatric Nursing Dec/Jan 11(10):18–21

Inclusive Technology. Online. Available: http://www.inclulsive.co.uk 12 March 2006

McGaw S, Sturmey P 1993 Identifying the needs of parents with learning disabilities. Child Abuse Review 2:101–117

McGaw S, Ball K, Clark A 2002 The effect of group intervention on the relationships of parents with intellectual disabilities. Journal of Applied Research in Intellectual Disabilities 15:354–366

Miller N B, Sammons C C 1999 Everybody's different; understanding and changing our reaction to disabilities. Paul Brookes, Baltimore

O'Brien J, O'Brien C L 1995 A little book about person centred planning. Inclusion Press, Toronto

O'Hara J, Martin H 2003 Parents with learning disabilities: a study of gender and cultural perspectives in East London. British Journal of Learning Disabilities 31:18–24

Pitonyak D 2006 How can we help the person to expand and deepen his/her relationships? Online. Available: http://www.dimagine.com 2 November 2006

Race D G 2002 (ed) Learning disabilities — a social approach. Routledge, London

Roffman A J 2000 Meeting the challenge of learning disabilities in adulthood. Brookes, London

Sanderson H, Kennedy J, Ritchie P, Goodwin G 1997 People, plans and possibilities. SHS, Edinburgh

Shevin M 1999 On being a communication ally. Online. Available: http://www.shevin.org 2 November 2006

The Special Parenting Services in Cornwall. Online. Available: http://www.cornwall.nhs.uk/specialparentingservices 13 June 2006

Thompson J 2005 The challenges of person centred planning. Learning Disability Practice 8(3):18–20

Tymchuk K A, Andron L 1994 Rational approaches, results and resource implications of programmes to enhance parenting skills of people with learning disabilities, practice issues. In: Craft A (ed) Sexuality and learning disability. Routledge, London, p 237–256

Ward L 1995 Part one, Chapter 1. Equal citizens: current issues for people with learning difficulties and their allies. In: Philpot T, Ward L (eds) Values and visions: changing ideas in services for people with learning difficulties. Butterworth Heinmann, Oxford, p 3–19

Wharton S 2005 Assessing parenting skills when working with parents who are learning disabled. Learning Disability Practice 8(4):12–14

Wheeler P 2003 Patients' rights; consent to treatment for men and women with a learning disability or who are otherwise incapacitated. Learning Disability Practice 6(5):29–37

# 6 Midwives' skills, knowledge and attitudes: how they can affect maternity services

*Stella McKay-Moffat*

## INTRODUCTION

This chapter addresses maternity services, and although there is some unavoidable overlap with other chapters, especially Chapter 4, the content explores issues from a broader perspective and links more into professional concerns. The basis of this chapter is formulated from my qualitative and quantitative research project. Qualitative studies were used to elicit the experiences of five mothers accessing maternity services, and eight midwives' experiences of providing services for mothers with disability. The quantitative part of the study was introduced to discover what amount of experience a greater number of midwives had in providing care for women with disability. Additionally an aim was to discover what their attitudes to people and women were; how confident they felt with communication, midwifery care and parent education; and what their learning needs might include. Examples of some women's experiences are used to illustrate relevant points in the issues identified as pertinent to the care midwives offer women.

## STANDARDS OF CARE

Significant data from the limited number of recent UK (Thomas 1997, McKay-Moffat 2003) and American (Lipson & Rogers 2000) studies indicates a degree of failure in health professionals' ability to provide an effective maternity service for many women with disabilities. Key factors associated with sub-standard care were professionals' inadequate knowledge and

skills reflected in poor information giving, inappropriate help and ineffective communication; and the negative attitudes of some professionals. For some women these created dissatisfaction with maternity care.

These themes echoed those highlighted earlier by nurse-midwife lecturer Elaine Carty (1995) following her review of mainly American and Canadian literature and some key UK work related to pregnancy and motherhood for women with disabilities. She too had highlighted the negative attitudes of health professionals towards women with disabilities undertaking pregnancy.

An earlier publication offered insight from the consumer's perspective. Campion's book 'The baby challenge' (1990) was innovative at the time of publication, and still offers mothers and professionals considerable insight into her own experiences of pregnancy and motherhood and those of the many women with whom she had contact. She aimed to raise awareness of women's concerns in order that the services they received met their needs. In the chapter focusing on health professionals' support, she identified three main points. First, the negative attitudes that created damaging barriers; second, professionals' discomfort with and misconceptions about people with disabilities; and finally how people felt intimidated by professionals. Campion's knowledge and understanding prompted her to highlight the importance of treating women as individuals who possibly need some specialist advice, not as helpless people. As Crow (2003) more recently relates, the maternity services she received gave her the highest as well as the lowest moments in her life.

On a positive note, there are indications from the research and the literature of a way forward to improve care and ultimately provide a more appropriate, effective maternity service for people with disabilities. This could be achieved by raising disability awareness through education both during training and after qualification to raise the overall consistency of the quality of care.

## EVOLVING MATERNITY SERVICES

Midwifery care for women with disabilities in the UK needs to be considered both within the context of maternity services today and how those services have evolved. This enables an appreciation of the circumstances within which mothers find themselves when accessing help during pregnancy and childbirth.

There has been a move away from the medicalisation of childbirth that evolved over the last 100 years, to the present holistic model that focuses on midwifery-led woman-centred care: a key point in the government's *Changing Childbirth* report (DoH 1993). The holistic paradigm views pregnancy and child-bearing as a normal life event, encompassing a greater acknowledgment of psychological, social, cultural and religious influences on maternal and infant well-being. Recognition of these elements is clearly defined within the role of midwives (NMC 2004).

A woman's experiences of accessing and using health services, and life and people in general, will have influenced her attitudes, responses and expectations from midwives and other health professionals. Similarly, midwives' own attitudes may be influenced not only by their own preconceived ideas but their lack of specific knowledge of the needs of people with disabilities. It could be argued that the recent indications for the need for a specialist midwife to support women with disabilities during their childbirth experience (Brown 2001, Rotheram 2002) implies that midwives in general are not in a position to offer the right type of care. Indeed, even accomplished midwives may have limited experience of providing services for women with disabilities therefore encountering minimal opportunities for experiential learning.

On the other hand, the maternity service in the twenty-first century aims to offer *all* women respect for their individuality and enable them to have choice in, and take control over the care they receive. Whilst it could be argued that the aims are idealistic and not always achievable, service providers should continue to strive to fulfil those aims for women with or without a disability. Yet even in the highly advanced, sophisticated United States of America '...high quality health care for women with disabilities remains inconsistent and difficult to achieve' (Turk 2004, p 5). However, in the UK there is the advantage over the USA of a National Health Service enabling (in theory) equal opportunities for all to benefit from the whole spectrum of healthcare.

## MIDWIVES' ATTITUDES TOWARDS PEOPLE WITH DISABILITIES AND THEIR CONFIDENCE IN CARE PROVISION

Either implicit or overtly referred to in the literature, the attitudes of some health professionals towards people and mothers with a disability give cause for concern. There is also some indication that there is a lack of effective helping skills which may reflect inadequate knowledge and confidence in service provision. As midwives in the UK are the lead professionals in the majority of maternity cases, midwives' attitudes towards people and mothers with disabilities could have a profound influence on the quality of maternity services that women receive. Psychological barriers resulting from mothers' perceptions of service providers' negative attitudes towards them may lead to less effective or sub-standard maternity care.

### Qualitative study

The importance of midwives' attitudes as the key service providers was highlighted in my study that involved semi-structured interviews with eight midwives and five mothers with either congenital or acquired physical disabilities (McKay-Moffat 2003, McKay-Moffat & Cunningham 2006) (see Boxes 6.1 and 6.2 for guide questions used as the basis for the interviews).

Although the number of women in the study was small, and none of the women had sensory impairment which could have enhanced the quality of data, their experiences were similar to those described in the literature.

## Box 6.1 Questions used to guide semi-structured interviews with midwives

**1)** Biographical details

How long have you been a midwife?

What are your qualifications?

Where did you do your midwifery training?

How many hours do you work per week?

What is your main area of practice?

**2)** General details

During your training were you taught about pregnancy and childbirth for women with disabilities?

Have you attended any in-service education or study days about pregnancy and childbirth for women with disabilities?

**3)** Experience

How many women with disability have you provided midwifery care for within the last 5 years?

What was the nature of the woman's disability?

Could you tell me about each case?

**4)** Prompts to elicit key points

Was there anything you felt was particularly important about the care you gave?

How did you feel about providing care?

How do you feel about women with a disability having babies?

Do you think that all women with a disability should be offered a termination of pregnancy?

How would you feel about offering a woman with a disability antenatal screening for fetal abnormality? (Explore specific conditions e.g. spina bifida and sensory disability when a woman has that condition.)

Where do you consider women with a disability should give birth?

Have you been involved in parent education/ classes for disabled women? Have you any thoughts on how midwives can best fulfil their education role for women with disability?

Do you have any ideas that could help improve midwifery services for women with a disability?

## Box 6.2 Questions used to guide semi-structured interviews with mothers

**1)** Biographical details

How old are you?

What type of education have you had?

Do you go out to work? If 'yes'—occupation and qualifications.

Are you married/have a partner? If 'yes'— occupation of husband/partner.

**2)** General details

Could you tell me about your disability?

Prompts: Do you use any special equipment/ aids/need any help from an assistant?

Are there any areas that you find particularly difficult with self-care, child-care or as a mother?

**3)** Obstetric history

How many children do you have and how old are they?

Were your pregnancies planned?

What type of delivery(s) did you have?

Have you had any other pregnancies?

**4)** Experience(s)

Could you tell me about your pregnancies during the last 5 years?

Could you tell me about your midwifery care for these pregnancies?

Prompts: How did you find your midwifery care?

Did you have the same midwife throughout?

Where did you have the majority of your midwifery care?

Where did you have your baby(s)? Was that your place of choice/did you have a choice?

What information did you receive?

Were you offered screening during pregnancy for fetal abnormalities? How did you feel about having the tests?

Were you offered termination of pregnancy? Explore feelings about.

Did you attend parent education classes? If 'yes' were they helpful?

What were your specific needs during pregnancy, labour, postnatal? Were they met?

How could your midwifery care have been improved?

*Mothers' results*

Despite the obvious limitations of the study there were five themes that emerged from the mothers' interviews that midwives need to consider to enhance the quality of maternity care they offer women. First, and similar to evidence from other mothers' experiences, it was evident that there was a 'Quest for normality and independence' by the mothers. They did not wish their disability to be the focus of attention but neither did they want it to be ignored. This resulted in a conflict with their need to acknowledge the disabling aspect of their impairment but unwillingness to do so. This often resulted in attempts to try to conceal or minimise a disability and not ask for help.

The second theme 'The disability as paramount', was identified as, without exception, the experiences of each of the mothers was influenced by her disability. They had feelings of self-consciousness and embarrassment as their disabilities drew others' attention. They all had misgivings about their ability to fulfil their roles as mothers and felt that professionals, family and friends would perceive them as inadequate in that role. One mother was convinced that this had led to her postnatal depression.

Theme three was labelled 'Midwives lack of knowledge'. This theme echoes much of the existing related literature. The mothers felt that there was a lack of knowledge because their specific needs were not recognised and discussed, therefore they remained unmet. Additional evidence from four mothers indicated that midwives lacked skills to be able to offer practical help with infant care to overcome the disabling effects of their impairment. This appeared to be a contributory factor to the mother's postnatal depression in her opinion.

The label for theme four was 'Disability awareness and positive attitudes'. Disability awareness and positive attitudes towards the women was demonstrated by receipt of care that was sensitive and respectful, and privacy and dignity was assured. This resulted in satisfaction with maternity care. But this did not always take place and there were some examples of incidences demonstrating poor awareness and negative attitudes. This occurred when disability was not acknowledged or when a woman felt watched because of her disability; when essential medication to alleviate symptoms from the condition was not given on time; and

when there was insensitivity or intolerance of the mother's inability to do things. This latter element of interaction with midwives caused some mothers distress.

Of particular note was the postnatal experience of a mother with multiple sclerosis (MS) during her hospital stay. Because her 'invisible' condition caused her to have poor muscle strength she had difficulty in pushing her baby in the heavy cot cabinet. Unwilling to leave her baby unattended, she carried her baby a few yards out of the four-bed ward to the staff work station to ask for a formula feed. She received angry chastisement from a midwife because she had failed to push the baby in the cot: a procedure recommended to all mothers to minimise the risk of dropping a baby. She felt humiliated and angry by such insensitivity and felt that there was a lack of understanding about the consequences of her condition.

Conversely, a mother who had a leg amputated below the knee during early pregnancy had felt midwives were very positive in their approach and offered her sensitive care that met her needs for the majority of the childbirth continuum. This resulted in her feeling very satisfied with the care she received. These examples indicate that there is difficulty in achieving the right balance between acknowledging and disregarding a mother's impairment. If someone is not overtly disabled i.e. the impairment is invisible, it is possible, as Lipson & Rogers (2000) postulate, that they are more likely to receive insensitive care because their disability goes unrecognised or unacknowledged. Nevertheless, reflecting on their experiences the majority of mothers in the study indicated that they had, on the whole, actually felt that they had been treated the same as other mothers, rather than being singled out as different. They appreciated this approach.

The final theme 'Effective communication', indicates how vital this process is to successful and satisfying maternity care. When midwives communicated well with mothers they were less likely to be afraid or anxious and individual needs were recognised and met. When interdisciplinary communication was evident, particularly over information about a mother's history and especially about her disability, then there was less embarrassment and frustration for the mother. However, this process did not always take place and three mothers felt that if an occupational therapist or specialist midwife/disability advisor had been contacted their expertise would have enhanced the quality of their care and additional needs would have been more effectively met.

### Midwives' results

Despite the small number of midwives, their experiences of providing care for mothers with disability offered an insight into how midwives feel about their ability and confidence to provide this group of women with maternity services, and their attitudes towards the mothers and people with disability in general.

Three themes emerged from the interviews. Theme one was 'Midwives' lack of knowledge'. Although the midwives had provided care for between two and six mothers with a variety of mobility and sensory disabilities, they were concerned about their lack of knowledge and experience in some aspects of care provision. This led to feelings of inadequacy in some cases and anxieties about their ability to provide women with the services and care they needed. One said she felt out of her depth.

'Midwives' attitudes' formed the second theme. Reflecting on their experiences, the professionals demonstrated that their attitudes were generally positive towards mothers with disability. It was clear from what they said that care they offered was sensitive, respectful and individualised. They also believed that every woman with a disability should receive the same high standard of service as other women. Additionally words like partnership in care, choice, advocacy, flexibility, adaptability and sensitivity were indicators of underlying attitudes. Furthermore, all midwives who participated in the interviews were adamant that every woman whether disabled or non-disabled has the right to choose to have a baby if she wishes. Termination of pregnancy just because of a mother's disability was judged not to be something that should be considered. This is in stark contrast to the experiences of some mothers in the past where the attitudes of professionals (and often a woman's family and friends) were negative. This presented as opinions that women with a disability were incapable of being effective mothers or that having a child would be a burden to the family and society.

The final theme was 'Effective communication'. As an aid to care planning, all midwives, either overtly or implicitly, indicated that effective communication with mothers and the multidisciplinary team were key elements in the process. Only two actually mentioned liaison with other professionals or support agencies. Communication with mothers in every situation was recognised as not always easy. They were generally concerned with the possibility of causing offence by either what they said or did not say, and what or how to ask a woman about her disability. Discussing screening for fetal abnormality, and the subsequent implications for termination of pregnancy because of an abnormality, gave some cause for concern as they did not wish to be seen as devaluing people with a disability. There was appreciation of the challenges with communicating with women who were deaf and the potential frustration for all concerned. Four of the group pointed out that sign language skill for midwives would be beneficial in some cases.

### Summary of the findings

Evidence from these interviews indicates that positive attitudes and effective two-way communication are pivotal elements in the successful provision of maternity services for women with disability. Negative attitudes appear to stem from a lack of knowledge, understanding and confidence on the part of professionals. This could be alleviated initially by more open communication. However, there seems almost to be mutual collusion between women and midwives to avoid highlighting a woman's disability and address the pertinent issues that underlie impairment. Therefore it is important that women and midwives are not afraid to be both honest and receptive in their approach to a woman's disability. With this approach, successful identification of additional or alternative ways of meeting specific individual needs is more assured. Midwives need to remember, nevertheless, that women may be reluctant to highlight concerns, therefore they need to be proactive in identifying and addressing the issues. There is, though, a fine line between offering help and making someone feel different and it is not always easy to obtain the correct balance.

## Quantitative study

A quantitative approach was used to gain further insight into the unresearched phenomena of midwives' attitudes, and to elicit information about their experiences of providing maternity services for women with disability. The responses of 224 north-west of England midwives to a postal survey were analysed (McKay-Moffat 2003). Background data were gathered to obtain a picture of their experiences and to ascertain any correlations between attitudes and experience or education as Gething (1992) had evidence that these variables were influential on individuals' attitudes. Data included:

- years of practice as a midwife;
- amount of disability-centred education (either as a student or since qualification);
- the number of mothers with disability cared for during the childbirth continuum (either as a student or since qualification) (see Box 6.3 for general list of disabilities);
- experience of being with or caring for anyone with a disability outside of midwifery practice.

Participants in the study had been in practice for a wide range of years giving a diverse group of respondents (see Table 6.1). Years of experience as a midwife ranged from 1 to 38: those over 25 years were in the minority. The mean was 13.15 years, the mode (i.e. most common) being 2 years, with 5 and 12 the next most common lengths of experience.

Lectures related to midwifery care for mothers with disability were rarely given during midwives' training for those midwives qualified over 10 years. Since qualification, almost two-thirds had made some effort to learn about pregnancy and childbirth for women with disability. Most of this had been by reading although the quality of the literature was not ascertained. Few had received any formal education, for example study days, since qualification.

*Table 6.1*   **Number of midwives completing the survey and years in practice**

| No. | Years |
|-----|-------|
| 44 | 0–4 |
| 39 | 5–9 |
| 52 | 10–14 |
| 25 | 15–19 |
| 31 | 20–24 |
| 7 | 25–29 |
| 13 | 30–38 |
| 3 | not stated |
| 224 | total |

Experience of people and mothers with disability was generally limited. Over a third of midwives had never had any interaction with people with disability outside of midwifery. Approximately 12% of the midwives had never provided midwifery services for women with disability. In the majority of cases those midwives who had provided care for women did so for just one woman during one aspect of the childbirth continuum. These data indicate a lack of experiential learning opportunities to develop knowledge and expertise to offer skilled help.

### Attitudes

To elicit midwives' general attitudes towards people with disability, the initial part of the survey comprised of an Australian questionnaire developed during the 1980s (Gething 1994). This internationally validated questionnaire measures discomfort, anxiety and uncertainty when interacting with people with disability (the Interaction with Disabled Persons (IDP) scale). The second section of the questionnaire contained questions that were formulated to focus specifically on midwifery and to ascertain respondents' attitudes towards mothers with disability and their confidence in providing this small group of women with maternity services (see Box 6.4). Answers to both of these sections and the background information were then correlated with the results of the IDP to identify relationships.

---

**Box 6.3**   **List of general disabilities used with questions in Box 6.4**

- Visual impairment.
- Hearing impairment.
- Upper limb.
- Lower limb.
- Wheelchair user.
- Learning difficulty.

---

### Box 6.4   Additional midwifery-focused questions

- I would feel confident in providing midwifery care.
- I would find communication with the mother difficult.
- I would be afraid of doing or saying the wrong thing.
- I feel I would be able to offer effective parent education.
- I would find it difficult to see beyond a mother's disability.

---

## The IDP questions and responses

The questionnaire consists of a set of 18 statements that require a response on a Likert scale i.e. from strongly agree to strongly disagree and is suitable for people from all walks of life, although it appears never to have been used with midwives before this study. As with previous studies, to make sense of results and discover their meaning a factor analysis was applied to data (Robson 2002). This correlated and grouped statements together depending on the answers obtained and was undertaken with the aid of computer software called the Statistical Package for Social Sciences (SPSS).

Results of analysis indicated the 12 statements that grouped into factors 1, 2 and 5 were the most reliable (see Table 6.2 with the list of these statements and factors) and therefore only these will be included here for discussion. The strongest correlation of statements formed factor 1 in both Gething's (1994) study and my own, and is labelled 'Discomfort in social interaction'. Additional groupings although not exactly the same as Gething's led to similar labels reflecting knowledge, sensitivity, coping and vulnerability. The meaning of the factors can be summarised. Factor 1 suggests that midwives would not find interacting with people with disability a major problem. This in turn points to positive attitudes. Factor 2 indicates that midwives felt knowledgeable about disability, and they had sensitivity to the situation of the person with the disability. Factor 5 indicates that although midwives may have had a sense of vulnerability about the possibility of becoming disabled themselves, they felt able to cope with the disability of other people.

The key factor that relates to comfort interacting with people with disability (factor 1) correlates with positive attitudes towards them. Gething (1992) argued that '......negative attitudes stem from

---

*Table 6.2*   **IDP statements adapted from Gething (1994) grouped into the three significant factors identified in the study of midwives (McKay-Moffat 2003)**

| Factor 1. Discomfort in social interaction | Factor 2. Knowledge and sensitivity | Factor 5. Vulnerable/coping |
|---|---|---|
| I am afraid to look the person straight in the face | I feel frustrated because I don't know how to help | After frequent contact I notice the person not the disability |
| I tend to make contacts only brief and finish them as quickly as possible | It hurts me when someone wants to do something and can't | I wonder how I would feel if I had this disability |
| I feel overwhelmed with discomfort about my own lack of disability | I feel ignorant about disabled people | Contact with a disabled person reminds me of my own vulnerability |
| I feel uncomfortable and find it hard to relax | | |
| I feel unsure because I don't know how to behave | | |
| I can't help staring at them | | |

a perception of people as being strange or unfamiliar and that this creates the uncertainty or anxiety' (p 26). The higher an individual's score, the greater the discomfort and therefore the negativity towards people with disability.

Over 90% of midwives in the study appeared to hold positive attitudes towards people with disabilities. When results of the IDP from midwives were compared with a range of community and professional groups from Gething's study (Gething 1994) (see Table 6.3) there were fewer midwives with extreme negative attitudes or feelings of discomfort as represented by the lower standard deviation scores. Additionally it is clear that the overall mean (average) score of midwives in the study group was lower (the lower the score the more positive the attitudes). They were even lower than that of physical therapists and rehabilitation professionals who would be dealing with people with disabilities as part of their daily work. Caution must be used when interpreting these data as it must be noted that Gething's data were gathered some time ago between 1988 and 1992. Therefore the present study results *may* point to changes over time in the general attitudes of society and professionals towards people with disabilities, rather than necessarily that midwives have more positive attitudes than other groups.

## The midwifery-focused responses

### Confidence in maternity service provision

Two questions were included in the questionnaire to elicit midwives' confidence in providing maternity services for mothers with disability as this may be influenced by underlying attitudes. One question was asked about general midwifery care and the other about confidence to offer parent education.

Most midwives felt confident to provide general midwifery care although confidence with women with physical disability was lower than for women with sensory disability or learning difficulty. Experience of people and mothers with disability appeared to have no influence on their confidence to provide midwifery care. Confidence to provide parent education was less evident and was only expressed to any degree with mothers with lower limb disability or those using a wheelchair. This reflects the visual, auditory and 'hands-on' aspects of parenting, and thus parent

**Table 6.3** Comparison between IDP scores of selected Australian groups during 1988–1992 (Gething 1994) and the midwives studied (McKay-Moffat 2003)

| Sample | Sample no. | Mean[a] | SD[b] |
|---|---|---|---|
| General population | 4180 | 64.1 | 12.2 |
| Members of the judicial system | 59 | 67.5 | 12.2 |
| Government employees | 541 | 63.0 | 12.5 |
| High school students | 181 | 69.3 | 11.3 |
| University education students | 272 | 72.8 | 10.8 |
| University nursing students (1st year) | 104 | 67.3 | 10.1 |
| University nursing students (2nd year) | 136 | 65.5 | 9.8 |
| University nursing students (3rd year) | 372 | 63.3 | 10.4 |
| Registered nurses | 376 | 62.3 | 10.3 |
| Enrolled nurses | 123 | 60.0 | 11.0 |
| Physical therapists | 121 | 58.6 | 9.7 |
| Medical physicians | 171 | 61.1 | 10.2 |
| Rehabilitation professionals | 351 | 58.8 | 12.3 |
| Members of disability agencies | 63 | 60.8 | 12.8 |
| **The present study** | | | |
| Midwives | 224 | 54.6 | 6.3 |

[a]Mean = average score. The lower the number the more positive the attitudes.
[b]SD = standard deviation. The smaller the number the greater the similarity of responses i.e. less extreme opinions.

education. Midwives qualified for less than 15 years appeared the least confident.

### Attitudes towards mothers

Confidence in communication with mothers with disabilities reflects confidence with interaction.

Three questions addressed this issue: one specifically asked about communication, another asked about being afraid of doing or saying the wrong thing, and the third asked about fear of being patronising. A further question was included to ascertain any negative attitudes by identifying if midwives had difficulty seeing beyond a mother's disability, i.e. a woman's disability was their prime concern.

It was evident from the midwives' responses to the questions that their general beliefs about people with a disability were transferred. The majority felt that they would not find communication difficult, although not unexpectedly, more envisaged problems communicating with mothers with hearing or visual impairment and learning difficulty than with physical disability. Few midwives felt afraid or uncertain about doing or saying the wrong thing or of being patronising. This indicates a general lack of feelings of discomfort in interaction. A large majority felt that they would not have difficulty in seeing beyond a mother's disability, thus indicating that the disability was not paramount, which in turn reflects a positive attitude.

It must be acknowledged nevertheless, that what people say and what they do are not always the same. Additionally, it would appear that approximately 10% of the midwives did indeed hold some negative attitudes. This is unacceptably high. Furthermore, although the survey response rate was approximately 52%, this left about 48% of midwives in the study area whose opinion was not obtained. There is, then, the possibility of a positive bias in the data gathered.

## Summary of data and correlation

Not unexpectedly, experience in providing midwifery care for mothers with a disability correlated with greater comfort in interaction (and thus more positive attitudes) as indicated by the IDP results, in particular factor 1. Less discomfort in interaction positively correlated with less perceived difficulty in communication. As the midwives felt more knowledgeable and became more sensitive towards women with disability they felt less afraid of doing or saying the wrong thing. Disability education clearly influenced attitudes as midwives who had received some education felt more comfortable during interaction. This factor is comparable

with Gething's findings in 1992 when she studied a cohort of student nurses during their 3-year training. As their education and interaction with people with disability increased during their course, their attitudes towards them became more positive. Here, then, is evidence from two diverse populations of participants for the way forward to aid the development of practitioners' positive attitudes towards people and women with disability.

Results of the IDP indicated that although the midwives appeared to feel knowledgeable about disability generally, some appeared to have feelings of personal vulnerability to impairment. Three per cent of the group indicated through the IDP that they would see an individual's disability as paramount. Midwives who felt vulnerable, and those seeing someone's disability as dominant are likely to have formed part of the negative 10% element of the results. It could be assumed that ingrained attitudes developed from familial and societal exposure to negative attitudes may not be easily changed.

Midwives who felt comfortable interacting with mothers with disability were more likely to see a person with a disability as 'an individual' rather than a 'disabled person'. Years in practice and experience of people with a disability outside of the midwifery profession appeared to have little or no influence on their attitudes. This latter element contradicted findings from a study by Paris (1993) who used the Attitude to Disabled Persons Scale which is similar to the IDP used in the study with midwives. However, this result from the present study must be viewed with caution as the amount of individuals' disability experience is difficult to quantify.

Whilst not generalisable to all midwives in the UK because of small numbers and a regional response, results from the questionnaire offered understanding of some midwives' general attitudes towards people with disability, and mothers with a disability in particular.

## MIDWIFERY CARE

The move to a psycho-social model of care helps professionals view people as individuals and could prove of great benefit to mothers with disabilities. However, women with disabilities remain in the minority, although numbers are apparently increasing

(RCM 2000). This means that midwives have only recently begun to gain more experience and expertise in meeting these mothers' additional needs. Indeed, approximately 12% of the midwives in my study had never cared for a mother with a disability (McKay-Moffat 2003). The majority of midwives who had provided care did so for just one or two mothers in one part of the childbirth continuum i.e. during pregnancy, *or* labour *or* the postnatal period. This led to feelings of uncertainty, inadequacy or being out of their depth about meeting a mother's additional needs, and was compounded by the lack of knowledge and understanding. Yet if midwives recognise that mothers are the experts in their own conditions and situations, and seek information from them to enable a partnership of care then challenges are more likely to be met successfully.

## Respect for individuals

Midwives are generally focused these days on providing individualised care for women. It is vital that all mothers are respected and treated as the unique person they are whether disabled or not, and that includes the choice of parenthood. Midwives need to be mothers' advocates in this and in all situations, for example with other members of the multidisciplinary team or women's families. This requires an even greater emphasis for women with a disability who are frequently entering motherhood having chosen the undertaking after considerable thought and planning.

Motherhood for all women is generally hard work, but for mothers with a disability it will present additional issues that need to be confronted. Those challenges will be specific for each woman and it must be remembered that for mothers with an acquired disability, especially if relatively recent, they may still have issues of acceptability and adaptability related to their impairment and disability, which could be compromised by pregnancy and parenthood.

Understanding of all of these issues will enable midwives to offer care that is non-patronising, sensitive and meets, as far as possible, both mothers' needs and wishes. Yet midwives may be in a dilemma about how to approach mothers. Women should be acknowledged as people before their disability but this may be easier said than done when it is clear that

there is impairment. Indeed some would argue that impairment should be readily acknowledged to avoid missing an opportunity to find solutions to meet requirements.

Nevertheless, midwives may be either afraid to acknowledge a mother's disability because of fears of causing offence, or express concern that they would be perceived as apparently ignoring her disability if they did not ask about it (McKay-Moffat 2003, McKay-Moffat & Cunningham 2006). When then should midwives mention a woman's disability? There is no *right* time to talk about it but it should not be ignored because her impairment is part of the person she is (Morris 1991, 1993, Oliver 1991). Open, honest questions that are obviously aimed at obtaining factual information is likely be the best approach, probably after the general questions asked of all mothers during the booking interview in early pregnancy. A comprehensive record of the answers at this time will go a long way to ensuring that women are not repeatedly asked for the same information by other professionals at subsequent visits. This ensures that women themselves and then their pregnancy, not their disability, remain the main focus of conversation.

The crucial factor is to remember that these are women, and women who are or going to be mothers. Additionally, that they have a disability that *may* give them physical or cognitive limitations for which they need help or advice or alternative strategies to fulfil additional needs. Primarily women will want the same information and service initially as all mothers. A genuine, open approach to discussion about their *abilities* as well as their disabilities is indispensable. The challenge is not only to see a mother as an individual but to also be aware of the impact impairment may have on her life.

## Antenatal screening

Choice in antenatal screening is a significant area of information exchange during the antenatal booking interview. An issue that may cause some considerable discomfort for the midwives is that of offering antenatal screening for fetal abnormalities, particularly if a mother's disability is genetic in origin (McKay-Moffat 2003). In all probability this is because of the implication for termination of pregnancy if an abnormality is identified with the concurrent potential to be seen as devaluing people with disabilities. For some mothers, whatever their situation, there is no right time to discuss this topic and sensitivity is required when broaching the subject. Mothers with disability are entitled to the same standard of service and screening facilities as any other mother. Therefore if midwives discuss such issues tactfully, women are unlikely to be offended.

Although a vital component of all midwifery care, possession of effective communication skills is particularly necessary at this time. If midwives lack knowledge about the implications related to mothers' specific disabilities they will feel disadvantaged in this situation. However, midwives need to remember that women could have greater appreciation of possible issues related to their own situation and therefore are able to share that with midwives. But if they have no existing knowledge midwives have a duty of care to seek that information from other experts or the literature. In some situations little will be known, and even what is known is unlikely to be applicable to all mothers. Therefore a 'wait and see' strategy may need to be utilised which is not without potential for stress and anxiety for all involved.

To minimise unnecessary anxiety, the issue of lack of evidence to inform mothers' choices needs to be freely and frankly discussed. This will ensure that they understand that the lack of offered information is not deliberate but is in response to unknown factors. In the end women may choose not to accept the offer of screening either because of the information received or due to the uncertain nature or absence of information.

## Communication

Appropriate, effective two-way communication is fundamental to success with service provision for all mothers. This means the sharing of information and the discussion of issues between mothers, midwives and members of the multidisciplinary team. Inter-professional communication, with the sharing of important details about a mother's disability is crucial. This will minimise the need of mothers to reiterate particulars about their condition and thus avoid repeatedly drawing attention to their disability. The value of this can clearly be ascertained

from the experience of a mother that I interviewed who had a congenitally abnormal pelvis. All her life she had received medical and nursing attention and had repeatedly had to give her history. She felt disempowered by this. However, she commented that she had found it 'refreshing' that midwives shared important information about her circumstances thus ensuring that for the first time in her life she did not have to keep repeating her details. History-giving time after time can cause women considerable frustration and distress. Shared information will also enable advanced preparation for a mother's attendance at an appointment, for example to ensure appropriate facilities are available.

Midwives need to be proactive in liaison with other specialist health professionals, for example physiotherapists and occupational therapists, but this appears not to be commonly undertaken (McKay-Moffat 2003). It is unclear whether midwives lack an appreciation of the help that these professionals may offer, or if they assume that they will already be involved in the provision of services for a mother. As pregnancy is a state of altered physiology alternative techniques may need to be found for mobility, lifting and personal hygiene. Physiotherapists are the experts able to offer advice about specific exercises and movements, while occupational therapists may have suggestions for specialised equipment or adaptive techniques.

Physiotherapy and occupational therapy may enhance a mother's ability to find alternative methods of approaching everyday situations related to pregnancy and parenthood enabling independence to be at the highest achievable level. If possible joint professional working with mothers and the sharing of expertise will not only benefit mothers, but enhance midwives' understanding of how to continue to support each individual mother. Alternative ways of mobilising, positioning for examinations and the birth, strengthening of muscles and self-lifting, and lifting baby can be identified and practiced in a 'dry run' long before they become essential.

However, it must not be assumed that all physiotherapists and occupational therapists have the knowledge, experience and expertise to offer the type of help and support that women need. They too may have little or no experience of helping women with disability during the child-bearing process.

This means that expertise and help must be sought elsewhere. Specialist and charitable organisations may offer the best option for relevant help and support, for example the organisation Disability, Pregnancy and Parenthood International. Additionally, other mothers may be useful sources of information and support.

Other members of the multidisciplinary team may be able to offer their specialist information and advice to both mothers and midwives. For example physicians, neurologists or orthopaedic consultants could have suggestions that solve problems, for example medication to relieve muscle spasm. Specialist continence nurses may be able to offer help if continence issues need alternative solutions because of pregnancy-related changes. It is important therefore, that midwives liaise with specialists as appropriate and if necessary refer mothers for appointments. Attendance at the appointment with a mother would enable a midwife to be a mother's advocate and could enhance her own knowledge and helping skills. In reality a lack of time and low staffing levels may not permit this to happen.

If a midwife is knowledgeable about a mother's condition and feels comfortable with social interaction with a mother with a disability she is more likely to find communication unproblematic (McKay-Moffat 2003). If communication with a mother is difficult midwives may feel stressed as they strive to maintain valuable discourse. This is of particular note when mothers are hard of hearing or deaf. In this situation midwives need to identify a mother's choice of method of communication (Iqbal 2004) which may be text, lip-reading, or British Sign Language (BSL) (see Chapters 4 and 7 for further discussion).

Much of the information that midwives generally offer women is potentially complex therefore it is vital that it is presented in a format that is readily understood. Without, or in addition to, the help of professional interpreters, midwives may make use of other methods of communication. Visual aids such as pictures and models can clarify specific information, particularly of a midwifery or medical nature. These can be especially useful for mothers with learning difficulties where the written word or even simplified details present comprehension difficulties. Three-dimensional models (Figs. 6.1, 6.2) are additional useful aids for mothers with visual

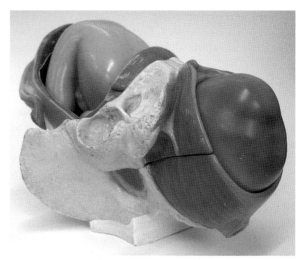

*Figure 6.1* This is an example of a series of true-to-life anatomical models (see Chapter 9) of a fetus in the uterus and progress during birth which are useful visual and tactile teaching aids. Photograph by Martin Baxter, with kind permission from Adam Rouilly Ltd.

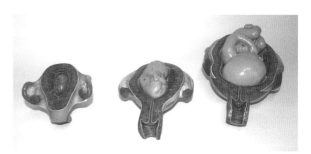

*Figure 6.2* These are examples of a series of true-to-life anatomical models (see Chapter 9) of fetuses in the uterus which are useful visual and tactile teaching aids. Photograph by Martin Baxter, with kind permission from Adam Rouilly Ltd.

impairment. Midwives may need to be innovative in enhancing their communication skills and develop their own visual aids, or it may be a simple matter of using pen and paper for writing.

Mothers themselves also have a responsibility to communicate with midwives. However, they may be unwilling to focus attention on their disability and additional needs, or to seek help particularly if they feel that the help might not be beneficial (see Thomas 1997). Women may be striving to be seen and treated as 'normal' and able to cope, to be socially acceptable and to counteract criticism (Grue & Tafjord Lærum 2002). Therefore there is the quest for normality versus the need for help. This theme (see above) was evident from interview data with the five women in my study (McKay-Moffat 2003).

Experience of professionals' non-receptiveness to two-way communication in the past may prompt a reluctance to chance possible rejection again. The 'does she take sugar' scenario, where a helper is spoken to rather than the person with a disability, is a profound statement of rejection, albeit inadvertently. Woman may have 'white coat syndrome' where individuals feel inferior to professionals offering care and thus feel inhibited to offer information or ask for assistance. To counteract these potential issues midwives need to be open, approachable, encouraging and receptive to mothers, and indeed their partners and families. They also need to be perceptive in order to recognise when mothers have unspoken needs or when they are finding difficulty articulating their feelings or wishes. Recognising a mother's non-verbal signals in such situations can be invaluable.

## Parent education

Midwives' parent education role appears to present some anxieties, concerns and lack of confidence for a large number of midwives in relation to mothers with a disability (McKay-Moffat 2003). As noted earlier, this was particularly evident for those midwives qualified for less than 15 years and when needed by mothers with visual or hearing impairment or upper limb disability. However, when midwives feel confident to provide women with disability with general midwifery care, and feel comfortable in social interaction with people with disabilities, they are more likely to have confidence to offer parent education. Nevertheless, midwives' increasing knowledge about disability and sensitivity to potential needs appeared from the study to undermine that confidence. This may be because a greater awareness that mothers have additional needs emphasises midwives' own lack of skills in effectively being able to meet those needs, thus affecting self-belief in their ability to offer any parent education.

Evidence of the importance of midwives having effective helping skills and the need to acknowledge someone's disability came notably from one mother in my study. She described her feelings following the birth of her first child who was approximately two years old at the time of the interview (she was pregnant for the second time). She had one arm that was paralysed following a road accident some 10 years earlier. It was only when needing to take her blood pressure that her paralysed arm was acknowledged, and only then because she was unable to lift the sleeve of her clothes over her unaffected arm for a cuff to be applied. No questions were ever asked about why her arm was paralysed or how she adapted her way of doing things.

None of the midwives asked her if she had any specific needs or made any attempt to discuss infant care with her either during pregnancy or once the baby was born. She felt unsupported by the midwives throughout and this continued when she was under health visitors' care. She had felt totally bewildered about how to safely manage bathing, dressing and moving her baby which led her to feel inadequate as a mother. This she felt had resulted in her postnatal depression. She did, however, state that she had been reluctant to ask for help as she did not want to be seen as unable to cope because of her disability. She admitted this had been a mistake on her part. Trial and error had enabled her to find solutions to her dilemmas but she felt that if someone had taken time to work with her those solutions may have been more readily found. If nothing else she felt that at least someone would have been supporting her.

Early discussion with women during pregnancy will enable the exploration of a variety of approaches to meet specific needs. Additionally, liaison with other members of the multidisciplinary team and outside agencies, for example occupational therapists, physiotherapists, and makers of special equipment, will aid problem-solving. Midwives could have a significant impact on the quality of a mother's experience by facilitating one or more 'dry runs' using alternative strategies to meet unconventional needs. This will not only benefit an individual mother but also midwives, as they too learn different ways of doing things that may be useful for other mothers in the future.

Whilst individual strategies on a one-to-one basis are likely to be essential to meet alternative needs, some mothers may be happy to attend formal parent education classes. Indeed they may welcome the opportunity, as most mothers attending do, of sharing pregnancy experiences, concerns and anxieties within a mutually supportive group. But physical access to a classroom situation may be difficult and *disabling*, as it is hard to ensure facilities meet the needs of all mothers. This is because individuals' requirements vary tremendously and the number of women with disability is relatively low. Yet, with the 1995 Disability Discrimination Act the deadline for all public places to be accessible by people with a disability was 2004. It is up to midwives then to put pressure on the Fund Holder of the facility to comply with the Act.

Classes need not only to be physically accessible but they need to be psychologically accessible also. One major cause of women not attending general classes is likely to be their reluctance to highlight their difficulty or inability to participate as other mothers do. An example from my study was a mother with cerebral palsy. She was a well-educated single mother employed by a local authority. Her baby was 6 weeks old at the time of the interview. She felt nervous with unfamiliar people and situations and knew this made her tremor worse which compounded her self-consciousness. Although she understood the potential benefit, she had felt unable to attend parent education and relaxation classes. This was because she knew her self-consciousness would increase, she felt that she would be stared at and would be unable to participate effectively because of her palsy and tremor. Little opportunity for parent education had been offered to her, and what she had revolved mainly around basic infant care and formula feeding whilst in hospital. She left hospital with her baby earlier than she wanted, despite limited support from her non-resident partner, because she felt that midwives and support staff were watching her to see how she was managing her infant's care. She found this disempowering.

For this mother and many mothers with disability, individual sessions that are either planned or ad hoc and include partners may be the most appropriate. A programme of planned sessions in the home setting may be the ideal solution but this requires time and commitment on the part of midwives and service providers; this is not always easy when staffing levels are low.

Planned sessions should include a visit for mothers and their partners to the maternity unit, especially the delivery suite if hospital birth is planned. A visit will enable familiarisation with the facilities and equipment. Additionally, it affords the opportunity for mothers and midwives to try alternative methods of approaching different situations, for example examinations and birthing positions. For visually impaired mothers this will enable them to touch the equipment and have an idea of the layout of both the delivery suite and the postnatal ward. Mothers with learning disability will have time to assimilate a new, possibly frightening environment. For mothers and midwives this exercise, which may need to be repeated, offers a valuable learning opportunity with the potential to minimise anxiety and enhance confidence in themselves and each other.

## MIDWIVES' LEARNING NEEDS

Many mothers look to midwives to provide practical solutions to their problems during and after pregnancy. These may be childbirth related or otherwise, so midwives need a large and broad repertoire of answers or information about where or from whom to find those solutions. However, midwives must acknowledge their limitations (NMC 2004) and also that not all problems are resolvable. This may be difficult for both midwives and mothers to accept. Women may well have concerns about any of the common maternity-related matters or they may have very different issues. This then means that midwives need to enhance their knowledge in order to ensure they provide an effective maternity service.

Formal educational opportunities related to pregnancy for women with a disability appear, however, to have been limited to date. It has only been during the last 10 years or so that some student midwives have received even a minimal number of lectures related to midwifery care for mothers with a disability (McKay-Moffat 2003). It has not been a subject universally included in curricula. In-service education and study days have been rare.

The quality of published literature, that has steadily begun to emerge over the last 10–15 years, varies from a few specific research papers to magazine articles describing mothers' experiences. Some internet websites related to specific conditions have been developed but are primarily aimed at the general public. They may contain limited information about fertility, pregnancy and child-care, however they do offer insight into issues related to living with the condition that professional literature often fails to address. Overall then, the subject of women with disability and the issues related to pregnancy, childbirth and child-care have been relatively poorly addressed topics from theoretical, practical and professional perspectives. Coupled with a lack of experiential learning opportunities in practice, it is not surprising that some midwives' knowledge base and skills are inadequate.

In my survey approximately half of the midwives felt that they lacked knowledge about mothers' additional needs, with achondroplasia (55%) and multiple sclerosis (MS) (55%), the conditions with the highest percentages (see Table 6.4 for a list of conditions and midwives' responses) (McKay-Moffat 2003). (Table 6.5 provides an overview of possible additional needs. See Chapter 8 for more detail.) This admission of lack of knowledge contrasted with the high numbers of midwives who expressed confidence in providing midwifery care for mothers with a disability generally. It therefore calls into question the effectiveness of some of the maternity care women with a disability receive. Midwives' confidence to provide midwifery care does not necessarily mean that mothers' additional

specific needs were, in reality, being met. It could be argued that midwives may lack perception of the fact that they were not essentially providing optimum individualised care.

Nevertheless, contemporary midwives do generally have skills of adaptability and flexibility, and additionally a great knowledge and appreciation of related topics with transferability to new situations. There is much midwives can do to enhance their learning and understanding of the subject and the issues involved. Without the relevant knowledge and skills midwives may feel anxious and inadequate in their ability to provide mothers with appropriate care. Therefore, enhancing disability awareness has the potential to promote more positive attitudes towards people with a disability (Gething 1992).

## The interaction between physical impairment and pregnancy

Many areas need to be considered by midwives in order that they can provide accurate information and advise women on strategies to minimise difficulties (see Table 6.5 for an overview and Chapter 8 for more detail). They not only need an appreciation of how individual mothers use adapted methods to cope with the activities of daily living, but how the altered physiology of pregnancy and childbirth may influence those adaptive mechanisms. The day-to-day issues involve mobility, personal care and sexual relationships. A mother with a congenital disability will have her own natural way of doing things. Mothers with an acquired impairment may still be coming to terms with their physical changes and be less well adapted.

Alterations in body weight and centre of gravity may make mobility more difficult, and an already compromised mobility may no longer be possible without additional aids, for example a wheelchair. Joint mobility and pain may be affected due to the hormonal effects of progesterone and relaxin that increase throughout pregnancy. Mobility may further be influenced by the physiological haemo-dilution that normally occurs during pregnancy where there is a relative fall in oxygen-carrying red blood cells as plasma levels rise, which may cause breathlessness. This may be further aggravated by the enlarging uterus inhibiting respiratory capacity (see Chapters 4 and 8).

*Table 6.4* **Percentage of midwives identifying a lack of knowledge about mothers' additional needs related to specific disabilities (McKay-Moffat 2003)**

| Disability | % Midwives |
|---|---|
| Visually impaired | 47.8 |
| Hearing impaired | 43.8 |
| Spina bifida | 51.8 |
| Achondroplasia | 55 |
| Lower limb disability | 45 |
| Upper limb disability | 44 |
| Multiple sclerosis | 55 |
| Arthritis | 53 |
| Cerebral palsy | 44 |
| Wheelchair user | 45 |
| Learning disability | 43 |

*Table 6.5* Overview of possible issues relating to specific conditions during the childbirth continuum and possible solutions (see Chapter 8 for greater detail)

| Type of disability | Potential issues/difficulties | Actions/possible ways of overcoming difficulties | Additional help |
|---|---|---|---|
| Visual impaired/blind | If genetic origin | Genetic screening preconception; chorionic villus sampling in early pregnancy | Genetic counselling |
| | Finding way round hospital/clinic/ward | Guided tour—mother may wish to rest a hand on guide's arm, guide dog allowed, tactile signs | 3D map model |
| | Usual leaflets/written information and records | Braille alternatives, audio tape of leaflets/information, written records reported verbally | Royal National Institute for the Blind (RNIB) (for resources see Chapter 9) |
| | Unable to see visual parent education tools e.g. videos, demonstrations e.g. preparing infant formula | Individual sessions, verbal description of events, tactile models to explain processes e.g. labour, encourage mother to touch & participate in simulated demonstrations. Ready prepared infant formula may be best | |
| | Ultrasound scan pictures | In-depth description of pictures | |
| | Baby's appearance/behaviour | As mother touches baby describe what is happening | |
| Hearing impaired/deaf | If genetic origin | Genetic screening preconception; chorionic villus sampling in early pregnancy | Genetic counselling |
| | Hearing name called at appointments | Direct contact with the mother aided by information from receptionist | Information from GP/advanced booking forms about needs |
| | Information exchange during face-to-face contact | Identify mother's chosen method of communication e.g. sign language, lip-reading, pencil & paper, visual material to explain complex concepts e.g. labour & pain relief Gentle touch on arm to attract attention For lip-reading speak at steady pace, ensure face is lit & clearly visible at all times Individual parent education sessions, use of videos with subtitles | Learn some basic signs (see Chapter 7) Book specific interpreter as required/chosen by mother in advance Royal National Institute for Deaf (RNID) (for resources see Chapter 9) |
| | Information exchange from a distance | Minicom equipment, text equipment, in writing e.g. completion of an information form prior to booking in | |
| | Communication during labour | Epidural avoids drowsiness from narcotics & sedatives; forward planning ensuring mother knows processes & procedures; plan visual signs e.g. face expressions for 'push' & 'pant' | |

*table continued*

*table continued*

| Type of disability | Potential issues/difficulties | Actions/possible ways of overcoming difficulties | Additional help |
|---|---|---|---|
| | Hearing the baby cry | Vibrating or flashing equipment that responds to audible cry | (See Chapter 9) |
| Spina bifida | Mobility/accessibility, wheelchair access | Forward planning; larger room with large en suite facilities/wheel-in shower etc.; height-adjustable examination couch/bed | |
| | Increased risks of: | | |
| | Fetal spina bifida | Folic acid 4 mg 3 months before and after conception | |
| | UTI[a] | Increase oral fluids & cranberry juice; regular screening; early treatment | |
| | Genital tract/area infection | Scrupulous hygiene, early recognition & treatment | |
| | Pressure sores | Increase pressure-relieving activities will also reduce DVT risk | |
| | DVT[b] | Examination for visual indicators e.g. swelling & inflammation | |
| | Anaemia | Early recognition & treatment; diet modification; prevent UTI[a] | Dietician |
| | Continence issues | Review existing management; diet modification e.g. fibre content | Continence advisor |
| | Breathing difficulties late pregnancy | Strengthening & breathing exercises | Physiotherapist |
| | Labour issues: | | |
| | Painless—onset missed | 'Wind-like' sensations, uterine fundus rising | |
| | SRM[c]—missed | Liquor odour different to urine | |
| | Urge to bear down absent | Uterus may expel baby or advise Valsalva[d] manoeuvre | |
| | Autonomic hyperreflexia | Avoid stimulation, early recognition & management (see Chapter 8) | |
| | Handling baby | Height-adjustable cot; slings for carrying baby; pram/buggy that attaches to wheelchair; bath on stand | Specialist suppliers (see Chapter 9) |
| Achondroplasia counselling | Genetic condition | Preconception genetic screening; chorionic villus sampling in early pregnancy; ultrasound scan to measure fetal limbs | Genetic counselling |
| | Short limbs affect mobility & reach | Additional time to complete tasks; height-adjustable couch, bed, cot; 'dry run' with equipment/facilities; step stool | Mother likely to have her own equipment for daily activities of living |
| | Spine abnormalities—back & neck pain; difficulty intubating & to site epidural | Additional rest; analgesia as required; avoid over-extension of neck | Neck X-ray |
| | Small/abnormal pelvis | Caesarean section—possibly continuous epidural | Skilled anaesthetist for intubation/ epidural |

*table continued*

*table continued*

| Type of disability | Potential issues/difficulties | Actions/possible ways of overcoming difficulties | Additional help |
|---|---|---|---|
| | Reduced lung capacity & breathing difficulty | Breathing exercises; additional rest; early delivery | Pulmonary function tests |
| | Poor coordination/dexterity; lifting & moving | Muscle strengthening exercises; adapted equipment; additional support for breast-feeding | Physiotherapy; occupational therapy |
| | Reduced pelvic organ sensation | Screen for UTI[a] & early treatment; vigilance for signs of labour & early admission to hospital | |
| Lower limb disability | Mobility; balance; prosthesis; walking/mobility aids | Forward planning; time for manoeuvres; larger room with large en suite facilities/wheel-in shower; height-adjustable examination couch/bed; strengthening & balance exercises; 'dry run' with equipment e.g. delivery suite & infant care | Physiotherapist Specialist equipment suppliers (see Chapter 9) |
| Upper limb disability | Activities of daily living/self-care during pregnancy/postnatal | Work with mother to adapt her usual ways of doing things | Specialist equipment suppliers (see Chapter 9); occupational therapist |
| | Moving, handling, bathing baby; fine movement | 'Dry run' with equipment/positioning for infant care & breast-feeding during pregnancy; minimise distance between transfer points; alternative strategies e.g. mother lifts baby using her teeth to grip a sling/sheet/baby's clothing Velcro fastenings—babies learn to be still or 'help' in time | Helper may be needed in some situations—mother should remain in control |
| Multiple sclerosis | Drug regime | Preconception advice | Specialist medical advice |
| | Weakness; balance affected; excessive tiredness; muscle spasm & pain; inability to abduct legs; poor nerve sensation | Time to complete activities/movements; additional rest periods; timing of appointments when less tired; height-adjustable couch & bed; left lateral for vaginal examination if leg spasms; self-medication in hospital will ensure usual drug regime followed | |
| | Anaemia compounds tiredness | Screening; consider prophylactic iron therapy; diet & nutritional advice | Dietician |
| | Urinary tract, bowel & continence problems | Cranberry juice; screening & treatment for UTI[a]; consider prophylactic antibiotics; pelvic floor exercises; diet modification | Physiotherapist; dietician |

*table continued*

*table continued*

| Type of disability | Potential issues/difficulties | Actions/possible ways of overcoming difficulties | Additional help |
|---|---|---|---|
| | Teratogenic effects of some drugs | Preconception advice to change medication; ultrasound scan to identify potential fetal abnormalities | Specialist medical advice |
| | Risk of hypertension, diabetes, premature labour, infection with steroids | Screening for the conditions; steroid boost needed during labour or any illness/excessive stress | |
| | Intolerant of hot environments | Modify environmental temperature especially in delivery suite | |
| | Onset of labour/second stage unrecognised | Teach mother to recognise uterine fundal rise during contractions, admission to await labour/in early labour to avoid precipitate labour; midwife vigilant for signs of second stage | |
| | Poor energy levels for second stage of labour | Epidural may relieve muscle spasm & result in less tiredness; consider instrumental delivery/prophylactic episiotomy | |
| | Depression/mood changes | Information about possibility of occurrence; counselling & support; early recognition/treatment for postnatal depression | Liaison with health visitor for long-term support/ monitoring for postnatal depression |
| | Difficulty with speech | Avoid overtiredness; patience with communication | |
| | Breast-feeding—drug contraindication; tiredness | Avoid contraindicated drugs if possible otherwise infant formula used; additional rest/help/support | |
| | Moving & handling baby | Additional rest to avoid excess tiredness; main baby activities e.g. bathing when least tired; minimise distance between transfer points; lightweight equipment | |
| Arthritis | Drug regime | Preconception advice regarding drugs | Specialist medical advice |
| | Pain/restricted mobility; tiredness | Adequate analgesia; time to complete activities/movements; additional rest periods; timing of appointments when less tired; height-adjustable couch & bed; identify most comfortable position for vaginal examination/ delivery e.g. with a 'dry run'; self-medication in hospital will ensure usual drug regime followed | Physiotherapy; walking aids |

*table continued*

*table continued*

| Type of disability | Potential issues/difficulties | Actions/possible ways of overcoming difficulties | Additional help |
|---|---|---|---|
| | Hypertension; premature rupture of membranes; IUGR[e] | Routine screening; raise mother's awareness & seek hospital admission; caesarean section more likely | |
| | Reduced fine movement dexterity; difficulty moving & handling baby | 'Dry run' with moving & handling baby; Velcro fastenings on baby wear | Occupational therapist |
| | Symptoms may worsen with breast-feeding | Discuss possibility with mother; analgesia 30–60 minutes after feeding | |
| Cerebral palsy | Drug regime | Preconception advice regarding drugs | Specialist medical advice |
| | Pain/muscle spasms; mobility; tremor; swollen ankles; tiredness | Adequate analgesia; massage/limb bracing; time to complete activities/ movements; additional rest periods; timing of appointments when less tired; height-adjustable couch & bed; identify most comfortable position for vaginal examination/delivery e.g. with a 'dry run'; frequent position changes avoiding joint damage; attention to pressure areas; self-medication in hospital will ensure usual drug regime followed | Physiotherapy |
| | Communication if speech affected | Patience with communication | Partner/family member may help communication |
| | Control of fine movements | 'Dry run' with moving & handling baby; Velcro fastenings on baby wear | |
| Wheelchair user | Access to clinic/rooms/ facilities; transfer from chair to couch/bed | Forward planning; large room with en suite facilities/wheel-in shower; height-adjustable couch, bed, cot; positions for labour & delivery depending on specific situation | |
| Learning disability | Exchange of information; poor understanding of what is going on may cause fear/ anxiety/poor cooperation | Patience; consider language/ terminology used; use of models & visual aids to explain/teach; introduce new information in small stages, repetition & participation in simulated practice; visit to hospital during pregnancy | Models (see Figs. 6.1, 6.2), diagrams & pictures |

[a]UTI = urinary tract infection.
[b]DVT = deep vein thrombosis.
[c]SRM = spontaneous rupture of membranes which may indicate the onset of labour.
[d]Valsalva manoeuvre = to use diaphragm to press on uterine fundus: take a deep breath, hold and bear down.
[e]IUGR = Intrauterine growth restriction.

Personal hygiene and elimination may become more difficult to cope with without help, due to the increasing size of the growing uterus and thus difficulty bending. In some cases the increased susceptibility to urinary tract and vaginal infections that all pregnant women experience may be exacerbated by a mother's condition. Therefore midwives need to pay attention to the increased need for screening for infection and to offer appropriate advice to lower the risk of infection developing (see Chapters 4 and 8 for more details).

All of these physiological factors need to be taken into consideration when planning antenatal and intranatal examinations and care, and positions for labour and birth. Additionally, postnatal comfort, for example if there is pain from an episiotomy or surgery, and positions for breast-feeding and strength and dexterity for infant care need to be contemplated. Plans need to be formulated with mothers to minimise complications and discomfort and thus enhance successful outcomes. Women often want factual information to enable them to make plans and choices, and tips or ideas to offer alternative ways of doing things. Experienced midwives may be able to adapt existing skills to offer appropriate suggestions or seek help from other mothers who have developed different ways of doing things.

It is not only how the pregnancy may influence the impairment but how the cause of the disability may influence the pregnancy (see Chapter 8). From the medical and obstetric perspectives this may only be of importance if the condition has a genetic origin, if the condition is likely to change, or if any medication that is being taken is significant. Midwives need to have knowledge of these implications in order to be able to effectively discuss women's choice of actions.

Ideally, preconception care should be available for health promotion advice, for genetic screening or to balance the need for the medication against any potential risks. But in reality few women (although women with a disability may be the exception) attend before pregnancy. Additionally, although preconception care is integral in the role of midwives, few are in a position where they are able to offer information and advice at this time. Therefore early pregnancy may be the first opportunity to plan any investigations, treatment or life-style changes. Investigations may include chorionic villi sampling at about 8 weeks gestation or

amniocentesis at 16–18 weeks, ultrasound scan, and blood tests. Medication changes may involve the dose or the actual drug used and will be specific to each individual woman. Specialist medical and obstetric advice is probably the most appropriate in these situations but midwives need to know what may or may not be suitable to enable rapid referral. Life-style changes will be similar to those for most women i.e. diet, nutrition and smoking cessation.

## The multidisciplinary team

Midwives need to know about all referral procedures in their area so that they are able to rapidly seek the expert assistance of other members of the multidisciplinary team to offer their skills to mothers. Knowledge and understanding of those specialists' roles will additionally aid midwives in recognising how mothers may be helped. Further assistance could be obtained from other support workers e.g. from the Social Services, and specific organisations. In all of these elements midwives should not only be proactive in seeking that additional support but could formulate a new, or update an existing database of contact people. People on the database may even be mothers in a similar situation although caution must be exercised as what works for one mother will not always be suitable for another. Early liaison during pregnancy will enable solutions to be found as early as possible and enhance a woman's quality of life.

A database might also contain a selection of relevant literature that informs readers of pertinent aspects or issues, thus affording all members of the midwifery team the opportunity to enhance their own knowledge. But of course, often the best source of information is the women themselves, or their partners and helpers, therefore midwives need to recognise that a partnership of care with all those involved is likely to be the most successful.

## Psychological and social aspects

Midwives need to accept that, as with all pregnancies, for mothers with disability pregnancy is a psycho-social event. In this sense mothers with disability are subject to all the emotional highs and lows that having a baby evokes in every woman's life and the lives of the people around her. However, there are potentially other issues that midwives may need to take into consideration. These revolve around the impact that pregnancy and the desire for parenthood may have on the response of women's families, friends and society because of their disabilities (see Chapter 1).

People may respond to a woman's pregnancy negatively not only because of her obvious sexual activity, but their perception of her as irresponsible for undertaking a pregnancy when they feel she may not be able to cope with bringing up a child (Rogers et al 2004). Reports from the women themselves through the literature and television programmes confirm this negativity to what they consider 'good news'. Here, then, is an opportunity for midwives to exercise their role as mothers' advocates and endorse the 'can-do' attitude promoted by Rogers et al (2004, p 169).

Even with support, pregnancy is a time of anxiety to a greater or lesser degree for all mothers. If midwives appreciate the possible additional anxieties that a mother with a disability may have they will be in a far better position to offer appropriate support. Mothers may feel embarrassment about their disability, for example gait, dexterity and communication skills. Evidence for this came from the mother in my study with the amputated leg. She felt extreme embarrassment about midwives having to handle her stump during labour and had worried about this for her whole pregnancy. Unfortunately she felt unable to discuss it with the midwives participating in her care which also offers a clue to how women may find communicating their feelings and anxieties difficult.

Women's anxieties may encompass thoughts about general health and the impact having a baby may have on their condition during and after pregnancy. They may be concerned about fetal well-being and their abilities to cope with labour and birth. Women may even be concerned about interacting with midwives and other health professionals, especially if previous experiences have been unsatisfactory or if they have heard of other mothers' inadequate encounters with maternity service providers. If midwives employ a sensitive, respectful manner with effective communication skills much of mothers' anxieties may be alleviated.

## CONCLUSION—KEY POINTS

- Midwives' positive attitudes towards mothers with a disability are likely to enhance the quality of their childbirth experiences. Development of those positive attitudes is enhanced by knowledge and experience.
- A sound knowledge about disabling conditions and their interaction with pregnancy aids midwives' confidence and helping skills. Feelings of uncertainty may lead to a reactive approach to care provision therefore education about disability is essential.
- Midwives need to be proactive in identifying and meeting mothers' additional needs which may mean effective liaison with other professionals or support agencies. Midwives may need to develop a greater understanding of the roles of members of the multidisciplinary team.
- To date midwives' experience of providing care for mothers with disability appears limited. Therefore the sharing of expertise and experiences could enhance midwives' ability and confidence with communication, and in the provision of general midwifery care *and* parent education.

## References

Brown B 2001 The introduction of a special needs advisor. British Journal of Midwifery 9(6):348–352

Campion M J 1990 The baby challenge: a handbook on pregnancy for women with physical disability. Routledge, London

Carty E 1995 Disability pregnancy and parenting. In: Alexander J, Levy V, Roach S (eds) Aspects of midwifery practice. Macmillan Press, Basingstoke

Crow L 2003 Invisible and centre stage: a disabled woman's perspective on maternity care. Midwives: the Official Journal of the Royal College of Midwives 6(4):158–161

Department of Health (DoH) 1993 Changing Childbirth. Report of the Expert Maternity Group. HMSO, London

Disability Discrimination Act 1995 HMSO, London. Online. Available: http://www.drc-gb.org 1 March 2006

Gething L 1992 Nurse practitioners' and students' attitudes towards people with disabilities. The Australian Journal of Advanced Nursing 9(3):25–30

Gething L 1994 The interaction with disabled persons scale: psychosocial perceptions on disability. Journal of Social and Behaviour and Personality, A Special Issue 9(5):23–42

Grue L, Tafjord Lærum K 2002 'Doing motherhood:' some experience of mothers with physical disabilities. Disability & Society 17(6):671–683

Iqbal S 2004 Pregnancy and birth: a guide for deaf women. RNID & National Childbirth Trust, London

Lipson J G, Rogers J G 2000 Pregnancy, birth and disability: women's health care experience. Health Care for Women International 21:11–26

McKay-Moffat S 2003 Midwifery care for women with disabilities. MPhil thesis. Liverpool John Moores University, Liverpool

McKay-Moffat S, Cunningham C 2006 Services for women with disabilities: Mothers' and midwives' experiences. British Journal of Midwifery 14(8):472–477

Morris J 1991 Pride against prejudice: transforming attitudes to disability. The Women's Press, London

Morris J 1993 Women confronting disability. In: Clarke J (ed) A crisis in care? Challenges to social work. Sage Publications, London, p 122–131

NMC 2004 Midwives rules and standards. Nurses and Midwives Council, London

Oliver M 1991 The politics of disablement. 2nd edn. Macmillan Education, London

Paris M J 1993 Attitudes of medical students and health-care professionals towards people with disabilities. Archives of Physical Medicine and Rehabilitation 74:818–825

Robson C 2002 Real world research. 2nd edn. A resource for social scientists and practitioner research. Blackwell Publishers, Oxford.

Rogers J G, Tulega C V, Vensand K 2004 Baby care preparation: pregnancy and postpartum. In: Welner S, Haseltine F (eds) Welner's guide to the care of women with disabilities. Lippincott Williams & Wilkins, Philadelphia, p 169–184

Rotheram J 2002 The maternity needs of disabled women. Disability Pregnancy and Parenthood International 40:10–11

Royal College of Midwives (RCM) 2000 Position Paper No. 11a February. London, RCM. Online. Available: http://rcm.org.uk 1 March 2006

Thomas C 1997 The baby and the bath water: disabled women and motherhood in social context. Sociology of Health and Illness: a Journal of Medical Sociology 19(5):622–643

Turk M A 2004 Health care challenges for clinicians and clinical researchers In: Welner S, Haseltine F (eds) Welner's guide to the care of women with disabilities. Lippincott Williams & Wilkins, Philadelphia, p 5–8

# 7 Sensory impairment

## Pam Lee

## INTRODUCTION

Sensory impairment has a major effect on people's lives: it affects them physically, socially, emotionally and financially. However, it is often a part of who they are, the way they operate and negotiate the world they live in, and often that world disables them more than the impairment itself (Butler 2004).

Women with sensory impairments who become pregnant may find dealing with the maternity services very frustrating (Iqbal 2004). Generally speaking the healthcare professionals they are referred to—the midwife, doctor or health visitor—are not trained to meet the needs of a deaf or partially hearing person, blind or partially blind person, or someone who is deaf-blind. Specialist services are required to facilitate their care during the child-bearing process. Communication is often the main problem and simple strategies can help improve the situation for all concerned. The aim of this chapter is to highlight some of the issues around caring for people with sensory impairment and to provide some practical advice.

## DEAF AND HARD OF HEARING

There are different degrees of deafness ranging from people with a mild hearing loss to those who are profoundly deaf. Unlike a blind person who usually has some form of aid which will indicate that they cannot see it is very difficult to identify someone who is deaf. Different categories of deafness can be described:

- Mild hearing loss—which may be helped by a hearing aid or the ability to lip-read and a quiet environment for conversation.

- Moderate hearing loss—which may be helped by a hearing aid, lip-reading and a quiet environment but following a conversation with more than one person at a time, could prove difficult.
- Severe hearing loss—where a person may have great difficulty following a conversation even if they have a hearing aid; many lip-read and some use sign language or electronic resources to aid communication.
- Profound hearing loss—where hearing aids are of little or no benefit and the person uses sign language, lip-reading and other electronic resources to help them communicate (Iqbal 2004).

The Disability Discrimination Act 1995 (DDA) defines disability as: 'A physical or mental impairment which has a substantial and long term adverse effect on the person's ability to carry out normal day to day activities' (Iqbal 2004, p 104).

An inability to hold a conversation with someone talking in a normal voice or to hear a telephone conversation constitutes an adverse effect and so deaf people are covered by the DDA 1995. Some people see themselves as part of the deaf community and are therefore referred to as the 'Deaf', with a capital 'D' as opposed to someone hard of hearing being called 'deaf'.

There are a wide range of resources available to deaf people to enhance their communication with each other and with healthcare professionals. Hospital Trusts have a duty under the DDA 1995 to provide access to some of these services. Midwives should check what this provision is in their own units and how the services can be accessed if required. The services may include a British Sign Language (BSL)/English Interpreter, lip-speaker, and various electronic/telephone services such as Videophone,

Minicom (textphone), RNID Typetalk (national telephone relay service) or BT TextDirect (Butler 2004). Mobile phones are good for sending texts, but their use is frowned upon in hospitals and the mobile phone may cause severe interference with some hearing aids.

## INTRODUCTION TO BRITISH SIGN LANGUAGE (BSL)

BSL is the primary language of the deaf community of Britain, but not all deaf people use sign language (see Chapter 1 for history of this). Policies determined by non-deaf people continue to promote 'oralism' (speech) rather than signing. People need to be bilingual for BSL and English if they were born profoundly deaf or lost their hearing before the age of 2 years. It is unlikely that these people will become proficient in speech, having had no hearing experience of it. Nevertheless BSL is an essential and valued tool for communication which has visual, spatial and gesture components (Smith 1990).

BSL has no written form; signs are normally represented by English words or *glosses*, e.g. RUN. As RUN has more than one meaning this can be confusing but the sign for RUN in BSL means the physical act of running (Miles 1988). On the other hand one sign may have to be glossed by several English words, for example 'A FORTNIGHT AGO'; there is one sign for these three words. Words can be spoken at roughly double the rate at which signs can be produced, yet it is possible to interpret from one language to the other in the same space of time without loss of meaning, nuance or intent (Smith 1996).

Sign language relies less on words and more on the inventive use of space and movement: the handshapes that are used combined with non-manual information carried by the head, face and body (Smith 1996). All of these factors are taken in by the eye at the same time—things can happen simultaneously in the visual language. BSL has grammar but not like spoken English, although many features of sign language structures are found in other spoken languages (Kyle and Woll 1985). For instance, a sentence such as 'Est-ce qu'il vient d'arriver?' translates literally as 'Is it that he comes to arrive?' not 'Has he arrived yet?' so the order of the sentence might be different, e.g. we might say 'turn right at the traffic lights'; a deaf person would sign traffic lights, right turn. Deaf BSL users find signed English difficult because of its linear approach, although sign-supported English—a form of English with key signs added—may suit some deaf people in some situations. However, it does not meet all the linguistic needs of those deaf from infancy for whom English is not their first language.

When signing to each other deaf people do not just look at the hands but at the face and body as well. BSL is part mime, it exists in a visual-spatial mode with iconic signs (resembling what they say) such as GIVE: hands together, palm upwards moving towards the other person, or FOOD: fingers bunched together moving towards the mouth, and signs such as EASY and ALLOW which have no clear iconic origins (Kyle and Woll 1985). The sign for LOOK: two fingers in V shape pointing forward near eye, can be modified for 'YOU LOOK AT ME', 'LOOK AT EACH OTHER' or 'KEEP LOOKING AT ONE ANOTHER' by using both hands, one to sign look and the other to sign the different instructions i.e. at me, at each other, or keep looking. Mime is used to enhance story-telling rather than to give meaning, much the same as a hearing person who uses their hands to make a point when talking to another person. The use of space is important and the story-teller adopts a different posture or orientation to indicate a change of speaker or perspective. At the same time as signing, the signer silently mouths the words so that they can be lip-read to aid understanding.

BSL is used in England, Scotland, Wales and Northern Ireland. However, the Republic of Ireland, in the Roman Catholic deaf community, uses Irish Sign Language which is one-handed finger spelling. Other Roman Catholic communities in the United Kingdom may use this form of sign language. From a historical perspective it depends on which school someone was educated at (see Chapter 1). Deaf communities in Australia and New Zealand use a recognisable form of BSL, but American Sign Language is a different language based on French Sign Language which is also one-handed. Sign languages from different countries have more in common than the spoken language. Deaf people, when coming together for the first time at international conferences, quickly establish a common ground and understanding of the different forms of sign language (Smith 1996).

The Dictionary of BSL contains about 2000 signs; the Oxford Dictionary contains approximately 600 000 words (Smith 1996). Signs can have different meanings depending on the situation, e.g. BATTERY/ELECTRIC, FAMILY/AUNTIE. In different parts of the country there will be variations on signs, similar to different dialects in the spoken language. If a deaf person is having problems understanding an interpreter it may be that they come from different areas, although they can soon adapt to the different form (Iqbal 2004). Sign language evolves as does any language and modern BSL is different from that of the nineteenth century (Miles 1988).

## BSL—a useful guide

Although it is preferable to have an interpreter or someone who can sign present during interaction with a deaf person, it may not always be possible. A basic knowledge of the British two-handed finger spelling might aid communication temporarily.

Words can be spelt out using this alphabet (Fig. 7.1). The right hand is shown making shapes

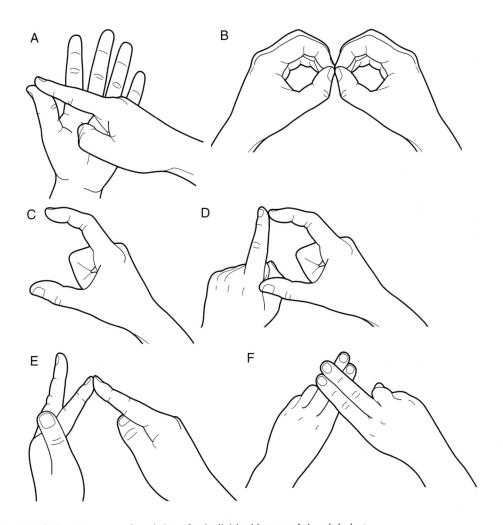

*Figure 7.1*  British Sign Language hand signs for individual letters of the alphabet.

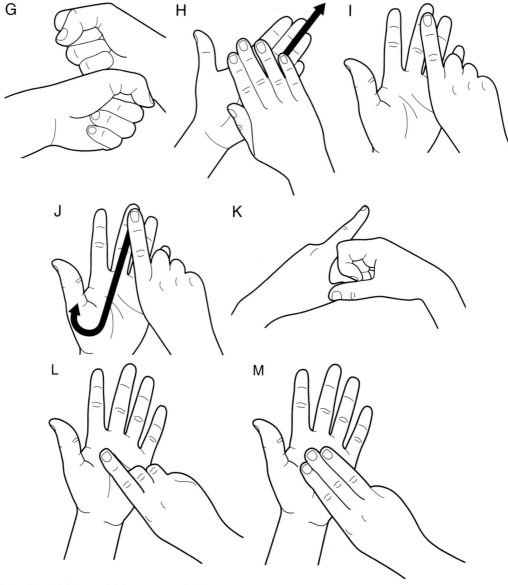

*Figure 7.1 —Cont'd.* [Note with letters H and J the right hand moves in the direction of the arrows.]

with the left hand to create the letter. If a person is left handed they would sign the opposite way round. Names can be spelt out this way, and if the deaf person cannot understand an individual sign then finger spelling might help. However, it must be remembered that English may not be their first language so long sentences should be avoided to prevent confusion.

When signing conversation, different parts of the hand are used (Fig. 7.2). Terms are used to describe the directions in which the hands are facing, pointing and moving (Figs. 7.3a, 7.3b) and the hand is also put into different shapes (Fig. 7.4). These variations are used to modify a word or make a phrase (see below).

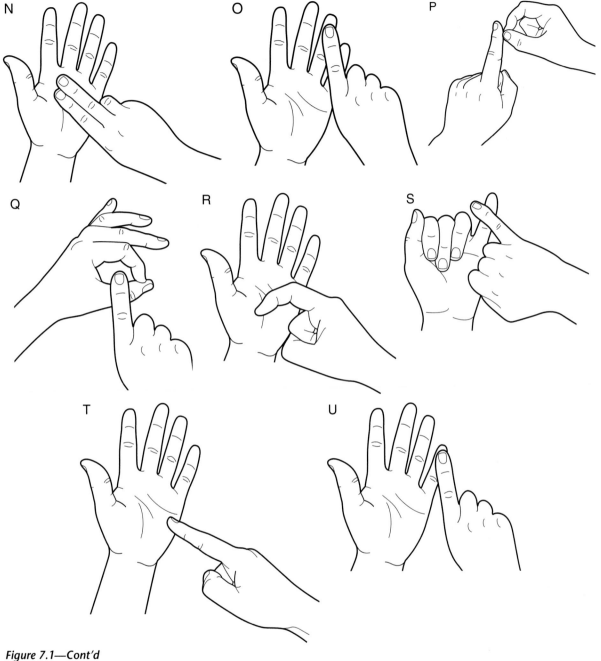

*Figure 7.1—Cont'd*

Some useful words/phrases are described:

- GOOD—closed hand with thumb extended—we are all familiar with the 'thumbs up' sign meaning 'good'. Variation in expression can

give the impression of 'quite good' or 'excellent'. The GOOD hand shape can be modified in a number of ways:

- KNOW—the thumb, clenched fingers facing outwards, touches the side of the forehead.

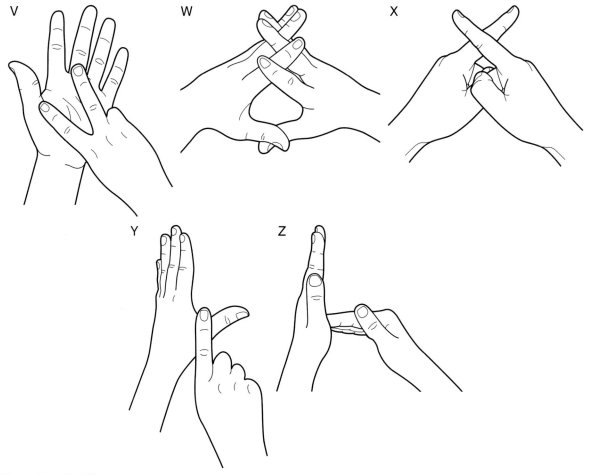

*Figure 7.1—Cont'd*

- CLEVER—the right thumb, clenched fingers turned inwards, moves across the forehead in a sharp movement.
- NICE—the thumb, clenched fingers facing inwards, moves across the chin from left to right.
- BRAVE—the right hand is flat against the chest, it moves forward closing the hand and extending the thumb in a sharp movement.
- WELL—both hands 'thumbs up' move down upper chest and twist forwards.
- BETTER—both hands 'thumbs up', the right thumb strikes the left thumb in a forward motion.
- BAD is formed by a clenched fist with the thumb on top of the fingers and the little finger extended. Again, a sign that you may have seen in general use (but is generally rude!). There are

many variations on this sign, most with negative connotations.
- ILL—both hands in BAD shape, move simultaneously down the chest with the little fingers against the body. This sign can also be 'tiredness' or 'general malaise'.
- WEAK—BAD shape, move right little finger down left arm. An alternative involves the index finger pointing into the cheek with a twisting movement.
- WRONG—BAD shape and bring the edge of the right little finger down onto the left open palm.
- WORST—both hands BAD shape, right little finger tip brushes sharply forward down against the left little finger. A single movement is worst, but repeated movements mean WORSE.

Parts of the hand

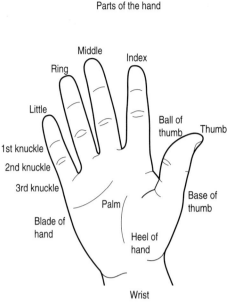

**Figure 7.2** Different parts of the hand illustrated here are used for conversation in British Sign Language.

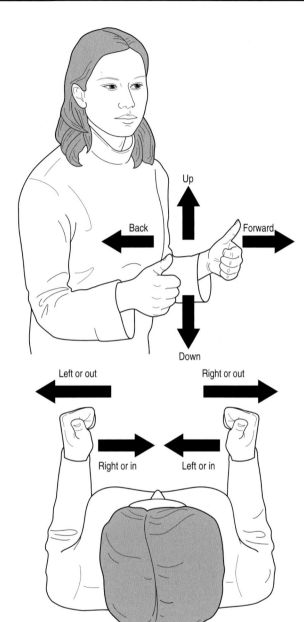

**Figure 7.3** The direction of hand movements is used to modify or emphasise a word or create a phrase in British Sign Language.

A clawed hand, fingers and thumb bent but open, expresses tension or agitation.

- WORRY—clawed hand makes circular movement near temple.
- MISERABLE—clawed hand pulls down in front of face.
- ANXIOUS—both hands clawed, move in alternate circles over the stomach.
- SCREAM—claw hand, palm near face, moves forward and up away from mouth.

Fluttering fingers relate to number in some form.

- MANY—open hands move apart, fluttering fingers.
- WHEN—fingers of right hand flutter at side of chin.
- HOW OLD—fingers of open hand flutter in front of nose with questioning facial expression.

Different areas of the body are used for specific types of signs i.e.:

The forehead is the mind area and KNOW has already been described.

- THINK—the right index finger is put against the forehead: a sign you may have seen used in general use.
- REMEMBER—clawed hand closes sharply to fist at temple.

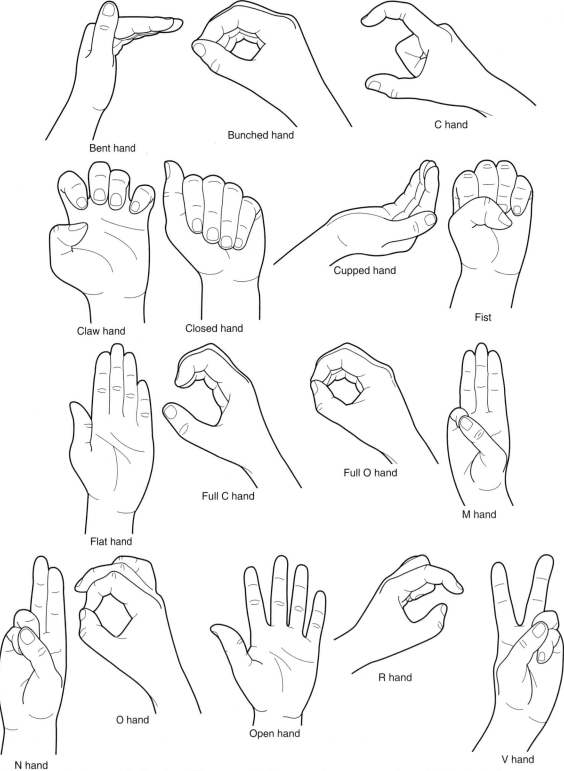

**Figure 7.4** The shape of the hand modifies or emphasises a word or creates a phrase in British Sign Language.

- FORGET—right hand closed to make an 'O' shape, moves away from the forehead and opens up.
- CONFUSE—point to temple with right index finger, then two open hands, palms down, cross sharply.

Eye or eyes:

- a V hand represents the direction in which the eyes are looking and for READ—the right hand moves from the eye to sweep twice along the left palm.

The ear is usually related to signs about hearing:

- HEAR—is a cupped hand behind the ear and HEARING—is the 'good' hand shape moving from the ear to the chin.
- DEAF is signed using two fingers of the right hand (as in finger spelling 'N') touching the ear.
- NOISE—the index finger on the right hand makes circular movements around the ear.

Sounds connected with speech usually start at the mouth:

- SPEAK—the index finger of the right hand moves backwards and forwards from the mouth.
- TALK—both hands are closed with the index finger extended. The right hand moves to the mouth then bangs on top of the left hand twice, at right angles to it.
- EXPLAIN—the right index finger touches the mouth, then two flat hands rotate around each other in forward circles.

The nose is often connected with signs about age. The nose is also used when signs about falseness and pretence are made:

- HOW OLD or AGE—fluttering fingers in front of nose.
- FALSE—closed hand with middle finger extended touches the nose, then twists and points forward.

The side of the chin relates to days and date:

- DAY—the index finger touches the side of the face.
- YESTERDAY—the right index finger is held on the side of the chin and then drops down backwards over the shoulder.
- TOMORROW—the right index finger touches the side of the chin, then the hand swings forward and down, finishing with the palm up.

The bosom or breast is often associated with feelings of passion. The chest is often the area where affection can be expressed, also desires, physical and emotional feelings.

- FEEL—index fingers of both hands brush up the body from waist to upper trunk.
- LOVE—open hands crossed at wrists are held on the chest.
- LIKE (prefer) flat hand taps chest twice.
- NEED—right flat hand, held on right side above waist, brushes down, twisting to palm down.
- HUNGRY—the right hand moves round in circles over the stomach.
- PLEASED—flat hand rubs in a circular movement on the chest, not to be confused with:
- SORRY—where a closed fist is moved round in circles on the chest.

A more detailed account of signed vocabulary can be found in the books referenced at the end of the chapter and the RNID website has an interactive section on signing which can be accessed from the home page (RNID 2006).

## An appropriate environment

Deaf people who rely on lip-reading and signing as their main method of communication will require an environment appropriate to their needs. Chris Harrowell, an architect and access consultant (Deafworks 1999) suggested the following:

- Clear, well-lit and safe routes to buildings and car parks.
- Video entry phones with acknowledgement light to show the door has been activated (may be used for entry to maternity unit/birth centre at night).
- Avoid car parking barriers which require a spoken request to raise the barrier.
- Minimise extraneous noise in a room, e.g. air-conditioning, electric fans or equipment.
- Minimise glare so people's faces can be seen clearly, use blinds or screens to block out glare.
- Avoid surfaces that reflect light such as highly reflective glass counters.
- Do not use very highly patterned wall coverings that impair the ability to see clearly.

- Avoid very harsh light which makes facial features flat and shadowless—this interferes with lip-reading and signing.
- Balance access with confidentiality, for example use frosted glass or screens to prevent a lip-reading person from overseeing the conversation.
- When selecting paints or surfaces during refurbishment, choose a matt surface.
- If people are wearing hearing aids, use a loop system to enhance their hearing.
- Make sure there are visual indicators in lifts, and use electronic display systems rather than information over a Tannoy system.
- Use visual fire alarm systems.
- Subtitles on screens and emergency textual information.

These strategies would be advantageous to any person entering a hospital/clinic environment and not just the deaf or hearing impaired.

## MAKATON

BSL is not the only sign language used in this country. Makaton began as a research project which aimed to find an effective method of communication between deaf adults who also had learning difficulties. The name stems from the three people who devised it: *Ma*rgaret Walker, a Speech Therapist, *Ka*thy Johnston and *TON*y Cornforth, both visitors at a Psychiatric Hospital. Makaton is related to BSL but is not a natural development of sign language as it was created for a particular purpose. Kyle and Woll (1985) cite Walker and Armfield (1982) who said that Makaton was designed to provide a controlled method of teaching 350 signs to people who were language compromised, for example children with Down's syndrome or cerebral palsy, and other children/adults with learning disabilities where BSL could not be used (see Chapter 9). It is used to provide a basic means of communication; to encourage expressive speech where possible; and to develop an understanding of language through signs, where there would not otherwise have been one. This aid to communication has often been demonstrated to be a critically important step towards interaction and to spoken language.

Makaton is at heart a training programme and to date over 50 000 people from all walks of life have taken the Makaton programme. Makaton does share some common signs with BSL, being based on it in the UK. There are, however, many differences and the two should not be confused: BSL or Makaton are recognised by the user, whether with special needs or deafness.

A woman with learning disabilities who becomes pregnant will probably have her own support worker and issues around the care of such a woman have been discussed in Chapter 5.

## MIDWIFERY CARE

Communication services are available to help deaf and hearing people communicate with each other. When a deaf woman arranges a booking appointment make sure that she is asked what type of support she would prefer. As you may have to book the services some time in advance, make sure that the appointment is given in time for the services to be put in place. Allow extra time for interaction at appointment.

A BSL/English interpreter interprets from one language to another and has been trained to do this. A deaf woman may also bring a signing partner with her but it is better if an interpreter is present as she may be in an abusive relationship that is not known about. If an interpreter is not available, the Royal National Institute for the Deaf (RNID), which represents nine million deaf or hard-of-hearing people in the UK, can provide video interpreting (RNID 2006). This service allows organisations to comply with the DDA 1995, part of which came into force on 19th July 2003. This service is like using any interpreter but they will appear on a video screen.

There are over 50 000 people who use BSL as their first or preferred method of communication and only 200 trained interpreters. Previously it might have taken a week or more before an interpreter could have been accessed whereas now with this method the service can be accessed at short notice. The service connects a deaf and hearing person by videophone to an interpreter at RNID offices. Signing can then be seen and interpreted to the hearing person, whose response can then be signed back to the deaf person. RNID has placed 42 videophones in sites around the country including police help desks, medical settings, Social Services departments and Citizen's Advice Bureaux (RNID

2006). It would be worth checking if such a service is available in the area you work. Some deaf people have purchased their own videophones and some mobile phones can be used in a similar way.

Lip-speakers may be used if the hard-of-hearing or deaf person can lip-read. The lip-speaker repeats what a person is saying without using their voice. They produce the shape of the words clearly on their lips, using facial expression and gestures (Butler 2004). If the deaf person does not understand what is being said, the lip-reader may also use finger spelling if asked. The lip-speaker can also speak what the lip-reader is saying and this can aid communication. A lip-speaker must be trained and is bound by rules of confidentiality. As normal speech is very fast, a lip-speaker will only speak what is relevant, without losing sense of what is being said. A highly qualified lip-speaker manages more than 120 words per minute (see Box 7.1 for tips for using a lip-speaker). Lip-speakers are in short supply, as are interpreters, and may need booking a few weeks in advance.

If the hard-of-hearing woman who uses a hearing aid wishes to attend parent education classes with or without her partner, then a loop system may be made available. This entails a cable that circles the listening area and a loop amplifier to reduce or cut out background noise. This may enable the deaf person to keep up with what is being said. It is also better if a woman sits near the front and there is a clear view of the speaker's mouth so that speech can be lip-read (Iqbal 2004).

It is not only face-to-face communication that needs to be considered but contact is often needed from a distance. Many deaf people have textphones which have a small screen and keyboard so that their message can be typed and sent as words rather than speech. If a woman has her lead midwife's mobile phone number she can communicate using text either with her own mobile phone or her textphone. Whichever method is used, it is important that a woman can contact her midwife for advice, especially when in labour or if she develops problems. Midwives can telephone the maternity unit and inform the hospital team of the situation so that they are prepared for a woman's admission. In an ideal situation every hospital ward or clinic where the public may need to contact would have a textphone as part of standard equipment. Until then mobile phones present the best option.

An additional source of help for deaf women during their childbirth experience is a book called 'Pregnancy and birth a guide for deaf women' by Sabina Iqbal (1996). This is a comprehensive guide similar to other pregnancy books with contact numbers that women might find useful. It has some good diagrams and photographs to meet the needs of women who are profoundly deaf and have BSL as their first language. It also contains stories from deaf women about their birth experiences which makes interesting reading. The book is also a useful resource for healthcare professionals as it offers information and insight into issues that deaf women and their professional helpers may need to address.

## Issues to consider when providing midwifery care

Common sense should prevail in the birthing room. There should be good lighting and as little extraneous noise as possible. Midwives should be familiar with each woman's individual situation and how best to communicate with her. If signing is needed, the presence of birth partner/relative who can sign is required as many women do not want an interpreter present at this intimate time (Iqbal 2004). If a woman lip-reads, then midwives and other carers should ensure that their face can be seen clearly when talking. If a woman's partner is also deaf then his needs must also be considered.

---

### Box 7.1 Useful tips when using a lip-speaker

- You prepare the lip-speaker first with a little background information, particularly if specialist words or phrases are being used.
- The deaf or hard-of-hearing person meets the lip-speaker in advance so that they can find the preferred method of communication and the deaf person can get used to the lip-speaker's mouth shapes.
- The deaf person and the lip-speaker sort out between themselves what finger spelling, if any, may be required. Also the ideal distance between the two for communication and good lighting needs to be discussed.
- The lip-speaker confirms rest breaks and mealtimes.

The conduct of the birth should have been discussed during pregnancy and birth plans devised accordingly. If an emergency arises it is important to talk to a woman and not just to her birth partner as she has to understand what is happening. Women have often complained about people talking to their partners and not to them which made them feel stupid (Iqbal 2004).

Postnatally it can be difficult for a deaf woman as she may be unable to talk to the other women in the ward, thus feeling isolated. There may also be problems with hearing her baby cry and this can lead to anxieties from other women and staff on the ward that the baby is not getting enough attention. Use of a vibrating pad that responds to a baby's cry can be helpful but would need a woman to be in a single room as it would respond to other babies' cries. Breast-feeding should be encouraged and it can allow women to feel in control. All help, support and information should be given as normal with use made of illustrations rather than too much written text.

Women will probably feel more confident in their own homes where they have access to their own deaf aids and support from family or partners. However, isolation may be an issue after a few weeks when visitors are less. Midwives should be aware of this and be alert for signs of post-natal depression. The services of an interpreter may be warranted to maintain confidentiality; women may not want to admit to feeling depressed in front of family or partners. The Deaf Parenting Project at DPPi (Disability, Pregnancy and Parenthood International—see Chapter 9) has a library service with information leaflets and books which are useful to deaf parents and there may be local deaf clubs which can provide support. Midwives may need to liaise with health visitors and family doctors to ensure continued care.

Further discussion about pertinent issues and a case scenario to illustrate what support is needed and how it can be given can be found in Chapter 3.

## DEAF-BLIND PEOPLE

It is estimated that there are 24 000 deaf-blind people in Britain (Butler 2004). But this figure is thought to be underestimated as there are potentially more deaf-blind people when the very elderly population is included. Many elderly people do not register as deaf-blind as they may be in nursing homes or just consider sensory loss to be a part of growing old (Butler 2004).

Someone who was born deaf-blind, or developed it at an early age, may not see their condition as sensory loss, just part of who they are. If deafness-blindness has developed over the years they may have had time to adapt to the condition, particularly if it is a hereditary disease and they can relate to other affected family members. A fairly common condition which results in deafness/blindness is Usher's syndrome which manifests with progressive hearing loss and retinitis pigmentosa (RNIB 2006) (see Chapter 8 for more details about retinitis pigmentosa). The person affected with this condition may have speech if their hearing was good enough in the early years and this can aid their ability to communicate. If the deafness/blindness happened as the result of an accident, then the situation is more difficult for the individual and it takes time to develop coping strategies.

Stigma is attached to sensory impairment and people are spoken to as 'though we are daft, not deaf/blind' (Butler 2004). Comments like 'people don't let me do things for myself — they think I'm incapable, but I'm not — I can do anything .....' are often voiced by those with sensory loss. People who have dual sensory impairment experience a degree of impairment far greater than the sum of the two individual impairments (Butler 2004). If they only have a hearing loss, they depend on other senses such as sight to compensate. If there is sight loss then development of more acute hearing is compensatory. But when sight and hearing are both lost then touch, taste and smell are the only senses left and compensation is more limited. There is a danger that the individual may become very isolated.

The accepted definition of deafness-blindness from the Department of Health is: 'Persons are regarded as deaf-blind if their combined sight and hearing impairment causes difficulties with communicating, access to information and mobility' (Butler 2004, p 11). Social Services have a duty to provide this specific support for deaf-blind people under the DDA 1995 and there are guide communicators who are professionals trained to support individuals with dual sensory loss (see Box 7.2 for

## Box 7.2 Areas where someone with dual sensory impairment may need help

- Communication.
- Information.
- Emotional support.
- Counselling.
- Mobility.
- Equipment.
- Independence.

areas of help that someone with dual sensory loss is likely to require). Guide communicators can help to relieve isolation, help the individual to retain independence, can act as an advocate and provide information and also provide respite for the family carers. The areas where a guide communicator can help are:

- Accompanying the deaf-blind person to the GP/clinic/hospital.
- Visiting friends and relatives or other social events.
- Assisting them with their shopping.
- Helping them communicate in a one-to-one setting or in a group.
- Supporting the deaf-blind person using aids such as a loop system and vibrating alarms.
- Helping the person make telephone calls.
- Assisting them with claiming benefits, receiving payments or paying bills.
- Reading and writing correspondence.
- Ensuring medication is taken accurately.
- Helping with exercise and healthy living (Butler 2004).

## Approaching someone with dual loss

It is difficult to imagine what it is like to be deaf and blind. However, it is worth remembering that visual impairment does not necessarily mean living in total darkness as in some cases the vision is very distorted or 'bits of the picture' are missing (as in diabetic retinopathy). It is similar for hearing loss. A deaf person may be able to hear very loud noises or have tinnitus or other abnormal noises in their ears.

If someone has dual sensory loss and is dependent on other people for care it must be difficult sitting waiting for something to happen. When a person has a visitor they may have no idea who is visiting or what is going to happen which may give a sense of vulnerability. However, visiting people with dual sensory loss helps to prevent them from becoming isolated. Some tips on approaching people with dual sensory loss are provided by Sarah J Butler (2004):

- Approach the person from the front or side so that if they have any vision they can see you.
- Try using clear speech first, speaking closely to the person.
- If there is no response, try a light touch on the upper arm and leave your hand there so that they can feel it.
- If they do not want to communicate with you, they may 'shy away'.
- If clear speech does not get their attention, try block—'writing' capital letters on the person's hand to spell out words (manual alphabet for the deaf-blind discussed later).
- They will usually have some method of communicating so try and get them to explain what it is (depends on extent of visual/auditory loss).

Approaching someone for whom touch is culturally inappropriate, for example Muslim women, may be best done by asking a member of the family to tell them you are there. Working with the family may help to overcome the deaf-blind person's reluctance to communicate with anyone outside the family.

## Communication using deaf-blind manual and block

As a teenager I used to cycle with the Manchester and District Tandem Cycling Club for the Blind. The sighted person was in front and the blind person at the back, often with their feet up! There were two deaf-blind people in the club. Both had developed their sensory loss after they had learned to speak. Because they could respond to the finger spelling with speech it made it easier for the person communicating.

It may be that a deaf-blind woman who presents at antenatal clinic will have a similar method of communicating. If a woman with dual sensory loss becomes pregnant she will need a lot of support from her guide communicator and also from midwives and maternity services. Many women will be used to communicating with other people using the deaf-blind manual. This entails spelling out words on a person's fingers and hand. It is quite easy to learn but requires patience and is fairly time-consuming. If a deaf-blind person has been using this method of communication for many years they become very fast at spelling the words out which may be difficult for someone receiving the message.

## Deaf-blind manual alphabet

Block is simply spelling block capitals on a deaf-blind person's palm (Fig. 7.5). There is a set way of writing the letters i.e. making smooth movements with contact on the hand at all times. It is easy to learn but relies on the deaf-blind person being able to feel the writing on their palm. If the person has an illness which interferes with this sensation then communication may be difficult and another

method must be found. Another problem is that the user and the person trying to communicate need to be literate and able to spell. Another consideration is that some people do not like being touched or having their personal space invaded by someone sitting close to them and holding their hand. Sarah Butler (2004) describes one such case where a compromise was reached by using plastic alphabet letters to spell out words instead. The deaf-blind person could feel the shape, decipher the message and then spell out a response which seemed to work quite well.

Whatever the form of communication it is important that a deaf-blind person knows when you are leaving otherwise they are left trying to communicate with someone who is not there which could lead to embarrassment. Individual agreements can be made as to what this sign might be. It could be a squeeze of the hand or pat on the shoulder, as long as each party understands what it means. Whilst communication may be limited, it is essential that

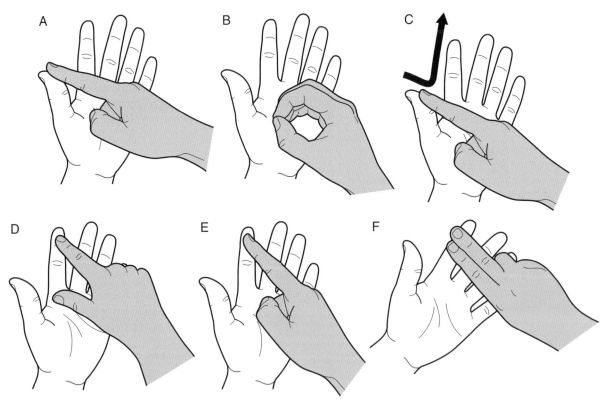

*Figure 7.5* Signs for deaf-blind people similar to British Sign Language but of necessity they have to be tactile on the palm of the recipient's hand.

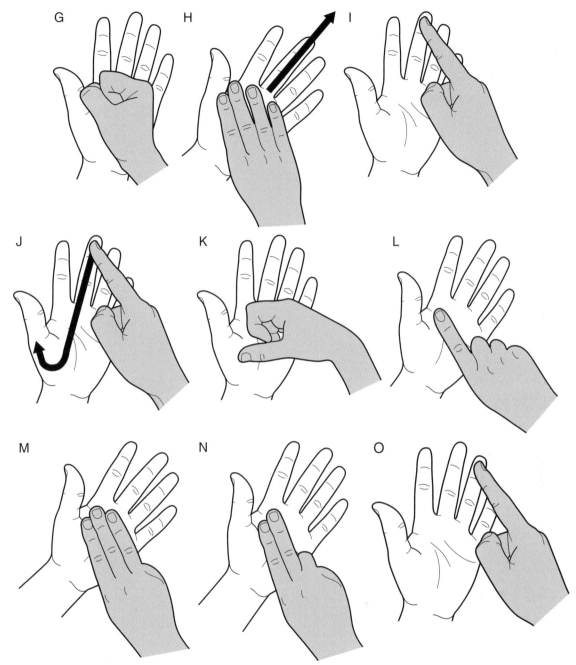

*Figure 7.5—Cont'd*

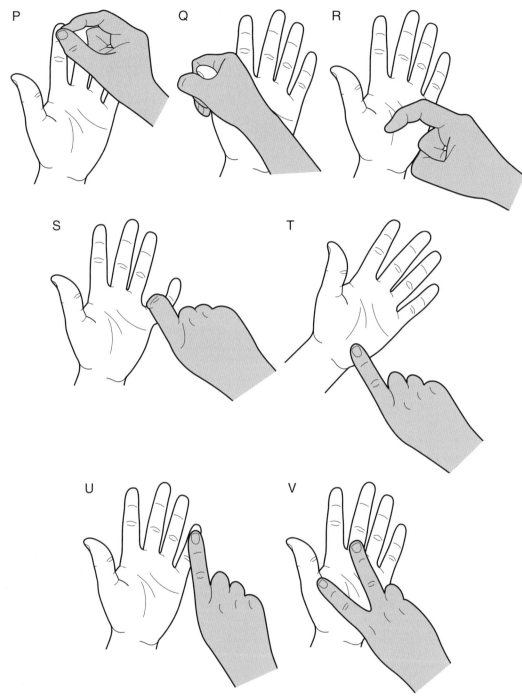

*Figure 7.5—Cont'd*

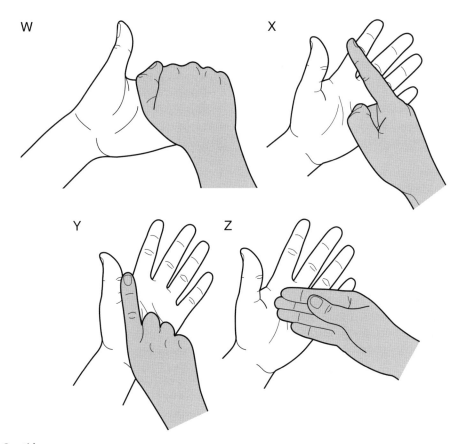

*Figure 7.5—Cont'd*

an attempt is made to stop deaf-blind people from feeling isolated.

## Midwifery care for women with dual sensory loss

Midwifery care that is provided for all women is meant to be holistic and 'woman-centred' (DOH 1993). It is important that midwives understand what women need and desire so that appropriate care can be given. Home visits to a woman with dual sensory loss would be helpful as a midwife could see what facilities she had to help her with her day-to-day living, and also meet her partner, carers or guide communicator. This would then facilitate a team approach to care which would provide a woman with the best and most suitable service.

Place of birth should be discussed and a woman offered home birth if thought appropriate. This would enable her to give birth within an environment in which she is familiar, with her partner and family present if desired. If home birth is not an option, then a visit to the birthing area would be useful to assist her in becoming familiar with the environment to help allay fears. If she is attending antenatal clinic a guide communicator should be present, especially to explain all the screening tests which may be offered and any procedures which may be carried out. Imagine being deaf-blind and having to undergo a vaginal examination: unless the woman understands what is being done and why, it would feel like an assault. Sensitive care with the appropriate support should enable the deaf-blind woman to have a fulfilling birth experience.

## BLIND AND PARTIALLY SIGHTED

Visual impairment is caused by a range of diseases and conditions which may or may not have been present at birth. It is difficult to imagine total darkness and never having been able to see if one is sighted. For the person blind from birth it is all they have ever known and therefore is part of who they are.

People who have progressive loss of vision will have been able to learn what colours are and what things look like, and will retain a memory of this unless they were too young to understand when sight was lost. It may be difficult for sighted people to explain what they can see as sight is a very individual thing; people with visual loss due to varying conditions may see things differently (Butler 2004).

Some eye conditions can be treated and cured while others can be controlled and deterioration prevented. Others may become progressively worse as there is no available treatment. It is important that visual impairment is properly diagnosed so that an affected individual is aware of the potential prognosis.

The Royal National Institute for the Blind (RNIB) is a national organisation that provides practical ideas and advice for people visually impaired. They can be accessed on their website where different pages offer information and support. One such page is called 'Parent's Place' (RNIB 2006) and is for parents who are visually impaired or have children with sight problems. They are currently offering information about a pack that is useful for women and midwives called 'Having a baby resource pack' which has been available since March 2006. The pack was produced by Disability, Pregnancy and Parenthood International (DPPi) (see Chapter 9) and it is available in large print, Braille, audio and Daisy—Digital Accessible Information System— which offers standardisation of talking books.

Midwives may find useful information from the RNIB website when planning parent education. The site offers practical advice about making things easier to see such as making things bigger, using large print, or photocopying normal print and enlarging it. Text and graphics are easier to see if they are brighter than the background, and thick black felt tip pen will stand out if written on a white back-ground. Making things bolder helps those things to stand out so looking at the colour of backgrounds can be important when designing posters, or putting things on notice boards.

Lamps which can move directionally will aid reading as the reader can shine the light directly onto the page to make it clearer. Better lighting generally can improve vision, as can avoidance of shadows. Magnifying glasses are particularly useful in the home as they help a visually impaired person do many of their daily chores, e.g. sorting out the washing into appropriate loads, setting the oven to the correct temperature and undertaking minor repairs, reading small print on labels, instructions on domestic appliances or correspondence. But they may also be useful during clinic or hospital attendance, enabling a woman to read information and clarify understanding while a midwife or doctor is still present.

Clocks and watches with large numbers can be bought and the availability of such timepieces during labour may be invaluable for a woman enabling her independence in timing her contractions and monitoring her progress in labour.

Another good RNIB web page (RNIB 2006) which midwives may find useful provides information with photographs to help a sighted person guide someone who is blind. Although some visually impaired people carry a white stick while others have a guide dog to assist them in walking safely, they may appreciate help particularly if they are in unfamiliar surroundings. Sighted people may be hesitant about offering help to a blind person but the best way is to ask how they would like to be guided and comply as far as is safe. It is important, however, that anyone offering help introduces themselves as a blind person may not be aware that help is on hand.

If there is enough room, walking side-by-side with a helper taking a person's arm is effective. In a crowded place or on a narrow pavement walking single file is needed and in this case the helper moves an arm back so that he/she can be held onto. If there is a kerb or step up or down, this must be explained first before negotiating it. When climbing or descending stairs a blind person needs to hold the hand rail to help with steadiness. An arm tucked into the helper's as the stairs are used will indicate the steepness of the stairs as the arm moves. When reaching the top or bottom care must be taken to ensure the person knows that ground level has been reached.

Lifts are probably easier than escalators to negotiate and many public places have 'speaking lifts' which announce when the doors are opening, closing or at which floor the lift has stopped. Doorways can be difficult to negotiate and if guiding a person it is important to tell them whether the door opens towards or away from them. Putting the flat hand against the door and sliding it along until the handle is felt will help on this aspect and helps with closing the door. If going through a door together it is best if the helper is away from the hinge side of the door.

Many doors in hospitals are automatic and make considerable noise which can be off-putting. A guide should explain this, and the need to stand back until the doors are fully open. Swing and revolving doors and turnstiles are best avoided particularly if a guide dog is used as it may be confused by the barriers posed by these types of entrances.

## Midwifery care for blind or partially sighted women

Communication may be easier with a blind or partially blind woman as they can hear, speak and engage in a conversation. However, visiting an unfamiliar building with many hazards can prove challenging and it is helpful if a sighted person can attend with them. When a woman visits hospital it is important that whoever meets her, receptionist, maternity assistant or midwife, introduces themselves and stands near enough that she knows where they are. She should then be guided, with her partner or companion, to a seat and made comfortable. If she has to move to another area in the clinic, or give a urine sample for testing, someone should be available to offer help.

Any procedures, even taking blood pressure, must be explained in greater detail than normal when a woman is unable to see. Women may require assistance onto an examination couch with guidance as to the width to prevent rolling off. During an abdominal examination it will help a mother to feel her baby if the midwife moves a woman's hands with her own, explaining what she can feel and using a sonicaid so that the mother can hear her baby's heart rate. This is often a valuable experience for all mothers but may be particularly useful to help mother-baby bonding for a mother who is unable to see an ultrasound picture of her baby. Following the examination assistance may be needed to get off the couch and be comfortably seated before discussing any necessary issues.

A woman may want to attend parent education classes although any visual elements e.g. a baby bath or different positions for labour may be better addressed in a one-to-one session where she could feel what was being shown. A guided tour of the unit visiting the birthing room in particular would be useful. Taking her to an empty room to enable her to feel the bed and have a demonstration of some of the equipment, for example the Entonox, may help alleviate any fears. However, a blind or partially sighted woman may feel more confident in her own home that is familiar to her with her own equipment, and home birth may be a feasible option. This would enable her to have the people she wants around her which would also promote her confidence during labour and birth. Even if she has a hospital birth, transfer home as soon as possible would allow her that control at home.

---

### CONCLUSION—KEY POINTS

- Forward planning is essential as soon as a woman is referred for services.
- For women with sensory impairment a high standard of communication is essential.
- Partners should be included in care as they will often be the most appropriate person for communication but the need for confidentiality must be considered.
- Midwives may find an ability to use simple BSL signs beneficial for everyone.
- Special services are available e.g. interpreters, text by phone.
- Alternative ways of providing information may need to be planned e.g. in Braille or pictures.
- One-to-one parent education is likely to be the most effective.

- A visit to the place for birth will enable a woman and her partner to become familiar with the environment and enable forward planning.
- A woman's own home is likely to be the place where she feels most confident but may elicit feelings of isolation—midwives need to be aware of this and seek appropriate help and support for women.

## References

Butler S J 2004 Hearing and sight loss—a handbook for professional carers. Age Concern, London

Deafworks 1999 'Opening Up' in association with London Borough of Camden, Arts & Tourism, Deafworks, London

Department of Health (DoH) 1993 Changing Childbirth. Report of the Expert Maternity Group. HMSO, London

Disability Discrimination Act 1995 HMSO, London. Online. Available: http://www.drc-gb.org 12 September 2005

Iqbal S 2004 Pregnancy and birth—a guide for deaf women. RNID in association with the National Childbirth Trust, London

Kyle J G, Woll B 1985 Sign language—the study of deaf people and their language. Cambridge University Press, Cambridge

Miles D 1988 British Sign Language—a beginners guide. BBC Books, London

RNIB 2006 Internet website. Online. Available: http://www.rnib.org.uk 8 November 2006

RNID 2006 Internet website. Online. Available: http://www.rnid.org.uk 7 & 9 November 2006

Smith C 1990 Signs make sense—a guide to British Sign Language. Human Horizons Series. Souvenir Press (Educational and Academic), London

Smith C 1996 Sign language companion—a handbook of British signs. Human Horizons Series. Souvenir Press (Educational and Academic), London

## Further reading

Taylor G, Bishop J 1991 Being deaf: the experience of deafness. Pinter Publishers in association with the Open University, London

# 8 The interaction between specific conditions and the childbirth continuum

*Stella McKay-Moffat*

## INTRODUCTION

In the past women with certain medical or disabling conditions would have been advised by their doctors not to undertake pregnancy for fear of making their condition worse, having a damaged child because of the condition or the medication, or not being able to cope with caring for a baby or growing child. With increasing knowledge about conditions, improved care and medication, and the greater freedom individuals have to make informed choices, women are deciding to have children. However, medical understanding and evidence to offer women to help them to make choices is not always available.

This chapter contains details about specific disabling conditions that women undertaking pregnancy and childbirth may have. The list is not exhaustive and by necessity the section on each condition is just an overview, therefore you are strongly advised to read further. Table 8.1 displays key issues for easy reference.

Not included are general medical conditions, for example diabetes, epilepsy, heart, renal or respiratory disease, or psychiatric conditions. Although they may be debilitating and therefore cause '*disability*', they are outside the scope of this book and are generally addressed adequately in other texts. Learning disability is not dealt with as the spectrum of cause and effects are vast and are well covered in readily available specific texts. Chapter 5 comprehensively discusses issues for women with learning disability in relation to pregnancy and childbirth. If you come across a woman with a condition not mentioned in this chapter it is essential that you perform your own literature review to learn as much about the condition as possible in order to offer evidence-based care.

Midwives with or without a nursing background may know little about the common disorders that lead to disability therefore brief information is given about the actual condition, for example how it may affect the individual and the medication that may be used. Included are details about the possible influence the condition or medication may have on a pregnant woman and the fetus, as well as how the pregnancy may affect the condition. It must be remembered however, that each person is an individual hence these details should be considered as a guide only, as some women will have less complications, whilst others will have more than expected. Additionally, what one person considers unacceptable, another will feel is tolerable and worthwhile, for example levels of pain or disability.

Some conditions are congenital or may have developed in early childhood and have therefore been long standing. Others may be relatively newly acquired, for example following an accident. The way someone perceives their situation, lives their life and copes with domesticity and new situations is unlikely to be the same in the two groups. Moreover, how one person adapts to a specific circumstance will not necessarily be the same as someone else even if their condition or disability is the same. It must also be understood that 'invisible' disabilities need to be acknowledged i.e. even if someone outwardly looks well they may still have difficulties in some aspect(s) of daily living. Additionally, some

*Table 8.1*  Disabling conditions with significant factors associated with pregnancy

| Condition | Cause | Possible impairments/issues | Medication/management | Significance in pregnancy & childbirth |
|---|---|---|---|---|
| Cerebral palsy | Perinatal compromise/lack of oxygen | Motor function/paralysis<br>Limb spasticity<br>Swollen ankles<br>Fatigue<br>Speech & sensory loss<br>Epilepsy<br>Urinary incontinence | Skeletal muscle relaxants<br>Anti-epileptics e.g. carbamazepine, phenytoin, valporate—combined treatment sometimes used | Increased risk of NTD[a] with anti-epileptics—single therapy less so—consider regime preconception & advise folic acid 5mg daily<br>Tiredness & muscle spasm may worsen in pregnancy & triggered by labour<br>In labour attention to pressure areas, massage may relieve muscle spasm, poor leg abduction may mean adaptable positions for examinations & birth<br>Mother may need vitamin K prior to labour with some anti-epileptics (as well as neonate)<br>Breast-feeding possible depending on type of medication e.g. avoid with phenytoin & if fatigue is managed<br>Combined hormonal contraception may not be suitable if poor mobility as risk of DVT[b] |
| Fibromyalgia | Unclear | Muscle pain<br>Joint pain & stiffness<br>Tender points on the body<br>Fatigue<br>Gastro-intestinal disturbance<br>Depression/anxiety common | Aerobic exercise<br>Sleep treatment<br>Anti-depressants | Preconception advice regarding medication & folic acid<br>Tender points on body may increase<br>Uterine cramps similar to pre-term labour<br>Alternative positions, mobility, hydrotherapy during labour will ease muscle/joint pains<br>Breast-feeding if fatigue managed |

*table continued*

*table continued*

| Condition | Cause | Possible impairments/issues | Medication/management | Significance in pregnancy & childbirth |
|---|---|---|---|---|
| Multiple sclerosis (MS) | Autoimmune condition Loss of myelin sheath over nerves | Weak muscles, spasm, pain Paraesthesia Imbalance Fatigue Loss of sensation Impaired bladder & bowel function Vision & speech affected Cognitive changes Depression Symptoms worsen in the heat/fever | Immune suppressants e.g. cyclophosphamide, methotrexate, azathioprine Steroids e.g. prednisolone Muscle relaxants | Preconception—risk of fetal abnormality with some immune suppressants (see text) Condition may improve during pregnancy or fatigue, pain & paraesthesia may worsen PIH[c], pre-eclampsia, diabetes & infection risk when on steroids— loading dose needed in labour Avoid UTI[d] & anaemia Labour—spasms may be triggered by pain, examinations & full bladder; epidural may prevent spasms; onset of labour may not be perceived & precipitate birth (teach mother how to palpate uterine contractions); second stage expulsive urge may be absent; abduction of legs may be difficult— flexible examination & birth positions Postnatally—fatigue/ weakness may inhibit self-care, infant care & breast-feeding; drugs do not appear to be contraindicated in breast-feeding although high doses may be; MS relapses in some cases; combined hormonal contraception may be unsuitable if poor mobility (risk of DVT[b]) |

*table continued*

*table continued*

| Condition | Cause | Possible impairments/issues | Medication/management | Significance in pregnancy & childbirth |
|---|---|---|---|---|
| Myalgic encephalo-myelitis (ME) | Unclear—possible post-viral syndrome | Overwhelming fatigue for over 6 months<br>Muscular pain<br>Paraesthesia<br>Headache/migraine/vertigo<br>Sensitivity to light, noise, odours<br>Sleep disorder<br>Altered cognitive ability<br>Altered temperature control<br>Food allergy<br>Depression | Exercise programme<br>Complimentary therapies<br>Cognitive behavioural therapy<br>Diet modification with allergies<br>Serotonin re-uptake inhibitors e.g. fluoxetine & mild anti-depressants | Preconception advice—drugs contraindicated (sudden withdrawal must be avoided); ensure optimum general health/well-being; forward planning<br>Pregnancy may trigger a relapse/worsening of symptoms<br>Chronic fatigue may reduce ability for self-care, coping with labour & infant care—forward planning; adequate rest & support<br>Risk of DVT[b] if mobility reduced<br>Reduced ability to understand/remember information<br>Labour—respond to need for light, noise & temperature controls if relevant; sensitivity to fatigue/avoid undue stress<br>Postnatally—drugs contraindicated; forward planning to avoid exacerbating fatigue |
| Rheumatoid arthritis (RA) | Autoimmune condition | Painful, swollen joints of hands & feet, sometimes neck<br>Damaged/deformed joints may affect mobility<br>Fatigue | Anti-inflammatory drugs e.g. non-steroidal i.e. paracetamol, ibuprofen, steroids i.e. prednisolone<br>Immune suppressants (see MS above) | See MS above regarding drugs; ibuprofen should be avoided until after the first trimester & from 34 weeks (early fetal closure of ductus arteriosus)<br>Some remission may occur in first trimester, but mobility & fatigue may increase later<br>PIH[c], pre-term rupture of membranes, IUGR[e] risk<br>Labour—care with joints & pressure areas; caesarean section rate higher because of risks above |

*table continued*

*table continued*

| Condition | Cause | Possible impairments/issues | Medication/management | Significance in pregnancy & childbirth |
|---|---|---|---|---|
| | | | | Postnatally—infant care e.g. lifting/carrying; flare-up of condition common within 6 weeks; breast-feeding may worsen symptoms but if performed advise analgesia 30–60 minutes after each feed (less secreted in next feed); no clear contraindications to hormonal contraception |
| Spina bifida | Congenital condition linked with folic acid deficiency—variable levels of severity | Leg control/mobility Lack of sensation Continence—urostomy/colostomy may be used Pressure area compromise UTI[d] risk Latex allergy Anaemia risk from chronic infection Autonomic hyperreflexia (see text) | Management of continence Prevention of pressure sores/treatment of infection Regular screening/management of UTI[d] | Preconception—folic acid at higher dose of 4 mg; general advice to reach optimum health including infection screening/management Pregnancy—infection screening/management—possible prophylactic antibiotics; identify/treat anaemia—possible prophylactic iron; extra care with pressure areas; compromised respirations in late pregnancy—risk of respiratory infection, advise physiotherapy; DVT[b] risk due to immobility Labour—onset of labour may not be perceived (or wind-like symptoms) & precipitate birth (teach mother how to palpate uterine contractions); second stage expulsive urge may be absent but vaginal birth possible; compromised respirations/anaesthetic |

*table continued*

*table continued*

| Condition | Cause | Possible impairments/issues | Medication/management | Significance in pregnancy & childbirth |
|-----------|-------|------------------------------|------------------------|-----------------------------------------|
| | | | | risk; epidural probably unsuitable; autonomic hyyperreflexia (see text) Postnatally—perineal hygiene & pressure area care; UTI[d] risk increased; no contraindication to breast-feeding; combined hormone contraception not recommended because of DVT[b] risk |
| Spinal cord lesions | Injury | Depends on injury site As with spina bifida High lesions compromised respiration/cough reflex Skill in managing activities of daily living will depend on how recent the injury | As with spina bifida | Preconception as for spina bifida although 0.4 mg of folic acid enough Pregnancy—risk of IUGR[e]; otherwise as with spina bifida Labour—significant risk of autonomic hyperreflexia (see text) therefore CVP[f] line & cardiac monitoring—if epidural possible it may reduce the risk; otherwise as for spina bifida |
| Achondro-plasia | Genetic mutation of short arm of chromosome 4 75% cases new mutation i.e. not inherited 25% cases autosomal dominantly inherited | Short stature & limbs; bow legs & abnormal gait; distinctive fingers; large head with distinctive features; joint mobility changes; spinal curvature & narrowing causing neurological symptoms & pain, airway obstruction/apnoea Hydrocephalus Small/abnormal pelvis Obesity Chronic ear infection & deafness Normal life span & intelligence | Anti-inflammatory drugs Life-style adaptations to minimise joint damage Environmental/life-style modifications to manage height issues Treatment to minimise chronic ear infection & deafness | Preconception—genetic counselling: mother only 50% chance of condition & 50% chance normality Mother & father 50% chance of condition, 25% normality, 25% lethal condition Pelvic X-ray Pregnancy—fetal screening i.e. chorionic villus & amniocentesis, ultrasound scan; mobility & back pain worse—analgesia; lung capacity falls—monitor respiratory function; neck X-ray to prepare for possible intubation at surgery Labour—forward planning; caesarean section likely; monitor |

*table continued*

*table continued*

| Condition | Cause | Possible impairments/issues | Medication/management | Significance in pregnancy & childbirth |
|-----------|-------|----------------------------|----------------------|---------------------------------------|
| | | | | blood gasses; avoid neck extension & care with spine to prevent nerve damage & paralysis<br>Vein cannulation may be difficult<br>Continuous epidural with careful dose control *not* spinal<br>Postnatal—monitor post-op. respirations; practical help & support with infant care<br>Paediatric referral if baby affected—avoid neck & joint damage, monitor breathing during feeds, look for signs of hydrocephalus |
| Muscular dystrophy | A group of inherited muscle degenerating disorders | Progressive voluntary & involuntary muscle weakness, including the heart | Limited treatment<br>Physiotherapy<br>Anti-inflammatory drugs & steroids | Preconception—ensure optimum health; review medication; genetic counselling; assisted reproduction with pre-implantation screening<br>Pregnancy—ECG & pulmonary function<br>Increased muscle weakness & fatigue<br>Risk of miscarriage, pre-term birth, polyhydramnios & intrauterine death<br>Labour—continuous cardiac monitoring & blood gases<br>Vaginal birth possible but if caesarean section epidural safer than general anaesthetic<br>Atonic uterus possible but responds to oxytocin<br>Rapid cervical dilatation possible<br>Risk of post-partum haemorrhage if uterus atonic—oxytocin for |

*table continued*

*table continued*

| Condition | Cause | Possible impairments/issues | Medication/ management | Significance in pregnancy & childbirth |
|---|---|---|---|---|
| | | | | third stage Postnatal—respond to energy levels with support & help; breast-feeding possible depending on fatigue; combined hormone contraception not advised if mobility reduced as risk of DVT[b] |
| Deafness/ hearing impaired | 50–60% of early onset deafness due to autosomal dominant or recessive inheritance | Total or partial hearing loss May be deaf with speech or without depending on age hearing lost | Deaf aids to enhance any available hearing Use of sign language or lip reading | Preconception—genetic counselling Pregnancy—genetic screening; forward planning for help with communication & allow additional time; parent education requires alternative methods; visit to the maternity unit Labour & postnatal— forward planning for communication Paediatric referral if necessary |
| Blindness/ visual impairment | Some conditions dominant recessive or X-linked e.g. retinitis pigmentosa | Visual loss may be total or partial | Aids for partial vision e.g. magnifying lens, large print text, white or ultrasonic stick Guide dog Braille Audible literature | Preconception—genetic counselling Pregnancy—information in appropriate format; guidance moving round clinic/hospital as required; parent education requires alternative methods; visit to the maternity unit Labour—forward planning; detailed information on layout of room, what is going on/who is in the room Postnatal—as for labour; help & support with infant care |

[a]NTD = neural tube defect e.g. spina bifida.
[b]DVT = deep vein thrombosis, commonly in a vein in a calf muscle but can be in pelvic veins.
[c]PIH = pregnancy induced hypertension.
[d]UTI = urinary tract infection.
[e]IUGR = intrauterine growth restriction.
[f]CVP = central venous pressure line.

people with impairment do their best to hide this wanting not to broadcast their disability. Husbands' or partners' feelings and helping skills need to be taken into consideration and respected. They may have issues surrounding their own health or abilities particularly if they are disabled themselves. Finally, help from family, friends and assistants need to be taken into account, and their opinions and feelings recognised, as these could make considerable difference to pregnancy outcomes.

## MUSCULOSKELETAL IMPAIRMENT

There are numerous conditions that affect the musculoskeletal systems and many of the principles related to each situation are the same. Some of the conditions have a neurological basis in their origin. A few of the more common ones are included below.

## Cerebral palsy

Cerebral palsy is a condition that midwives are familiar with in that there is always concern for the fetus and neonate related to potential risk factors that may lead to the condition developing. The main symptom of the condition is motor impairment, often with spasticity, but the range of possible symptoms is wide and each individual will have very different levels of severity of effects. Following an extensive literature review Odding et al (2006) offer a very comprehensive insight into the incidence of the condition, the impairments that may occur and the risk factors associated with the condition developing. Their findings are summarised below.

It appears that the worldwide incidence of cerebral palsy has increased since the 1960s probably due to the increased survival of pre-term and small babies. Prevalence is greater in babies from low socio-economic families. The UK figures discovered by Odding et al are 3.33 per 1000 births in the most deprived population compared to 2.08 in the most affluent groups of society. This difference in rate remains noticeable even when birth weight is normal.

There are many possible causes of cerebral palsy although the cause may not actually be known. Odding et al's findings are summarised as follows:

- Intrauterine infection (chorioamnionitis)—greatest significance in low birth weight babies.
- Low birth weight.
- In utero death of a co-twin.
- Multiple pregnancy—increasing with number of babies and when the babies are *over* 2500 g.
- Ante-partum haemorrhage especially from placental abruption.
- Cerebral ischaemia.
- Instrumental delivery.
- Birth asphyxia—although this is apparently controversial—low Apgar at 5, 10 and 20 minutes.
- Perinatal infections.
- Neonatal convulsions.
- Neonatal jaundice.
- Neonatal infection.

Odding et al state that 20–80% of people with cerebral palsy may have additional conditions. The following list of possible conditions has again been summarised from their literature review:

- Physical fatigue—probably due to the energy needed for motor movement.
- Weak muscles from lack of use.
- Hemiplegia—paralysis of one side of the body.
- Diplegia—paralysis of similar parts each side of the body.
- Tetraplegia—paralysis of all four limbs.
- Epilepsy.
- Cognitive ability diminished i.e. learning difficulty—often associated with epilepsy.
- Impaired sensibility of hands.
- Chronic pain—foot and ankle common.
- Speech impairment—as many as 80%.
- Hearing impairment.
- Low visual acuity—possibly due to cerebral visual disturbance.
- Urinary incontinence.

The organisation SCOPE focuses on the needs of people with cerebral palsy and offers information and support. Their online information sheet related to pregnancy and parenthood for people with cerebral palsy (Scope 2005) offers key information and advice. Preconception care and advice will enable the medication taken for muscle spasm or epilepsy to be reviewed prior to conception as some drugs may be teratogenic i.e. they have the potential to harm the fetus. General health and fitness can be improved through diet and exercise and folic acid supplements. The support of a physiotherapist may be beneficial in planning an exercise programme that helps to increase strength and flexibility of muscles and joints.

There appears to be no increased risk of miscarriage, premature birth or a baby with cerebral palsy. During pregnancy symptoms may improve. Swollen ankles are common in people with cerebral palsy and this may worsen during pregnancy. Some women find muscle spasms and tiredness increase, and labour pain may initiate muscle spasms. Frequent changes of position, massage or bracing may help to lower the number and frequency of spasms. Epidural analgesia can be used during labour in some cases but may not be possible if muscle spasms prevent the woman from keeping still during and after the procedure (Scope 2005). Attention to pressure and friction areas must be given to avoid damage to skin during times of immobility or spasms.

When motor function is affected transfer to the examination couch or bed may be difficult and will be improved if the equipment is height adjustable. Welner & Temple (2004) discuss the possible difficulty in examining a woman if her lower limbs are particularly rigidly flexed. This may have an impact during labour for vaginal examination and the birth if abduction of legs is compromised. Alternative positions need to be explored during pregnancy with a 'dry run' of positions that will enable these processes to take place. Lateral or even a modified knees-chest position may be useful. Midwives working in conjunction with a woman will enable the best solutions to be found. A key point is to ensure that any change of position is undertaken slowly to minimise the risk of initiating spasms (Welner & Temple 2004).

Following the birth additional rest and adequate family support may be necessary to combat fatigue. If lack of strength is an issue in the upper limbs alternative strategies may need to be developed for handling the baby. The help of an occupational therapist could be elicited during pregnancy and afterwards to work with a mother and her midwife to find alternative acceptable solutions. Breast-feeding is not contraindicated unless the medication a mother is taking is prohibitive. Again, if upper limb strength and dexterity are a problem changes in position

and use of strategically placed supports for the baby may make feeding successful. If dexterity is impaired breast-feeding may be an easier option than making bottles of formula.

Contraception advice postnatally is offered to mothers if they wish it. If dexterity is impaired the diaphragm is unlikely to be suitable. If lower limb immobility is present the combined oral contraceptive pill is probably unsuitable because of the risk of deep vein thrombosis (DVT), and is not suitable when breast-feeding. The progesterone-only pill or other progesterone methods may be suitable depending on any medication a mother is taking. An intrauterine device or system may be suitable, unless a woman is unable to abduct her legs due to spasticity which makes insertion problematic.

## Fibromyalgia

This is a complex non-inflammatory condition that leads to widespread muscular pain, joint pain and stiffness, and tender points on examination throughout the body. Csuka (2004) states that this tenderness is a cardinal sign for diagnosis of the condition, which is more common in women than men, and may have been present for many years prior to diagnosis. Csuka warns that diagnosis is difficult and misdiagnosis is common as symptoms are in many ways similar to osteoarthritis and rheumatoid arthritis, but the joints show no signs of damage. Additional symptoms include tiredness, non-satisfying sleep, gastro-intestinal problems, and swollen joint sensations (Csuka 2004, Schaefer & Black 2005). It is a relatively recently recognised condition that Cramer (1998) explains has similar symptoms to chronic fatigue syndrome (see myalgic encephalomyelitis below) and can cause the sufferer feelings of lack of control and loss of self-esteem. The American College of Rheumatology recognised the condition in 1989 (Schaefer & Black 2005).

The aetiology of the condition is unclear and medicinal relief of symptoms is patchy according to Csuka (2004). Aerobic exercise, treatment of sleep disorder, general health improvement and treatment of any concurrent depression or anxiety appear to be the best management (Cusak 2004). Cramer (1998) notes that, although short-term muscle activity that requires strength is affected during exercise, the cardio-vascular element of exercise is not. The most significant symptom is the fatigue that disrupts daily life, work and relationships, and the simultaneous depression (Schaefer & Black 2005). It is unclear if the depression is part of the syndrome or as a result of the debilitation that it leads to.

From their comprehensive literature review and Schaefer's studies of women with fibromyalgia Schaefer & Black (2005) offer some valuable information related to the childbirth continuum. Preconception care and advice should encompass discussion about medication; diet, including folic acid supplements; and recognition and management of any anaemia. Women, their partners and families need to discuss how the increased tiredness associated with pregnancy will impact on their lives in order to plan and develop coping mechanisms.

Spontaneous miscarriage appears not to be increased, but symptoms of the condition may increase and are similar to those experienced by many women during pregnancy, for example back pain, nausea and vomiting. Schaefer & Black advise women to consider these increased symptoms as pregnancy orientated although they do warn that uterine cramps may also occur similar to those of pre-term labour. Tender points in the body may become worse due to the increased pressure from the growing uterus and this may make lying on the side too painful. Analgesics may be needed.

During labour adequate analgesia is important and every effort is made to ensure a mother's comfort by using heat e.g. warm water, alternative positions and mobilisation, for example using a birthing ball and walking to maintain joint movements and lessen pain especially in knees, elbows and hips. Strategically placed cushions or foam wedges may help when lying down. Bright light and noise need to be avoided as these factors may increase pain perception and fatigue.

The postnatal period continues with the chronic fatigue and skeletal and muscle pain. Help and support from a woman's family is important and she needs to ensure that she has adequate rest. Breastfeeding is possible provided that the additional support is available and that a mother does obtain the additional rest. Varying a baby's position at the breast will help to alleviate pain on the sensitive points.

It must be remembered that this is an 'invisible' condition that can be excessively disabling therefore mothers need to receive sensitive care. Practitioners need to acknowledge that pain and fatigue are what a woman says they are, thereby showing respect for a mother's symptoms.

## Multiple sclerosis (MS)

This autoimmune condition may be 'invisible' as a disability in the early stages. It leads to a patchy loss of myelin that covers nerves of the spinal cord and brain, thus slowing nerve impulses. Although variable symptoms occur, it commonly presents with weakness, imbalance and fatigue. Additional symptoms may include bladder dysfunction e.g. frequency, incontinence or retention (Balzarro & Appell 2004) and bowel dysfunction, muscular spasms, stiffness and pain, difficulty with speech and vision, loss of sensation and depression. The depression is thought to have a physiological basis although the mechanism is unclear (Olkin 2004). Olkin also explains that people with MS may have cognitive difficulties and bouts of laughing or crying not associated with mood stimulation. MS symptoms can be made worse by fever or a hot environment (Neild 2006). The condition affects young adults (Lorenzi & Ford 2002) and is more common in women than men in a ratio of 2:1 (Olkin 2004). It is characterised by periods of relapse and remission but the disease is progressive over a number of years. However the prognosis appears uncertain and distinctive to the individual.

Neild (2006) explains that a woman's fertility appears to be unaffected by the condition and pregnancy has no long-term affects on the progress of the disease. Although not considered an inherited condition, there does appear to be a higher incidence of MS in the children of parent(s) with the condition (Neild 2006). Preconception advice would include discussion about the drugs taken to modify the condition or alleviate symptoms and these may need to be stopped for 3 months prior to conception. Drugs taken to modify the condition e.g. methotrexate and cyclophosphamide are not suitable during pregnancy (Ferrero et al 2004) while others are safer, including steroids e.g. prednisolone (Baschat & Weiner 2004). Higher rates of congenital abnormalities have been noted with methotrexate and cyclophosphamide

(Chakravarty et al 2003, Gordon 2004, Le Gallez 1999) and Gordon (2004) warns that steroids are associated with high blood pressure, pre-eclampsia, diabetes and infection risk. It must be remembered that if a woman has been taking steroids during pregnancy she is likely to need a loading dose during labour (Baschat & Weiner 2004) to enable her body to cope with the additional stress. Some drugs e.g. azathioprine and cyclosporine have a slight risk of causing intrauterine growth retardation (IUGR) and prematurity (Ferrero et al 2004).

During pregnancy the condition often improves or is stable (Ferrero et al 2004, Lorenzi & Ford 2002) especially during the third trimester (Vukusic et al 2004). This improvement is thought to be as a result of the altered immune state of the mother (that prevents rejection of the 'foreign' fetal protein) influencing the course of the condition (Lorenzi & Ford 2002) by some temporary re-myelination of the nerves. However, it must be acknowledged that this will not be so for some women. Additionally, as Neild (2006) warns, fatigue, balance and back pain may worsen during pregnancy due to the weight of the gravid uterus and the altered centre of gravity. In these circumstances a walking aid may help mobility and confidence.

If a mother's lower limbs are weak she may need time and help to get into position on the examination couch during antenatal visits. Existing bladder and bowel problems may be aggravated. Baschat & Weiner (2004) recommend the consideration of prophylactic antibiotics if urinary infection has been problematic. As one symptom of the condition is tiredness, anaemia should be avoided and prophylactic iron supplementation may need to be considered (Baschat & Weiner 2004).

The mode of delivery is not influenced by the condition (Ferrero et al 2004). Baschat & Weiner (2004) do warn that some women may not feel the onset of labour. It is important that midwives explain to women during pregnancy that there is a possibility that they may not perceive pain during contractions, and show them how to palpate the uterine fundus in order to feel the rise during a contraction. This will enable women to be alert to any hint of labour and seek admission to hospital or the attendance of a midwife. Otherwise there is a risk of a precipitate labour and an unattended birth occurring.

Muscle spasm and stiffness may be stimulated by the uterine contractions or a distended bladder during labour (Baschat & Weiner 2004) or discomfort from vaginal examinations (Welner & Temple 2004). It is important therefore, that women are encouraged to empty their bladder frequently during labour, and catheterisation may be needed if this is not possible. Vaginal examinations may not be easy to perform if a mother has leg muscle spasm or she has difficulty abducting her legs. It should be performed with care to avoid unnecessary discomfort, and if a mother has weakness in her legs help will be needed to hold them in position during the procedure (Welner & Temple 2004).

Epidural and general and local anaesthetics are safe to use (Ferrero et al 2004, Neild 2006, Vukusic et al 2004) as directed by the needs and wishes of individual mothers, or there are obstetric indices. Epidural has the advantage of possibly preventing any muscle spasm. However, Lorenzi & Ford (2002) were not entirely convinced that epidural does not increase the likelihood of relapse. Sevarino (2004) agrees that epidural is safe but advises against spinal because of the implication for making MS worse.

If there is poor or no pelvic feeling mothers may not perceive expulsive sensations (Baschat & Weiner 2004) so midwives need to be vigilant to recognise the onset of the second stage of labour. If a mother is unable to push during the second stage because of tiredness, instrumental delivery may be needed, or perhaps just an episiotomy. Midwives needs to use their skill in judging a woman's progress and the clinical situation.

It has been noted that relapse of the symptoms of MS have occurred in the first 3 months following childbirth (for example Ferrero et al 2004) or the condition may develop for the first time (Lorenzi & Ford 2002). To obtain clearer evidence of the developments of the condition Vukusic et al (2004) undertook a study of 227 women with MS postpartum for up to 2 years. There was indeed a greater chance of a relapse during the first 3 months following the birth, but on a brighter note rates were not actually high as 72% of the women did not have any relapses. Researchers were unable to predict who would have a relapse post-partum. However, there was some indication that the women more likely to have a relapse were those who had experienced a relapse(s) in the year before pregnancy, and those with greater disability at the time of onset of the pregnancy. After the initial 3-month period the risk of relapse reverted to the same as it had been prior to pregnancy. In the long-term the condition was not made worse by epidural, the mother's age, disease duration or age of onset, number of previous pregnancies, gender of the baby, or breast-feeding.

Vukusic et al (2004) found that women with less severe symptoms and fewer relapses were more likely to breast-feed. Breast-feeding is not contraindicated in women with MS unless they need to restart disease-modifying drugs (Neild 2006). If excess tiredness is a problem breast-feeding may be too much of an additional strain. These issues need to be discussed with mothers and the support and help of partners and families in the postnatal period need to be planned. Tiredness and weakness may make infant care challenging, particularly lifting and moving if there is weakness in the upper limbs. Alternative strategies may need to be developed for transferring the baby to and from the cot. Specific plans should be made for rest periods to ensure that mothers have as much energy as possible.

Part of the postnatal role of midwives is to offer contraceptive advice. Drey & Darney (2004) state that there is a lack of evidence on the safety of oral contraception and Chloe Neild (2006) highlights contradictory information about the benefits of oestrogen on the course of the condition. She does warn, however, that there is the potential for development of DVT with the combined pill if lower limb immobility is present. She further advises that the efficiency of the pill may be lowered by some MS drugs e.g. carbamazepine (Tegretol) (for the treatment of spasms and pain) and Modafinil used for fatigue. If progesterone alone is suitable this can be administered orally (the mini pill) or via implants and injections. The intrauterine system, i.e. a coil with a combined slow-release progesterone stem, may be suitable. This has the added advantage of lessening or inhibiting menstrual flow which may be an advantage to women. If a woman is prone to urinary tract infections the diaphragm (cap) is best avoided (Neild 2006).

## Myalgic encephalomyelitis (ME)

Like MS above, this condition may, in less extreme cases, be 'invisible' yet it is still debilitating. Often

labelled chronic fatigue syndrome or post-viral fatigue syndrome, this condition was originally called 'yuppy flu' during the 1980s because there were no diagnostic test indicators of an existing condition, and it only appeared to occur in people in well-paid employment. Considerable scepticism was present within the medical profession and society that it was actually a medical condition. The condition is increasingly being recognised as existing although some scepticism still exists. This is in part because the aetiology of the condition remains unclear and diagnosis is made on symptom history alone. The main indicator is fatigue that has been overwhelming and disabling for at least 6 months (Afari & Buchwald 2003).

The charitable organisation Action for ME (2006) estimates that there are 240 000 people in the UK with the condition, the majority developing the illness anywhere from their early 20s to mid-40s. It appears to be a complex multifactoral condition possibly with an individual genetic predisposition (Afari & Buchwald 2003). Physical and psychological factors seem to be involved. Symptoms and the severity of the disability vary with individuals which makes diagnosis challenging. There is often a history of a 'trigger' which for about a third of people is a viral infection but for others it develops following a vaccination or exposure to an environmental toxin, or as a result of severe physical trauma (Action for ME 2006). There are affects on the central nervous system, including the hypothalamus which is involved in the body's thermoregulation, sleep and appetite regulating. The body's immune system also appears to be affected.

There is a range of possible other symptoms related to these two body systems (Action for ME 2006). These include muscular pain and twitching; joint pain; neurological sensation e.g. paraesthesia (pins and needles); headaches and migraines; and sensitivity to bright lights, noise and odours. Sleep patterns are often significantly altered and cognitive abilities affected e.g. concentration and memory. The digestive system may be affected with irritable bowel syndrome presenting and increased sensitivity to certain foods, alcohol and medication. Central nervous system symptoms may include altered temperature control; sweating; vertigo and dizziness which affect balance.

These symptoms may last for a long time, even years, and for some individuals the condition never resolves but becomes progressively worse. For others they have times when they cope and others where there is a relapse. Coping mechanisms include managing physical and mental activity by structuring the day. This is helped by cognitive behavioural therapy which means that individuals understand their condition and how they can best manage sleep, nutrition, activities and goal setting. This aspect will also enable them to recognise their specific triggers for relapse and how to put in coping mechanisms to avoid or minimise the affects. Stressful times, concurrent illness, climate changes and even the menstrual cycle can all be triggers.

The nutritional aspect may be influential for an individual when there is an indication that certain foods are not being tolerated, for example wheat and dairy products, alcohol and sugar, but for others diet modification makes no difference (Action for ME 2006). Complimentary therapies e.g. aromatherapy and relaxation, and an exercise programme may be an additional mechanism that enables individuals to cope with daily life. Low doses of a selective serotonin re-uptake inhibitor and mild antidepressant such as fluoxetine (i.e. Prozac), and medication to alleviate muscle spasm and pain (BBC News 1998) may be prescribed to alleviate some of the symptoms.

It is not only the person with the condition that has to manage daily life but those around them must also develop coping mechanisms. For some with the condition they become increasingly dependent as their symptoms worsen. Women are more likely to have the condition than men, and they appear to remain fertile, therefore midwives may be required to provide maternity services for them.

The usual preconception advice related to optimising general health and well-being, for example through a well-balanced diet and taking folic acid supplements, will be the same for a woman with ME but additionally consideration needs to be taken related to any medication being used. Fluoxetine is contraindicated during pregnancy but should not be suddenly discontinued. Although a woman may be on a low dose, gradual reduction is advisable to avoid withdrawal symptoms. The drug is also unsuitable during breast-feeding.

If relapse of the condition is triggered by illness and stress it could be postulated that pregnancy may make the condition worse. The tiredness that pregnancy gives some women who are well may be enhanced. Women need to be aware of this and plan their day accordingly; this includes antenatal appointments. Many of the principles highlighted in MS above need to be taken into consideration, for example issues with mobility; transferring onto a couch or bed for examination; ability to cope with a growing pregnancy and the additional weight; coping with the exhaustion that labour may present; and self-care and infant handling and care following the birth. Issues such as analgesia during labour, the risk of DVT if leg mobility is reduced and the suitability of contraception all need to be explored and mechanisms put into place to enable coping and risk reduction.

## Rheumatoid arthritis (RA)

The aetiology of this chronic autoimmune disease is unclear. It is more widespread in older people although the onset can occur much earlier and it is more common in women than men, therefore it is of importance for women of child-bearing age. It presents as painful swollen joints with morning stiffness, commonly of the hands and feet but other joints may be affected, for example in the neck (Csuka 2004). Csuka explains that joint damage is an early complication with narrowing of the space between the bones and inflammation of the synovial membrane. The condition is progressive and results in joint deformity. Some neurological damage may occur if nodules form on the central nervous system or spinal cord (Baschat & Weiner 2004). Fatigue may be present. Exercise, anti-inflammatory and disease-modifying medication, for example methotrexate, and chemotherapy are used to control the progress of the condition (Csuka 2004).

Preconception advice is essential to optimise health and to change medication to those with little or no teratogenic possibilities at least 6 months prior to conception (Le Gallez 1999). Le Gallez advises that low doses of prednisolone are safe and may be useful if paracetamol is an ineffective analgesic. (See section on MS above for further drug information.) Non-steroidal anti-inflammatory drugs e.g. ibuprofen, are best avoided in the first trimester (Le Gallez 1999) but are suitable later during pregnancy until 34 weeks when they should be stopped as there is a danger of the neonate having heart problems (Gordon 2004). Fertility is unaffected in women under 30 years old, unless they have been on long-term oral cyclophosphamide therapy (Gordon 2004).

Although Le Gallez (1999) states that the condition may worsen during pregnancy, there appears to be a general consensus that more frequently there is some remission (Gordon 2004, Le Gallez 1999, Olsen & Kovacs 2002) in up to 70–75% of women (Baschat & Weiner 2004, Csuka 2004) usually in the first trimester. While there is a lack of understanding about the mechanisms, pregnancy hormones appear to lower the inflammation in the disease (Gordon 2004). Natural anti-inflammatory steroid hormones that rise during pregnancy may also account for the improvement (Barrett et al 2000) or it may be due to the rise in T cells of the immune system (Gordon 2004).

Gordon (2004) states that rates of miscarriage and stillbirth are no higher in women with RA. An American study of hospital admissions during pregnancy by Chakravarty et al (2006) noted that women with RA were more likely to have hypertensive disorder, premature rupture of membranes, intrauterine growth retardation and caesarean section. Bowden et al (2001) had noted earlier that the birth weight of babies whose mothers were not in remission tended to be lower.

Mobility may be affected during pregnancy because of the added weight of the gravid uterus. Excess weight gain is best avoided and advice from a dietician may be useful. Walking aids may be helpful particularly if confidence in balance is diminished. If mobility is affected, mothers need time to get into position for examination during pregnancy, labour and postnatal. Advice to take regular rest periods will aid energy levels if fatigue is a symptom. Afternoon appointments may be appreciated if joint stiffness is worse in the mornings. Advice from a physiotherapist may be useful to maintain mobility and minimise joint pain with strengthening exercises suitable during pregnancy. Midwives and occupational therapists ideally should work together with mothers to find and plan ways of managing infant care following the birth.

The usual labour care is needed, including analgesia as required. If epidural is the choice of analgesia,

it is important to consider the position of legs and feet to ensure that feet and ankle joints are not moved abnormally. Regular movement of limbs and affected joints will lessen stiffness. Vaginal examination may create no difficulties as large joints like the hips are generally unaffected by the condition. If a woman's legs need to be put into stirrups, position and movement must also be taken into consideration. If neurological symptoms are present, different positions may need to be tried to ensure comfort during labour.

Following the birth joints may be particularly stiff due to immobility during labour. RA tends to flare up postnatally within 6 weeks of the birth (Csuka 2004, Olsen & Kovacs 2002) and may be even more severe (Gordon 2004). Joint pain and stiffness cause restriction on the range of movement. If fine motor movements are affected there is a possibility that lifting or carrying any weight may be painful which would mean infant care requires alternative strategies.

Olsen & Kovacs (2002) state that RA appears to be made worse by breast-feeding possibly due to the high prolactin levels. Barrett et al (2000) undertook a study of 137 UK women with RA during pregnancy and the puerperium. They found that of the 88 women who breast-fed, of those who breast-fed for the first time for 4 weeks or more (N=38), significantly more had an arthritis relapse than those that had breast-fed one or more children before. Both groups experienced more symptoms than women who did not breast-feed at all. However, it is not inevitable that symptoms will occur as four of the first-time mothers reported no worsening of pain since the pregnancy. The authors postulated that genetic susceptibility explained those that did not have deterioration of symptoms. Le Gallez (1999) advises that if analgesics are required they are best taken 30–60 minutes after feeding. This enables the maximum metabolism and excretion by a mother's body prior to the next feed therefore minimising the amount of drug in the milk. As with pregnancy, adequate rest periods will help to alleviate fatigue and the help and support of family, friends and possibly social services would assist this, enabling a mother to cope and enjoy her baby.

There is some evidence that the combined oral contraceptive pill offers protection against RA but conflicting suggestions also exist (Drey & Darney

2004). Drossaers-Bakker et al (2002) suggest an indication that long-term use of oral contraception and several pregnancies may have some influence on the joints of women with RA, so that movement is less restricted, but not on the course of the condition. Conversely, Gordon (2004) seems unconvinced that the combined pill has any beneficial effect but does say that either the combined or progesterone-only pill is not precluded by RA. If a woman does want to take the combined pill then breast-feeding is contraindicated because of the oestrogen. Other methods of contraception may be selected according to personal choice and suitability.

## SPINAL CORD CONDITIONS

The two main conditions considered here are the congenital condition of spina bifida and acquired spinal cord lesions. The physical similarities mean that information offered for one condition and situation may also be transferable to the other. To avoid excessive repetition, some elements discussed with one condition may not be repeated in the other unless the differences are significant. The psychological issues and adaptation to daily living may be different for someone who has not been disabled before.

## Spina bifida

The cause of spina bifida is unknown although there appears to be a link with a lack of folic acid. There are three types of spina bifida where one or more of the vertebrae fail to form correctly leaving a gap or split (bifid) (ASBAH 2003). Spina bifida occulta is a mild form of the condition where although the vertebra is not completely joined there is no damage to the spinal cord. The individual may be unaware of the condition as the only sign is sometimes a tuft of hair or dimple over the site of the abnormality. Spina bifida cystica (cyst-like) has two types. The least serious one (meningocele) is where the cyst contains only cerebro-spinal fluid (CSF) and meninges (the spinal cord covering). With the other more serious condition (meningomyelocele) the cyst also contains nerves and spinal cord. This latter type generally results in some paralysis and loss of sensation (ASBAH 2003). Early surgery may be performed to close the back over.

Growth of the body and lower limbs below the more serious abnormalities is usually restricted. Some sensation may or may not be present depending on the nerve damage. Leg control and therefore mobility is usually a major problem and use of a wheelchair is commonly needed. Poor or inadequate innervation to the pelvic area means that bladder and bowel are affected, which leads to problems with continence. Perineal and pressure areas are susceptible to tissue breakdown without adequate precautions e.g. frequent lifting and keeping clean and dry.

Continence can be managed in a number of different ways. Constipation is often a problem because of the poor nerve supply to the bowel. Bowel training and regular toileting from childhood, attention to diet e.g. high fibre, and voluntary muscle help with evacuation may be successful. Training from infancy may successfully result in the ability to use digital anal stimulation to cause a reflex evacuation. If this does not work for an individual an enema or suppository, or even a bowel washout may be used. In the long-term if these procedures are unsuccessful surgery may be the answer. A stoma may be fashioned using large bowel (colostomy) or small bowel (ileostomy) so that faeces are collected in a bag on the outer abdomen. In the latter case the stool is often more fluid but in both cases diet modification, based on trial and error, may be needed to avoid excess flatus (wind) or excess diarrhoea (ASBAH 2001a).

There are several different ways of managing urinary continence according to the ASBAH internet website (2001b, 2001c) depending on the individual's circumstances. Incontinence due to spasms of the bladder may be lessened by anti-spasmodic medication. Clean intermittent catheterisation (CIC) can be performed, which the individual learns to do themselves using a disposable or reusable catheter, or an indwelling urethral or suprapubic catheter may be inserted. Surgery is another option and there are several procedures that may be performed depending on individual circumstances.

The ASBAH internet website offers some interesting details about the surgical procedures. Sometimes bladder augmentation is needed where a piece of bowel is used to enlarge a small or over-active bladder to increase its capacity. If the bladder sphincter is non-functioning, and therefore there is no control and urine retention, an artificial sphincter can be surgically implanted. This is composed of tubing, a cuff and an inflated balloon made of silicone elastomer. The balloon is inserted in the labia (in the male the scrotum) and pressed to open the sphincter every 4 hours enabling urine to be voided or CIC to be performed. Very occasionally a urostomy is fashioned where the ureters are implanted into a piece of bowel which forms a stoma on the outer abdominal wall. Urine then continually drains into a bag. The more recent mitrofanoff surgical procedure uses the appendix to form a stoma on the abdominal wall with a link to the bladder. This easily enables 4-hourly CIC. Bladder augmentation may be performed at the same time (ASBAH 2002).

Because of the risk of urinary tract infections (UTI) Welner & Temple (2004) emphasise the importance of annual renal checks. Regular screening for asymptomatic bacteruria should be part of well-women screening. As with anyone susceptible to UTI adequate oral fluid intake is vital. ASBAH recommend drinking cranberry juice daily to lessen the risk of infection developing. However, the urinary tract is not the only place where infection is likely. Damage to skin in pressure areas creating open wounds will be vulnerable to infection, therefore individuals need to take steps to prevent the development of skin lesions by changing position and using appropriate cushioned padding.

Another important health consideration for people with spina bifida is the potential for latex allergy (May 2005, Welner & Temple 2004). May states that this had first been recognised in America in 1984 where 18–40% of people with spina bifida have been recorded to have the problem. However, the incidence in the UK is unknown (May 2005) but may result in a wide spectrum of reactions, as with any allergy, from a mild skin rash to anaphylactic shock. Latex, a natural solution from rubber trees with added chemicals, can be found in many everyday products from gloves (surgical and household) to incontinence aids, condoms, urinary catheters, syringes and other medical equipment, chewing gum and adhesive tape (May 2005). If allergy is suspected a skin or blood test needs to be performed and non-latex products should be used.

It is not just these health considerations that need to be taken into account. In addition other well-women care is needed. If latex allergy is an issue, then contraceptives such as the diaphragm and condoms need to be latex free. The combined oral contraceptive pill may not be suitable if lower limb movement is minimal or absent, because of the increased risk of DVT formation.

Preconception care is an important consideration. A woman with spina bifida is at increased risk of having a baby with the condition. As a prophylactic measure to reduce the risk of spina bifida occurring, the Department of Health advises all women to take folic acid for 3 months prior to conception and the first 3 months of pregnancy. For mothers with the condition the dose of folic acid recommended is much higher i.e. 4 mg instead of 0.4 mg (400 mcg). As with all women, any medication needs to be reviewed to consider the potential influence on fertility and pregnancy. Additional considerations for women and their partners preconception will be the physical, social and psychological demands that a pregnancy and child will have and what support, if any, they will require to ensure that those networks be set up if needed.

Pregnancy, labour and postnatal considerations will be very much the same as for women with spinal cord injury (see below).

## Spinal cord injury

Once severed the spinal cord does not reunite, therefore there will be no sensory and motor function below the level of the injury and nerve supply to organs may be interrupted. Not all lesions are complete breaks therefore resulting paralysis is variable. Some interesting information can be found on the Spinal Injury Network internet website (2002–2004) related to the effects on body function with different positions of lesion. High cord lesions above T6 may affect respiratory control and above T12 cough reflex. A very high lesion in the neck, i.e. at or above C4, means that respiration requires assistance 24 hours a day. This is because intercostal muscles, diaphragm and abdominal muscles are paralysed. With lesions between T6 and C4 breathing is mainly with the diaphragm as the other muscles are weak. Any compromise on respiration and cough means an increased incidence of respiratory infection. Strengthening exercises for muscles that retain some function will improve respiratory and cough control.

Some reflex nerve responses may still be present below the lesion, as a reflex arc passes across the spinal cord rather than up to the higher centres in the brain. Some visceral sensation may still be present i.e. sensations of full bladder or bowel, wind pain and dysmenorrhoea (period pains). However, bladder and bowel activity is diminished. Bladder and ureters become atonic due to poor innervation and voluntary control to void urine is lost (Baschat & Weiner 2004). This means that stasis of urine and the need for self-catheterisation increases the risk of UTI which may result in chronic renal infection that leads to anaemia. Good local and catheter hygiene is essential to minimise the incidence, and frequent emptying of the bladder is necessary to prevent over-distension. Baschat & Weiner advocate screening for asymptomatic bacteruria and possibly prophylactic antibiotics for up to 14 days, especially if there is a history of pyelonephritis.

Another important health issue is the development of pressure sores. This is an ongoing risk and physiotherapy and exercises to change position and alleviate prolonged pressure will aid prevention. Attention to skin hygiene is vital because if skin breakdown does develop there is a risk of infection and chronic anaemia.

Further information about women's health and fertility is often anecdotal. Jackson & Sipski's (2005) extensive literature review as far back as 1957 found little research that focused on the sexual and reproductive issues of women with chronic spinal cord impairment. However there is one study by Jackson & Wadley (1999) of 472 women with spinal cord injury. They found that women had more UTI and vaginal yeast infections although other gynaecological conditions were no different than before injury. Additionally, they found that sexual function could be inhibited by dysreflexia (see autonomic hyperreflexia below) and bladder incontinence. Pregnancy is achievable even if a woman's partner has the same condition. A case report from Taiwan (Chen et al 2005) describes successful pregnancy outcome at 39 weeks in a couple who both have spinal cord injury. Sperm had been obtained by electro-ejaculation and then cryopreserved. Following ovarian stimulation and egg retrieval, intra-cytoplasm sperm injection (ICSI) resulted in five normal embryos. Four were transferred resulting in the normal vaginal birth of a healthy female infant.

Pregnancy is not without potential problems for women with a spinal cord injury. Achieving optimal health and well-being prior to conception, as with all women, will improve the chance of a successful pregnancy. Infection screening and a full blood count will enable any suboptimal results to be rectified, for example anaemia. Diet and nutritional advice may be required and physiotherapy to improve muscle tone and lessen any stiffness. Psycho-social issues may need to be discussed, in particular the help and support that will be required and the need for any aids or special/adapted equipment.

During pregnancy the risk of pressure sores increases due to the added weight, and UTI are more prevalent (Baschat & Weiner 2004, Jackson & Wadley 1999). It is important therefore that midwives offer to examine women to instigate early treatment if needed. There is a greater incidence of intrauterine growth retardation (Baschat & Weiner 2004, Jackson & Wadley 1999) possibly because of anaemia and poor nutritional status caused by chronic infection. Identification of iron and/or folate deficiency will need appropriate treatment to maintain general well-being and lower the risk of additional infection. Dietary advice may be needed.

Advice on breathing exercises and physiotherapy may be beneficial as lung capacity and residual volume decrease during pregnancy, which increases the risk of chest infection even further than usual (Baschat & Weiner 2004). An additional health issue is the potential for the development of a DVT because of lower limb immobility. Nevertheless, Baschat & Weiner recommend against giving prophylactic anti-coagulants unless there is a history of DVT or clotting problems. The movements encouraged for the prevention of pressure sores will also aid lower limb circulation.

Physical access to the antenatal clinic must be considered and time allowed for movement onto the examination couch. Parent education should be available for women and their partners the same as for other prospective parents. Home visits may be appreciated if hospital or health centre visiting is difficult. Individual parent education sessions may need to be organised.

General care offered to all women and their birth partners during labour remains the same with some modifications. Pressure area care must be high on the additional list of key considerations. If there is no pelvic organ sensation then the pain of labour contractions may not be perceived or they may give wind-like symptoms. Women will be able to palpate tension and a rise in their uterine fundus and antenatal preparation for this is needed. Failure to recognise the onset of labour means no prompt for the mother to obtain appropriate help or admission to hospital. This has implications for a potential unattended birth.

Indications from the literature prompt Baschat & Weiner (2004) to recommend that a woman with a high spinal lesion, i.e. about T6 is likely to require a central venous pressure (CVP) line and cardiac monitoring. This is because when there is an injury at this level there is a susceptibility to autonomic hyperreflexia (see below) particularly from an over-distended bladder, during vaginal examination or from the labour contractions. Therefore mothers need to be in a maternity unit where a senior anaesthetist is readily available 24 hours a day. Midwives need to understand the possible trigger mechanisms, how the condition can be minimised and how it is managed if it does occur. They should be confident and competent to provide special or intensive care should it be necessary. Baschat & Weiner (2004) recommend the risk be reduced by the use of epidural anaesthesia. This inhibits the nerve impulses from the stimuli thus preventing an abnormal reaction, although they admit the level of analgesia may be difficult to control and does not always offer complete block.

The urge to bear down and perineal stretching sensations during the second stage of labour may or may not be present. Therefore vigilance is needed by midwives to recognise when the second stage of labour has been entered. Baschat & Weiner (2004) advocate shortening the second stage with mid-cavity forceps or vacuum extraction. It must be acknowledged, however, that these are American authors. As UK midwifery is less medicalised, mid-wives may be more willing to wait and see if normal vaginal birth is possible providing there are no fetal or maternal indications to direct otherwise. The power of the uterus is capable of expulsion of the fetus without the help of secondary muscles i.e. the abdominal sheath. If women are able to control their own breathing they can use the Valsalva manoeuvre (breath holding that uses the diaphragm to exert pressure on the uterine fundus) and some may have voluntary control of abdominal muscles to bear down. An episiotomy may be necessary but should be considered from the clinical indications.

Postnatal care again should be basically the same as it is for every woman. Post delivery most women have a large diuresis as haemoconcentration occurs (i.e. plasma levels fall as the extent of the circulating blood volume decreases). Mothers need to be made aware of this as more frequent bladder emptying will be needed in the first 48–73 hours to avoid an over-distended bladder and autonomic hyperreflexia. Perineal pain may also cause this condition therefore appropriate analgesia should be offered if necessary.

Scrupulous perineal hygiene is needed to prevent infection and skin breakdown. Access to shower and bath may not always be easy unless facilities have been modified appropriately. Transfer home as soon as possible may be the best option as a woman's home will be suitably adapted. Unless a mother is on any unsuitable medication, there are no contraindications to breast-feeding if it is her choice. Additional rest and support at home may be necessary if excess tiredness is an issue.

## Autonomic hyperreflexia (dysreflexia)

This is a potentially severe condition resulting from an abnormal neurological response to a stimulus because the nerve impulses do not reach the brain to be tempered. Neurological signs and symptoms range from irritability, headache and seizures to coma. Those of the cardio-vascular system can include marked, but not labile, hypertension (as opposed to static hypertension in pre-eclampsia), cardiac irregularity and bradycardia, cerebral haemorrhage and facial flushing. Other signs may be dilated pupils, sweating and nasal stuffiness (Baschat & Weiner 2004). These reactions can be triggered by procedures as simple as changing a urinary catheter, vaginal examination and cervical stimulation, and rectal examination. Labour, an over-distended bladder or bowel, and a painful perineum are also potential stimulants.

## GENETIC CONDITIONS

## Achondroplasia

This condition is caused by a genetic mutation that occurs on the short arm of chromosome number four (Medicinenet 2005) which codes for growth (Grace Parker 2006, Trotter et al 2005). Information on internet site Medicinenet (2005) indicates that the word 'achondroplasia' means cartilage but the condition is actually a disorder of cartilage conversion to bone. It occurs as a new mutation in about 75% of cases i.e. for the first time (Grace Parker 2006, Trotter et al 2005) with the remainder of cases occurring as a result of an inherited autosomal dominant trait i.e. just one gene is needed from one parent. Babies born to older fathers are more at risk of a primary mutation (Medicinenet 2005). It is one of the oldest known birth defects occurring about once in 25 000 births worldwide, 1:10 000 in Latin America and 12:77 000 in Denmark, and occurs in both males and females (Medicinenet 2005). A milder form of the condition is called hypochondroplasia (Grace Parker 2006). Other variations of the gene mutation also occur with similar presentations.

The physical characteristics of the disorder are numerous. The inadequate conversion of cartilage to bone results in short stature and short limbs. Women are about 124 cm (49 inches) shorter, and the upper parts of their limbs are particularly short (Medicinenet 2005). People's torsos appear long as they are out of proportion to their body (Grace Parker 2006, Medicinenet 2005) while their heads are large with prominent forehead (frontal bossing), and underdevelopment (hypoplasia) of mid-face and cheekbones (Grace Parker 2006, Medicinenet 2005) and they have a narrowing of both the bridge of the nose and nasal passages. Their brains are large although their intelligence is normal (Medicinenet 2005, Trotter et al 2005).

People's hands are distinctive, fingers are short and the middle and ring fingers are splayed giving their hands a three-pronged (trident) appearance (Grace Parker 2006, Medicinenet 2005). Some joints are lax causing over-extension, in particular knees. However, hips and elbows may have restricted movement. People's legs are often bowed (genu varum) (Grace Parker 2006, Medicinenet 2005, Trotter et al 2005) particularly because the tibia is bowed. There can be either a lumbar lordosis (forward curvature of the spine) (Medicinenet 2005) or posterior curvature (kyphosis i.e. hump back) (Trotter et al 2005). The spaces between lumbar spine are narrow (Grace Parker 2006). This narrowing may cause spinal cord compression (Trotter et al 2005) resulting in pain; ataxia (poor muscle coordination); bladder, bowel and sensation problems.

In most people their foramen magnum (opening at the base of the skull) is small which may lead to compression of the spinal cord at the junction of the skull and cervical vertebrae (Trotter et al 2005). Trotter et al also note that hydrocephalus may be present. People have a small pelvis (Trotter et al 2005) with caudal narrowing (around the coccyx) and an abnormal ilium; narrow sacroiliac groove and flat acetabulum (Grace Parker 2006).

Some or all of these characteristics have the potential to cause mortality or morbidity. However, Trotter et al (2005) state that as few as 5–10% of people have serious problems and that life expectancy is normal. Nevertheless, potential life-threatening situations can develop. Upper airway obstruction may cause apnoea (Trotter et al 2005) in infancy and later in life. Apnoea can also be due to brain stem compression (Grace Parker 2006) or compression of arterial blood flow in the region of the foramen magnum (Trotter et al 2005) due to cervical vertebrae abnormalities and the narrow foramen.

Joint mobility, spinal curvature, and lower limb bowing potentially make walking difficult and gait is often abnormal. Continence and sensation problems may be present if innervation to the pelvic area has been compromised by spinal cord compression or damage. Obesity is a real danger because of small stature and this will aggravate mobility problems (Grace Parker 2006). Additional morbidity may develop as a result of a short eustachian tube (between the back of the throat and the middle ear) that leads to recurrent otitis media (middle ear infection) resulting in hearing damage or even deafness (Trotter et al 2005). If hearing problems occur early in life speech may be affected. The severity will depend on whether any language has developed or not.

There are some effective ways of managing or treating the complications to minimise morbidity. Not much can be done to improve stature other than costly limb lengthening (Grace Parker 2006, Trotter et al 2005) which is not without danger itself. Growth hormones and food or vitamin supplements appear from the literature to be of little use (Trotter et al 2005). Curvature of the spine can be corrected with a brace or spinal fusion, and lumbar laminectomy (removal of the posterior arch of the vertebra) can be performed to alleviate pressure on the spinal cord (Grace Parker 2006). Damage to joints can be prevented by avoiding impact movements e.g. excess neck tilting and jumping, and anti-inflammatory medication can be used when joints are painful (Grace Parker 2006).

People with achondroplasia, or the more acceptable term 'little people' ('dwarf' is used in the literature but this may not always be tolerable to individuals), can lead productive, independent lives. Environmental modifications may need to be made, for example making light switches and door handles lower and having a step stool available to reach things at everyday heights, and using gadgets, for example a 'wand' for cleansing following toileting. Little people form relationships and marry the same as everyone else. Those relationships may be with other little people or partners of normal height. Women are fertile (Trotter et al 2005) and therefore contraception and preconception advice will be needed. Trotter et al advise against long-term oral contraception because of the risk of fibroids developing, and they point out that using a diaphragm may be difficult because of short arms. That is not to say a partner could not insert a diaphragm if that method was acceptable to both parties. Partners could use a condom. An intra-uterine device or system may also not be suitable because of the size of the uterine cavity. It is unclear if a progesterone contraceptive would be suitable. Discussion with a specialist family planning doctor is probably advisable.

Preconception advice would encompass all the usual information and advice, for example about diet and nutrition, including folic acid; smoking cessation; and a review of medication and medical conditions. Weight control is particularly important for women with the condition as additional strain on joints needs to be minimised. If joints are already damaged the added weight of pregnancy needs to be taken into consideration with the potential to increase immobility and pain. Additionally, general health and social circumstances are other concerns that all women take into consideration when planning a pregnancy and parenting but these issues may be of greater importance for women in this situation.

Specifically for women with achondroplasia, Grace Parker (2006) suggests a pelvic X-ray to identify size and shape to see if a vaginal birth would be possible. Yet this would seem unnecessary as caesarean section appears to be standard procedure. Of significant importance for women with achondroplasia is likely to be genetic counselling. There is a 50% chance that a child will have the condition (heterozygous) i.e. one affected gene and one normal gene (as the gene is dominant just one gene will lead to the condition) and 50% chance of normality. If a woman's partner also has achondroplasia the risk of passing on the heterozygous condition remains at 50%; chance of normality falls to 25% but there is now also a 25% chance that their child will have a 'double dose' of affected gene (one affected gene from each parent = a homozygous condition) (Medicinenet 2005). This homozygous achondroplasia is lethal and results in stillbirth or early death (Trotter et al 2005).

During pregnancy women may wish to take up the option of screening for fetal anomalies. Chorionic villus sampling could be offered in early pregnancy, or later amniocentesis (Trotter et al 2005) particularly to diagnose a homozygous condition. Ultrasound scans can identify shortening of limbs and serial scans may be recommended to assist in growth monitoring. Alternatively, women may prefer not to have screening.

Mobility may be compromised and back pain may worsen during pregnancy because of the additional weight particularly if there is existing spine or joint disease. The advice of a physiotherapist may be helpful to suggest muscle and joint strengthening exercises. Women may need advice on sleeping positions and increasing rest periods to conserve energy and minimise joint damage. Mild analgesics such as paracetamol may be beneficial, but for some women stronger analgesics may be needed. As with all medication during pregnancy, the needs of a mother's health have to be balanced with the risks to the fetus. If mobility is problematic, home antenatal visits might be appreciated when hospital visits are non-essential. This would then offer midwives opportunity to see how a woman adapts her way of doing everyday activities enabling suggestions to be made for infant care later.

There is likely to be decreased residual lung capacity during pregnancy (Sevarino 2004) because of the short stature as the baby grows and fundal height increases. Trotter et al (2005) recommend monitoring baseline respiratory function early in pregnancy because of the high risk of respiratory compromise, particularly during the third trimester. An additional test recommended by Sevarino (2004) is related to the potential difficulties for intubation when administering general anaesthetic. She suggests a neck X-ray to ascertain the degree of abnormality and mobility of cervical vertebrae. This would be best performed in early pregnancy so that the pregnancy can readily be shielded during the procedure, and also rather than waiting until surgery is imminent. A consultation with an experienced obstetric anaesthetist during pregnancy would be beneficial in care planning.

During pregnancy parent education will be needed the same as for other women. Discussion about alternative ways of coping with infant care may be needed if fine motor movements and the potential for lifting and moving are affected. Visits to the labour suite and postnatal ward would be useful to enable mothers and midwives to have a 'dry run' with beds and equipment to ascertain what additional or adapted equipment might be useful e.g. a cot and bed that lower, and access to bathing and toilet facilities. The services of an occupational therapist may be helpful.

The plan of care is probably going to include birth by caesarean section (Trotter et al 2005). It is important that skilled and experienced obstetric anaesthetists who understand the possible anaesthetic concerns with someone with achondroplasia are present, and that they see women as soon as possible. If neck X-rays have not been taken previously then these should be arranged. Sevarino (2004) suggests pulmonary function tests and arterial blood gases should be performed and recommends the use of an intra-arterial catheter for blood pressure monitoring. Pulse oximetry is standard in all surgery to monitor oxygen saturation transcutaneously.

A skilled anaesthetist must be present for surgery. Intubation prior to general anaesthetic for caesarean section is likely to be challenging because of the neck problems. Di Nardo (1988) warns that neck extension may lead to quadriplegia or death, and movement of the back when there is kyphosis can compress the spinal cord leading to paraesthesia (tingling or numbness in hands) or paraplegia. Regional anaesthetic is not an easy option. Trotter et al (2005) point out that there is limited space in the spinal region therefore spinal anaesthetic should be avoided. Sevarino (2004) explains that if single-dose spinal anaesthetic

was used the effects would be unpredictable because of this narrowing of the canal. However, she does feel that continuous epidural or spinal using a catheter would be safe due to the slow dosing, although technically insertion may be difficulty. Care with dosing of all drugs needs to be taken to ensure they are size related (Trotter et al 2005). Intravenous cannulation may be difficult if elbow extension is not possible. Practitioners must be vigilant during surgery and when providing post-operative care because of the potential for breathing difficulties. Great care should be exercised when moving women to avoid joint and neck damage or even spinal cord compression.

Postnatal care will be required the same as for other women. Attention to mothers' additional or alternative needs will be required. They may need help or suggestions about how to handle and move their babies particularly post-operatively. Breastfeeding is possible, providing a mother is not taking any contraindicated medication, although help with positioning and supporting the baby may be necessary. Paediatric referral may be needed if a baby is known to have the condition or for diagnosis if confirmation is required, and for a long-term plan of care and advice. Information and psychological support may be needed by parents depending on how they feel about the situation.

The immediate care for parents if their baby has achondroplasia should be to offer specific advice to minimise early joint damage. Trotter et al (2005) advocate a baby carrier or chair with a firm back that supports an infant's back and neck. Unsupported sitting should be avoided until muscle tone is strong enough much later. Head movements should be controlled to avoid any sudden jerking that could potentially cause cervical spinal cord damage, particularly at the level of the foramen magnum. Damage to the spinal cord in this manner may lead to sudden death. Additionally, a baby should be observed carefully during feeding to monitor breathing. Observations should be made for signs of hydrocephalus e.g. bulging fontanelles and lethargy.

## Muscular dystrophy

This is a group of inherited disorders that result in muscle degeneration leading to progressive weakness. Lovering et al (2005) provide a comprehensive overview of the complex genetic nature of the 34 conditions, each caused by specific single gene abnormality from one of 29 genes. Many of these conditions are congenital or develop in early adulthood, for example Duchenne Muscular Dystrophy (DMD), or first present in adulthood. It is not only muscles of limbs and face that may be affected but heart and respiratory muscle involvement may occur. Some, like DMD, result in death in early adulthood, or severe disability therefore midwives are unlikely to see pregnant women with the condition. Others, where the onset is insidious or the symptoms are less profound, may mean that health and ability are only minimally compromised. Treatment is limited in its benefits and revolves around physiotherapy to minimise contractures and some medication such as anti-inflammatory drugs and steroids.

As these conditions are inherited, preconception advice and preparation for pregnancy from general health and psycho-social perspectives is vital. This involves ensuring optimal health and muscle strength through appropriate nutrition and exercise prior to conception; physiotherapy may be advantageous. Other considerations include medication, and planning for the appropriate help and support during pregnancy and after the birth. Offering women information about the potential danger to their health and their babies' well-being enables informed choice about the very real risks. Advice from a specialist in the field, a paediatrician and a genetic counsellor may be sought. If fertility is an issue or a woman wishes to ensure that her baby will not have the inherited condition, assisted reproduction technology may be the answer. This enables preimplantation genetic screening to diagnose embryos with a genetic disorder (Sermon et al 2004) so that normal embryos only are transferred in the hope of a successful pregnancy with a normal fetus.

Baschat & Weiner (2004) give a succinct overview of issues identified from the medical literature related to pregnancy. The risks include a likelihood that muscle weakness will increase during pregnancy especially in the third trimester, and miscarriage and pre-term labour are more common. Polyhydramnios may develop which may precipitate pre-term labour and increase the risk of intrauterine death. Pre-term labour may be rapid because of poor cervical strength. Conversely, labour may be prolonged because of poor uterine action although the myometrium will respond to oxytocics. If the uterus has a tendency to be atonic it must be assumed that there is an increased risk of post-partum haemorrhage. Baschat & Weiner do recommend active management of the third stage of labour with oxytocics.

Pregnancy management highlighted by Baschat & Weiner (2004) should revolve around monitoring a mother's well-being using electrocardiograph (ECG) and pulmonary function tests to identify any heart or respiratory compromise. General advice to mothers is that they should remain as active as possible to maintain muscle strength. If there are leg contractures additional physiotherapy may improve flexibility to enable vaginal examination and birth to occur more readily. To relieve symptoms, albeit a temporary measure, polyhydramnios may need to be treated by draining some of the liquor if it is severe.

Labour would be best managed in a consultant unit because of the risks. During labour cardiac and respiratory function may need to be observed using basic observations and continuous cardiac monitor and pulse oximetry. An experienced senior anaesthetist and obstetrician should be involved in a woman's care, and a paediatrician readily available. Baschat & Weiner (2004) state that a vaginal birth should be everyone's aim during labour. However, they do note that instrumental delivery may be needed for mothers who become tired or compromised. If caesarean section is necessary they advise against general anaesthetic because this has the potential to block muscle neurotransmitters resulting in further weakness. They recommend epidural as the safer option.

Postnatal care will be very much controlled by an individual mother's condition. Additional help and support may be needed if she is tired and weak to enable her to rest and conserve energy. Physiotherapy and muscle exercises should probably be continued to maintain strength. Handling and feeding her baby will need careful planning if muscle strength is limited. Family planning to ensure adequate spacing of children needs to be considered for mothers' general well-being. Some women may not wish to wait too long in case their condition deteriorates to such a level that the risks outweigh the desire to have more children. Contraception is not contraindicated although if muscle strength and fine movement dexterity are affected insertion of a diaphragm (the cap) may prove difficult. Additionally, if lower leg movements are limited the increased risk of DVT formation with the combined oral contraceptive pill will need to be considered.

## LIMB IMPAIRMENT

Limb impairment may be present for many reasons and will be part of many of the conditions discussed above. However, those conditions do not cover all of the possibilities that may result in a limb or limbs that do not function normally or at all. This section is included, therefore, to promote consideration of the diversity of reasons for limb impairment and to highlight some of the possible issues that women with an impaired or absent limb may have.

Limbs may be congenitally absent or they may have been amputated. Amputation may have been traumatic as the result of an accident, or because of a necessary surgical procedure due to injury, vascular failure, infection or bone disease. Limb function may be absent or impaired because of trauma especially if nerve damage has occurred, for example a brachial plexus (nerve junction at the base of the neck) injury will lead to weakness or paralysis of the arm. Although cerebro-vascular accident (stroke) is more common in older people it can occur at any age and may leave an individual with upper and/or lower limb weakness or paralysis often on one side of the body.

The physical, psychological and social consequences of that impairment will vary for every individual. Each person will find their own way of managing activities of daily living, socialising and the psychological issues that present. This is possibly easier for someone with a congenital impairment or absent limb(s), although Alison Lapper (2005) found that her quest to find her own way of doing things with upper and lower limb problems was impeded by non-disabled carers trying to insist that she use prostheses.

For someone who has lost a limb or the function of that limb, alternative ways of doing things have to be learnt. If a lower limb(s) is involved balance will be altered and gait changed, as well as having to learn to use a prosthetic leg(s) if that is relevant. This is an important issue for midwives to understand as the additional weight and altered balance of pregnancy could make walking problematic; increase back, sacro-iliac and pubic pain, and make choice of positions during labour less flexible. Any stasis of blood in the lower limb(s) will increase the risk of DVT for mation, therefore it is important that limb exercise is encouraged throughout pregnancy, labour and the postnatal period.

So many activities of daily living involve use of both hands or arms and creativity is needed to find alternative ways of performing them one-handed. This is particularly important for a new mother when learning to handle and care for her baby. Practice with a life-size and weight baby doll during pregnancy will enable alternative strategies to be planned. Some people have developed great strength in their jaw and are able to lift their baby using teeth gripping the baby's clothes. Hook and loop tape is easy for fastening clothes. Practice with different positions and supporting cushions will enable the best positions for infant feeding. Care will be needed selecting a bath and other equipment, and trying them out before buying is essential.

Psychologically someone with a congenitally abnormal or absent limb has to deal with the reactions of society from an early age and will hopefully have developed coping mechanisms. One often employed is minimisation, for example Carol Thomas (1999) describes concealing her congenitally missing hand, while others become publicly overt and enjoy celebrating their disability, for example Alison Lapper. Personal body image is a powerful psychological factor that may influence perception of self and will influence behaviour.

Women with a limb amputation may have body image concerns that cause them embarrassment when they undergo examinations or during labour, particularly if the amputation is relatively newly acquired. It is clear from Ide's (2004) investigations that body image causes amputees concerns and anxiety about partners' reactions to an absent limb which often diminishes libido. Although Ide (2004) does state little is known about amputees' perceptions of body image, and that although fertility and pregnancy are unimpaired, little research is available related to the sexual concerns of people with limb amputations. Therefore, it is worth midwives considering how a woman's body image may be influenced by her disability and how this may give her concerns about others' perceptions of her body. A sensitive yet professional approach will help to minimise a woman's embarrassment.

## SENSORY IMPAIRMENT

### Hearing

Absent or loss of hearing can be congenital or may develop at any time after birth. It can be genetic in origin or as a result of compromise, for example infection in utero, e.g. rubella, or at any time after birth. Burton et al (2006) and Phillips (2003) explain that studies have shown a genetic cause for 50–60% of congenital or early-onset moderate to profound hearing loss. Phillips quotes the occurrence as 1 in 1000 births. However, there appear to be some differences in the incidence depending on ethnic origin, and the different ages of onset of hearing loss can be attributed to gene mutation (Kokitsu-Nakata et al 2004).

Of the 30 000 genes in the human body about 10% are involved in controlling the development of the ear structure and formation of hearing (Burton et al 2006). The complex genetic origins of hearing impairment may be autosomal dominant, i.e. only one gene is necessary for the condition to occur (about 10% of cases) or autosomal recessive when two affected genes are needed. Over 400 different conditions have been recorded that have a genetic origin (Burton et al 2006). In 30–40% of cases the hearing loss is associated with genetic abnormalities causing a syndrome, i.e. other physical abnormalities (Burton et al 2006, Phillips 2003). This means that in 60–70% of cases the genetic abnormality is responsible solely for hearing loss. Interestingly, Dikkers et al (2005) describe a family case history of a rare congenital unilateral, i.e. one ear only, absence of hearing due to an abnormal formation of part of the auditory structures in one ear, but explain that the genetic aetiology is unclear at present.

Loss or absent hearing can inhibit or affect language and speech development, cognitive ability and psychosocial progress (Kokitsu-Nakata et al 2004). People who consider themselves 'Deaf', rather than deaf or hearing impaired, often view themselves as part of a linguistic minority particularly when they use British Sign Language (BSL) as their form of communication (for example Bramwell et al 2000). For midwives aiming to provide maternity services for a mother, and perhaps her partner too, there are challenges with communication. If the services of a BSL interpreter or a lip-speaker are to be commissioned with a mother's approval, someone acceptable to her must be used and they need to be booked well in advance (Iqbal 2004). Using family members, especially children, as interpreters is not suitable because of sensitive information that is exchanged and the need for confidentiality. Even a partner at times may not be the best person.

Midwives appear to lack confidence in offering parent education for mothers with hearing impairment (McKay-Moffat 2003). This is likely to be because of the communication difficulties, but it may be because of uncertainty about offering practical solutions to some infant care issues, e.g. hearing a baby cry. Effective use of visual material, including video material with subtitles, and written information will be useful to support communication and this is becoming more readily available than in the past. Complex midwifery or medical terminology may need special attention to ensure that mothers understand. Additional time may need to be scheduled for individualised parent education sessions unless the right support for communication is available for class sessions. Adequate time will also be needed at antenatal appointments for the sharing of information. It is also important to remember that the mother will not be able to hear her name called at appointments. Extra time will need to be taken during labour to explain what is happening, and it must be remembered that she may find it difficult to lip-read or sign during labour if analgesics cause drowsiness. The support of an interpreter acceptable to the mother may prove extremely beneficial.

Mothers may have concerns about their babies' ability to hear particularly if their condition is hereditary and may wish to have genetic counselling prior to conception. However, this may not be because women always want a child that can hear, they may actually wish to have a non-hearing child who will fit into their social circle and life-style. Early pregnancy genetic screening may be desired but on the other hand women may prefer early paediatric referral after the birth with specialist referral to an audiologist. It is their choice.

Mothers may be concerned about hearing their babies cry. There are devices on the market that vibrate or cause a light to flash alerting mother to baby crying. Information about where to obtain these devices and the availability of support agencies or local mothers may enhance confidence in infant and child-care.

## Visual

Leber hereditary optic neuropathy (LHON) is a condition passed through the mother that leads to optic nerve damage (IFOND 2005). Understanding of this condition is limited and relatively new. The incidence of the condition, which presents as sudden blindness, is unknown although it is known to occur 80% of the time in young men. It can develop in men and women of any age and has been recorded as early as 6 years of age (IFOND 2005). The International Foundation for Optic Nerve Disease's (IFOND) internet website offers some insight into the possible aetiology of the condition in that there seems to be a predisposition for some people with the genetic abnormality to develop blindness whilst others are unaffected. More investigation is needed in particular to develop effective treatment.

The more commonly known about genetic cause of visual impairment and blindness is retinitis pigmentosa. The Foundation Fighting Blindness (2006) provides a useful internet website with details about the condition. The foundation has discovered over 100 genes that are involved. These can be dominant, recessive or X-linked leading to a gradual degeneration of both the rod and cone cells of the retina. Initially the rods may be affected leading to night blindness, i.e. an inability to see in a dimly lit environment. As more rods are destroyed and cones are affected peripheral vision diminishes leading to tunnel vision. The onset of the symptoms occurs in the teenage years or early adulthood and the disease pattern is variable. As yet there is no cure for the condition although the foundation has had some success in slowing the disease with vitamin A supplements. Diagnosis is not easy and is usually made by a specialist ophthalmologist. Genetic screening can be of some help in identifying susceptible people.

Other causes of blindness or visual impairment may be due to a congenital abnormality, for example due to in utero infection, especially viral in early pregnancy or untreated infection acquired during the birth, for example chlamydia. Babies born prematurely are more susceptible to eye damage because they are pre-term and oxygen therapy has been linked to the development of retinopathy. Trauma at any time after birth may lead to loss of sight as may delay in treatment of poorly controlled diabetes. If a mother's visual condition is due to a genetic abnormality she may have concerns about passing it on to the baby. Genetic counselling may be required before or during pregnancy to identify the possibility of a baby being affected. Alternatively, early paediatric or geneticist referral may be required following the baby's birth.

Mothers may have concerns about recognising when their baby is unwell and about interacting with the baby. From a psychological perspective Niven (1992) made a significant point that a mother with a severe visual impairment may have difficulty perceiving her baby's signals. However, people with long-term visual impairment often have other senses that are highly developed, for example hearing, which would go some way in balancing the possible difficulties. Also mothers will get to know their babies through touch and will be able to recognise changes in the texture of their baby's skin and muscle tone. Their sense of smell will soon inform them of the need for a nappy change.

---

### CONCLUSION—KEY POINTS

- Generalisations about people with disabilities are inappropriate. Disabling conditions are not a static group of signs and symptoms of an aetiologically constant origin.
- The physical, psychological and social response of an individual to a specific condition is exclusive to that person. Additional or alternative needs are unique and individuals' environments will vary greatly. Thus the transactions between them and their environment will be distinctive and their self-perceptions and understanding of self will be diverse.

- Lack of appreciation about how an individual may perceive herself may mean the 'wrong' responses to that individual are initiated and inappropriate solutions for their requirements are identified.
- Pregnancy, birth and infant care may pose challenges for a woman, her partner and family and may not be without risk to her health. With the relevant information and appropriate support women will be in a better position to make choices related to parenthood.
- If midwives and other professionals and helpers are knowledgeable about specific conditions and how they interact with pregnancy and childbirth, they will be in a stronger position to offer accurate information, effective support, and skilled care that is required by women to enhance their experiences and minimise risks.

## References

BBC News 25 May 1998 Myalgic encephalomyelitis. Online. Available: http://newsvote.bbc.co.uk 13 November 2006

Action for ME 2006 Information centre for myalgic encephalomyelitis. Online. Available: http://www.afme.org.uk 13 November 2006

Afari N, Buchwald D 2003 Chronic fatigue syndrome: a review. The American Journal of Psychiatry 160(2):221–237

ASBAH Association for Spina Bifida and Hydrocephalus 2001a Get clued up on continence: colostomy, ileostomy and urostomy. ASBAH Online. Available: http://www.asbah.org 13 May 2006

ASBAH Association for Spina Bifida and Hydrocephalus 2001b Get clued up on continence: artificial sphincter. ASBAH Online. Available: http://www.asbah.org 13 May 2006

ASBAH Association for Spina Bifida and Hydrocephalus 2001c Get clued up on continence: bladder augmentation. ASBAH Online. Available: http://www.asbah.org 13 May 2006

ASBAH Association for Spina Bifida and Hydrocephalus 2002 Get clued up on continence: Mitrofanoff procedure. ASBAH Online. Available: http://www.asbah.org 13 May 2006

ASBAH Association for Spina Bifida and Hydrocephalus 2003 What is spina bifida? ASBAH Online. Available: http://www.asbah.org 13 May 2006

Barrett J H, Brennan P, Fiddler M, Silman A 2000 Breast-feeding and postpartum relapse in women with rheumatoid and inflammatory arthritis. Arthritis and Rheumatism 43(5):1010–1015

Baschat A A, Weiner C P 2004 Chronic neurologic diseases and disabling conditions in pregnancy. In: Welner S L, Haseltine F (eds) Welner's guide to the care of women with disabilities. Lippincott Williams & Wilkins, Philadelphia, p 145–158

Balzarro M, Appell R A 2004 Management of urinary incontinence in women with disabling conditions. In: Welner S L, Haseltine F (eds) Welner's guide to the care of women with disabilities. Lippincott Williams & Wilkins, Philadelphia, p 69–80

Bowden A P, Barrett J H, Fallow W, Silman A J 2001 Women with inflammatory polyarthritis have babies of lower birth weight. Journal of Rheumatology 28(2):355–359

Bramwell R, Harrington F, Harris J 2000 Deafness—disability or linguistic minority? British Journal of Midwifery 8(4):222–234

Burton S, Pandya A, Arnos K S 2006 Genetics and hearing loss: An overview. The American Speech-Language-Hearing Association (ASHA) Leader 11(1):31–33

Chakravarty E F, Sanchez-Yamamoto D, Bush T M 2003 The use of disease modifying antirheumatic drugs in women with rheumatoid arthritis of childbearing age: a survey of practice patterns and pregnancy outcomes. Journal of Rheumatology 30(2):241–146

Chakravarty E F, Nelson L, Krishnan E 2006 Obstetric hospitalization in the United States for women with systemic lupus erythematosus and rheumatoid arthritis. Arthritis and Rheumatism 54(3):899–907

Chen S, Shieh J, Wang Y et al 2005 Successful pregnancy achieved by intracytoplasmic sperm injection using cryopreserved electroejaculate sperm in a couple both with spinal cord injury: a case report. Archives of Physical Medicine and Rehabilitation 86(9):1884–1886

Cramer C R 1998 Fibromyalgia and chronic fatigue syndrome: an update for athletic trainers. Journal of Athletic Training 33(4):359–361

Csuka M E 2004 Disabling rheumatologic conditions affecting women. In: Welner S L, Haseltine F (eds) Welner's guide to the care of women with disabilities. Lippincott Williams & Wilkins, Philadelphia, p 45–68

Di Nardo S K 1988 Anaesthetic considerations for the achondroplastic dwarf. American Association of Nurse Anesthetists (AANA) Journal 56(1):42–48

Dikkers F G, Verheij J B G M, van Mechelen M 2005 Hereditary congenital unilateral deafness: a new disorder? The Annals of Otology, Rhinology & Laryngology 114(4):332–337

Drey E A, Darney P D 2004 Contraceptive choices for women with disabilities. In: Welner S L, Haseltine F (eds) Welner's guide to the care of women with disabilities. Lippincott Williams & Wilkins, Philadelphia, p 109–130

Drossaers-Bakker K W, Zwinderman A H, van Zeben D et al 2002 Pregnancy and oral contraceptive use do not significantly influence outcome in long term rheumatoid arthritis. Annals of the Rheumatic Diseases 61(5):405–408

Ferrero S, Pretta S, Ragni N 2004 Multiple sclerosis: management issues during pregnancy. European Journal of Obstetrics Gynecology and Reproductive Biology 115(1):3–9

Foundation Fighting Blindness 2006 Retinitis pigmentosa. Online. Available: http://www.blindness.org 1 June 2006

Gordon C 2004 Hormones, pregnancy and inflammatory arthritis. Arthritis Research Campaign. Online. Available: http://www.arc.org.uk 28 April 2006

Grace Parker J H 2006 Achondroplasia. Emedicine from WebMD. Online. Available: http://www.emedicine.com 18 May 2006

Ide M 2004 Sexuality in persons with limb amputation: A meaningful discussion of re-integration. Disability and Rehabilitation 26(14/15):939–943

International Foundation for Optic Nerve Disease (IFOND) 2005 Leber hereditary optic neuropathy. Online. Available: http://www.ifond.org 1 June 2006

Iqbal S 2004 Pregnancy and birth: a guide for deaf women. RNID and the National Childbirth Trust, London

Jackson A B, Wadley V 1999 A multicenter study of women's self-reported reproductive health after spinal cord injury. Archives of Physical Medicine and Rehabilitation 80(11):1420–1428

Jackson A B, Sipski M L 2005 Reproductive issues for women with spina bifida. Journal of Spinal and Cord Medicine 28(2):81–91

Kokitsu-Nakata N M, Guion-Almeida M L, Richieri-Costa A 2004 Clinical genetic study of 144 patients with nonsyndromic hearing loss. American Journal of Audiology 13(2):99–103

Lapper A 2005 My life in my hands. Simon and Schuster, London. Extracts online. Available: www.alisonlapper.com 9 June 2006

Le Gallez P 1999 The pregnant pause… Arthritis Research Campaign. Online. Available: http://www.arc.org.uk 28 April 2006

Lorenzi A R, Ford H L 2002 Multiple sclerosis and pregnancy. Post Graduate Medical Journal 78:460–464

Lovering R M, Porter N C, Bloch R J 2005 The muscular dystrophies: From genes to therapies. Physical Therapy 85(12):1372–1388

McKay-Moffat S 2003 Midwifery care for women with disabilities. MPhil thesis. Liverpool John Moores University, Liverpool

May P L 2005 Latex allergy and spina bifida: a medical view. ASBAH Online. Available: http://www.asbah.org 13 May 2006

Medicinenet 2005 Achondroplasia: health and medical information produced by doctors. Online. Available: http://www.medicinenet.com 20 May 2006

Neild C 2006 MS Essentials: for people living with MS. Women's issues—pregnancy, menstruation, contraception and menopause. Multiple Sclerosis Society. Online. Available: http://www.mssociety.org.uk 28 April 2006

Niven C A 1992 Psychological care for families before, during and after birth. Butterworth Heinemann, Oxford

Odding E, Roebroeck M E, Stam H J 2006 The epidemiology of cerebral palsy: incidence, impairments and risk factors. Disability and Rehabilitation 28(4):183–191

Olkin R 2004 Disability and depression. In: Welner S L, Haseltine F (eds) Welner's guide to the care of women with disabilities. Lippincott Williams & Wilkins, Philadelphia, p 279–300

Olsen N J, Kovacs W J 2002 Hormones, pregnancy and rheumatoid arthritis. Journal of Gender-Specific Medicine 5(4):28–37

Phillips M 2003 Genetics of hearing loss. Medsurg Nursing 12(6):386–411

Schaefer K M, Black K 2005 Fibromyalgia and pregnancy: what nurses need to know and do. Association of Women's Health Obstetric and Neonatal Nurses (AWHONN) Lifelines 9(3): 228–235

Scope 2005 Pregnancy and parenthood for people with cerebral palsy. Online. Available: http://www.scope.org.uk 28 April 2006

Sermon K, Van Steirteghem A, Liebaers I 2004 Preimplantation genetic diagnosis. The Lancet 363(9421):1633–1641

Sevarino F B 2004 Obstetric anaesthesia. In: Welner S L, Haseltine F (eds) Welner's guide to the care of women with disabilities. Lippincott Williams & Wilkins, Philadelphia, p 159–168

Spinal Injury Network 2002–2004 Complete spinal cord injuries Online. Available: http://www.spinal-injury.net May 29 2006

Thomas C 1999 Female forms: experiencing and understanding disability. Buckingham, Philadelphia

Trotter T L, Hall J G, Schaefer G B, et al 2005 Health supervision for children with achondroplasia. Pediatrics 116(3):771–783

Vukusic S, Hutchinson M, Hours M, et al 2004 Pregnancy and multiple sclerosis (the PRIMS study): clinical predictors of post-partum relapse. Brain 127:1353–1360

Welner S L, Temple B 2004 General health concerns and the physical examination. In: Welner S L, Haseltine F (eds) Welner's guide to the care of women with disabilities. Lippincott Williams & Wilkins, Philadelphia, p 95–108

# 9 Resources

*Jackie Rotheram, Stella McKay-Moffat,
Linda Moss, Pam Lee*

## INTRODUCTION

This chapter contains some of the possible resources that may be useful for both midwives and women with disabilities, their partners and families. The list is by no means exhaustive and a search of the internet will elicit many more. But the main ones are included and offer the opportunity for practitioners to browse internet sites or contact the organisations directly to seek further information. The second part of the chapter offers contact details of practitioners willing to discuss best practice related to services for people with disabilities in their locations. The next section gives a list of further recommended reading and the final section gives handouts that can be copied for individual women on contraception, sexual health and preconception care.

## EQUIPMENT

### Anatomical models

A useful selection of very realistic and life-size embryonic development and birth models are available from Adam Rouilly Ltd. which are useful teaching aids for someone with learning disability or where tactile exploration would enhance understanding.

*Contact details:*
Address:
Castle Road,
Eurolink Business Park,
Sittingbourne, Kent, ME10 3AG
Tel: 01795 471378
Fax: 01795 479787
Website: http://www.adam-rouilly.co.uk

### Giraffe® incubator

This high-specification incubator can be electronically adjusted for height appropriate for someone standing giving attention to the baby or for someone sitting e.g. in a wheelchair. Access can be obtained from both sides and a sliding drawer pushes either way to give knee space whist sitting. Supplied by the worldwide company GE Health Care.

*Contact details:*
http://www.gehealthcare.com—opportunity is given on the website to contact the firm by email.

### Height-adjustable couch

Supplied by:
Huntleigh Health Care Ltd, Akron Products Division
http://www.Huntleigh-Akron.com

## GENERAL RESOURCES

### Disability, Pregnancy & Parenthood International (DPPi)

This organisation offers information and support for disabled parents and professionals in the UK to promote fulfilling parenthood. They produce a quarterly journal suitable for parents and professionals alike.

*Contact details:*
Tel: 020 7628 2811
Fax: 020 7628 2833
Textphone: 0800 018 9949
Email: info@dppi.org.uk
Website: http://www.dppi.org.uk

## Disabled Living Foundation (DLF)

This organisation offers advice and information on equipment and assistive technologies to aid independent living. An appointment can be made to visit and have equipment demonstrated.

*Contact details:*
380–384 Harrow Road
London, W9 2HU
Helpline tel: 0845 130 9177 (Mon.–Fri. 10–4 pm)
Equipment centre tel: 020 7289 6111

## Disabled Parents Network

This is a national network of disabled parents helping other disabled parents (their definition of disabled parent is broad) and their families and friends.

*Contact details:*
Unit F9, 89–93 Fonthill Road,
London, N4 3JH
Tel: 08702 410 450
Website: http://www.disabledparentsnetwork.org.uk

## Joseph Rowntree Foundation

This organisation offers information and supports physically, sensory and learning disabled parents, and funds research.
Website: http://www.jrf.org.uk

## Sunderland Support for Parents with Disabilities

A charitable organisation offering support and advocacy for disabled parents.

*Contact details:*
Tel: 0191 566 2158

### RESOURCES FOR BLIND CLIENTS

## Foundation Fighting Blindness—Retinitis pigmentosa

http://www.blindness.org

## Royal National Institute for the Blind (RNIB)

This organisation offers practical solutions for people who are blind, fights for equal opportunities for blind people and funds research projects. They also supply reading material in Braille and talking books.

*Contact details:*
Helpline tel: 0845 766 9999
Website: http://www.rnib.org.uk

### RESOURCES FOR DEAF CLIENTS

## Baby monitors for deaf parents

These are vibrating baby alarms. Tomy has a digital vibrating baby monitor called Platinum Baby Monitor, which has a standard baby unit and portable parent unit with flashing lights and vibrating option which increases as the baby's crying increases. Boardbug Baby and Child Monitor has a digital watch for parents and a wristband for a baby or toddler that transmits sound, flashes and bleeps. Both are available from John Lewis and other outlets or online at http://www.boardbug.com

'Baby Monitors — information for deaf and hard of hearing people' is available from the RNID website (see below).

## British Deaf Association (BDA)

The BDA is the largest national organisation run by deaf people, for deaf people. BDA undertakes campaigning work and provides a range of vital services to the deaf community, including a helpline, publications, advocacy, and counselling, and youth services.

*Contact details:*
1–3 Worship Street
London, EC2A 2AB
Helpline tel: 0870 770 3300
Helpline textphone: 0800 6522 965
Fax: 020 7588 3527
Email: helpline@bda.org.uk
Website: www.bda.org.uk

## British Society for Mental Health and Deafness

This organisation promotes positive mental health for deaf people in Britain. They put on conferences, and provide books, videos and DVDs for professionals working in mental health and deafness. They have produced a Deaf Mental Health Charter Information pack to raise the awareness of the basic rights of deaf people when receiving mental health services and to help make services more inclusive.

*Contact details:*
Westwood Park, London Road,
Little Horkesley,
Colchester, CO6 4BS
Tel: 01206 274075
Textphone: 01206 274076
Fax: 01206 274077
Email: info@bssmhd.org.uk
Website: http://www.bsmhd.org.uk

## BSL software in general practice

SignHealth is a new computer program that healthcare professionals in general practice can use to assist communication with BSL users. The DoH is purchasing this software for all PCTs from January 2006. For further information access http://www.signhealth.com

## Chowdry S 2001 Deaf parents, gaps in services

This video was made by Sabina Chowdry in collaboration with Disability Pregnancy and Parenthood International (DPPi) (see below). It shows deaf women and their partners sharing their experiences of maternity services. (The video is not currently available to buy but check availability with your local health authority/hospital/university library.)

## CoDPUK (Children of Deaf Parents UK)

CoDPUK aims to inform, mentor and work with deaf parents in the UK, in broadening the horizons of their children and nurturing self-esteem. The organisation provides support via social events, as well as a quarterly newsletter.

*Contact details:*
PO Box 3272
Maidenhead
Berkshire, SL6 4WW
Email: info@codpuk.org.uk
Website: http://www.codpuk.org.uk

## Colville M 1985 Signs of a sexual nature. Forest Books, Coleford

This is available directly from Forest Books (see below) and gives illustrations and explanations of slang and educational sexual terms.

## Deaf Parenting UK (DPUK)

Deaf Parenting UK's objectives are to relieve all the needs of deaf parents (those who use BSL as their first language) and deaf parents-to-be in the UK. The organisation offers training and direct support services for deaf parents in partnership with several organisations across the UK.

*Contact details:*
Stephen Dering, Director
C/o Pertemps Mouzer, Fourth Floor, Charles House,
375 Kensington High Street, London, W14 8QH
Tel. 020 7471 6770
Textphone: 020 7471 6769
Fax: 020 7471 6768
Email: s.dering@disabilityserve.com
Website: www.deafparent.org.uk

## Disability, Pregnancy & Parenthood International (DPPi)

This international organisation provides a UK-based information service for deaf and disabled people who are already parents or considering parenting, health and social care professionals and others concerned with issues affecting the lives of deaf and disabled parents. DPPi produces a number of information sheets, available in various formats, and publishes an international journal. There is an ideas forum on the DPPi website where parents can share ideas and experiences. Small items of parenting equipment are on display in the National Centre.

Available from DPPi are two accessible resources on pregnancy, birth and early postnatal in BSL with subtitles and voice-over. They come with supplementary leaflets as well as a pack for visually impaired parents and parents-to-be and are available in large print, Braille, audio and Daisy (Digital Accessible Information System) formats. The resources can be used by professionals who work with parents with sensory impairment as well as by parents themselves.

*Contact details:*
National Centre for Disabled Parents
Unit F9 89–93 Fonthill Road,
London, N4 3JH
Helpline tel: 0800 018 4730
Helpline textphone: 0800 018 9949
Fax: 020 7263 6399
Email: info@dppi.org.uk
Website: http://www.dppi.org.uk

DPPi has facilitated a Deaf Parents Working Group. Contact the National Centre for Disabled Parents for details.

*Contact details:*
Becki Josiah
National Centre for Disabled Parents
Unit F9 89–93 Fonthill Road,
London, N4 3JH
Tel: 0800 0184730
Textphone: 0800 018 9949
Fax: 020 7263 6399
Email: becki@dppi.org.uk
Website: http://www.deafparent.org.uk

Disabled Parents Network (DPN) has published a series of briefings giving practical information and advice about disabled parenting: what the law says, getting needs assessed, planning care, direct payments, maternity services and support for new parents, making a complaint, advocacy advice and legal help.

*Contact details:*
Email: information@disabledparentsnetwork.org.uk

DPPi have also produced an information pack for blind and visually impaired people, which has been available since March 2006 called 'Having a baby resource pack'. It is available in large print, Braille, audio and Daisy, which offers standardisation of talking books. The pack is also available to healthcare professionals from:

Gill Lea-Wilson
Information Officer
DPPi
National Centre for Disabled Parents
Unit F9, 89/93 Fonthill Road
London, N4 3JH

## Forest Books

This bookseller specialises in resources about deafness and deaf issues. They provide a range of books, videos, CD-ROMs and DVDs, including BSL resources, books on language development and children's fiction featuring D/deaf characters.

*Contact details:*
The New Building, Ellwood Road,
Milkwall, Coleford,
Gloucestershire, GL16 7LE
Tel: 01594 833 858 (voice/minicom)
Fax: 01594 833446
Email: Forest@forestbooks.com.
Website: http://www.Forestbooks.com

## Free E-Group for Deaf parents and professionals working with Deaf parents

*Contact details:*
Website: http://groups.yahoo.com/group/Deafparenting/

## Iqbal S 2004 Pregnancy and birth: a guide for deaf women. RNID and National Childbirth Trust, London

This book is aimed at deaf women whose first or preferred language is British Sign Language (BSL) and other deaf, deafened or hard-of-hearing women. The book is useful for professionals and deaf parents alike. It covers a wide range of topics including planning for a baby, pregnancy, birth and afterwards, including care for mother, baby and father. It also includes some advice on maternity and paternity rights for working parents and legislation such as the Disability Discrimination Act (DDA) 1995. Additionally it includes stories by mothers and fathers. Available from Forest Books (see above).

## Parenting leaflets launched by DfES and Asda

A series of free leaflets addressing a range of parenting issues, created with input from charities ParentlinePlus, Fathers Direct, National Family and Parenting Institute.

http://www.parentscentre.gov.uk/

## Royal Association for Deaf People (RAD)

RAD promotes the welfare and interests of deaf people. The organisation works in the areas of deaf community development, employment, families and children, youth, information, advice and advocacy, learning disability, mental health, sign language interpreting and training.

*Contact details:*
Head Office
Walsingham Road, Colchester
Essex, CO2 7BP
Tel: 01206 509509
Textphone: 01206 711260
Fax: 01206 769755
Email: info@royaldeaf.org.uk
Website: http://www.royaldeaf.org.uk

## Royal National Institute for the Deaf (RNID)

RNID is a national membership charity, offering a range of services for deaf and hard-of-hearing people. The organisation provides information and support on all aspects of deafness, hearing loss and tinnitus. It is also involved in campaigning, training, providing equipment and undertaking medical and technical research.

*Contact details:*
19–23 Featherstone Street
London, EC1Y 8SL
Information line tel: 0808 808 0123
Information line textphone: 0808 808 9000
Fax: 020 7296 8199
Email: informationline@rnid.org.uk
Website: http://www.rnid.org.uk

## Smith C 1999 Signs of health. Pocket guide to medical signs. Forest Books, Coleford

Pocket-sized book containing over 200 signs relating to health and medical procedures. Available from the Forest Bookshop (see above).

## School B 1999 Signs for use in hospitals. Forest Books, Coleford

This booklet contains illustrations and explanations of signs useful in a hospital environment.

## Sign & Bond

This baby signing company offers services to both deaf and hearing children and parents, concentrating on how to teach signing. They supply DVDs and offer a consultancy and training service to enhance children's communication skills.

*Contact details:*
SMS: 07876 597974
Email: Yvonne@signbond.co.uk
Website: http://www.signbond.co.uk

## Two Can Productions

The company publishes low-cost leaflets on pregnancy, relaxation classes and antenatal clinic, labour and birth. They are written in plain English with pictures and BSL illustrations. They offer information on communication, sign language interpreters (SLIs) and deaf awareness. Under the Disability Discrimination Act (DDA), deaf people are entitled to communication support whilst in hospital. This means qualified SLIs. Unfortunately SLIs are in short supply and need to be booked well in advance. Arranging a hospital account with the local interpreting agency will make this easier. However, there will be times when it is not possible to have a SLI present.

*Contact details:*
Tel/fax: 01332 366 083
Textphone: 01332 371 750
Email: TWOCAN1@compuserve.com

## RESOURCES FOR LEARNING DISABLED CLIENTS

The Baring Foundation: www.baringfoundation.org. uk. This publication contains excellent information about resources available across the country for parents with a learning disability and for the professionals working with families. This is well referenced and up to date—a very useful document.

## Down's Syndrome Association

This organisation offers support, information and training for people with Down's syndrome and for parents with a child with the condition.

*Contact details:*
Langdon Down Centre
2a Langdon Park,
Teddington, TW11 9PS
Tel: 0845 230 0372
Fax: 0845 230 0373
Email: info@downs-syndrome.org.uk
Website: http://www.downs-syndrome.org.uk

## CHANGE organisation

This is a national organisation run by disabled people, including people with learning disabilities and people who are blind or deaf. They campaign and work for equal rights for disabled people.

*Contact details:*
Unit 19/20, Unity Business Centre,
26 Roundhay Road,
Leeds, LS7 1AB
Tel: 0113 243 0202
Fax: 0113 243 0220
Minicom: 0113 234 2225
Website: http://www.changepeople.co.uk

## Makaton

Sign language developed for people with learning disability who are deaf. Useful website: http://www. makaton.org

## MENCAP

This leading national charity works with people with learning disabilities, their families and their carers both nationally and locally by offering support and information.

*Contact details:*
123 Golden Lane,
London, EC1 0RT
Tel: 020 7454 0454
Fax: 020 7696 5540
Email: information@mencap.org.uk
Website: http://www.mencap.org.uk

## The Special Parenting Services in Cornwall

www.cornwall.nhs.uk/specialparentingservices

## RESOURCES FOR CLIENTS WITH SPECIFIC PHYSICAL CONDITIONS

## Spina bifida

Association for Spina Bifida and Hydrocephalus (ASBAH)

*Contact details:*
42 Park Road,
Peterborough, PE1 2UQ
Tel: 01733 555 988
Fax: 01733 555 985
Email: postmaster@ashab.org
Website: http://www.asbah.org

## Achondroplasia

Little People of America

*Contact details:*
PO Box 745, Lubbock, TX 79408
888-LPA-2001
March of Dimes
Information about achondroplasia on http://www.marchofdimes.com

## Medicinenet: Health and medical information produced by doctors

Website: http://www.medicinenet.com

## Arthritis

Arthritis Research

This charitable organisation offers information and support for people with the condition.

*Contact details:*
Copeman House, St. Mary's Court,
St. Mary's Gate, Chesterfield,
Derbyshire, S41 7TD
Tel: 0870 850 5000
Fax: 01246 558007
Email: info@arc.or.uk
Website: http://www.arc.org.uk

## Cerebral palsy

Scope

This is a national organisation that used to be called The Spastic Society. They offer information and support for people with cerebral palsy, and information for professionals.

*Contact details:*
Cerebral palsy helpline: Mon.–Fri. 9 am–9 pm; weekends: 2 pm–6 pm
PO Box 833
Milton Keynes, MK12 5NY
Tel: 0808 800 3333
Website: http://www.scope.org.uk

## Muscular dystrophy

Muscular Dystrophy Association

This is an American voluntary health association offering information on and undertaking research into the condition. The useful internet website includes a diversity of information and insight into the lived experiences of people with the condition.
Website: http://www.mdausa.org

## Multiple sclerosis (MS)

This is the UK's largest charity supporting people with MS, their families and friends. They provide support from all perspectives, including practical aspects, on a national and local basis. They also fund research.

*Contact details:*
MS National Centre
372 Edgeware Road,
London, NW2 6ND
Tel: 020 8433 0700
National freephone: 0808 800 8000 Mon.–Fri. 9 am–9 pm
Email: info@mssociety.org.uk
Website: http://www.mssociety.org.uk

## Spinal injury

Spinal Injury Network

This website provides information, including research data, fact sheets and a chat room.
http://www.spinal-injury.net

### CONTACTS FOR EXAMPLES OF GOOD PRACTICE

Liverpool
Liverpool Women's Hospital
Jackie Rotheram, Disability Advisor
Tel: 0151 702 4012 Mon.–Thurs.
Text: 07717517172
Email: jackie.rotheram@lwh.nhs.uk
Patricia Fairlamb, Midwife (special needs)
Tel: 01908 660033 × 3162
Email: pafairlamb@yahoo.co.uk

### FURTHER READING

Bramwell R, Harrington F, Harris J 2000 Deaf women: informed choice, policy and legislation. British Journal of Midwifery 8(9):545–548.

Brown B 2001 The introduction of a special needs advisor. British Journal of Midwifery 9(6):348–351

Brown J 2003 Tailor-made maternity services. Disability Pregnancy and Parenthood International (DPPi) 42:8–9

Campion M J 1995 An inclusive philosophy of care. Disability Pregnancy and Parenthood International (DPPi) 11:3–5

Campion M J 1997 Disabled women and maternity services. Modern Midwife 7(3):23–25

Carty E M 1998 Disability and childbirth meeting the challenges. Canadian Medical Association 159:4

Carty E M, Cohrine T, Holbrook A 1993 Supporting the pregnant woman who is disabled: guidelines for professionals. Disability Pregnancy and Parenthood International (DPPi) 3:8–11

Chowdry S 2001 Deaf parenting: raising a child—an initial study on deaf parents with children aged 0–11 years old in San Francisco, USA. Unpublished dissertation. To learn more about this research contact: deafparents@yahoo.co.uk or contact DPUK.

Department of Health Publications 2000 A jigsaw of services: inspection of services to support disabled adults in their parenting role. Online. Available: http://www.dh.gov.uk

Down's Syndrome Association Learning About Learning Disabilities and Health; what we know about parenting training. Online. Available: http://www.intellectualdisability.info 16 February 2006

Dunn D 2001 Sexual health. In: Thompson J, Pickering S (eds) Meeting the health needs of people who have a learning disability. Bailliere Tindall, London, p 211–234

Emerson E, Hatton C 2005 Deinstitutionalisation. Tizard Learning Disability Review, Brighton, Feb. 10(1):36

French S 1996 The attitudes of health professionals towards disabled people. In: Hales G (ed) Beyond disability, towards an enabling society. Sage, London, p 151–163

Galea J, Butler J, Iacono T, Leighton D 2004 The assessment of sexual knowledge in people with intellectual disability. Journal of Intellectual and Developmental Disability 29(4):350–365

Goodman M 1994 Pregnant and disabled? Don't assume the professionals will understand. Professional Care of Mother and Child Nov/Dec:227–228

Goodman M 1996 Action on disability and maternity: a report of progress towards good practice in the purchase and provision of maternity services for disabled women and their partners. Maternity Alliance London available from NCT

Josiah B 2004 Hearing the needs of deaf mothers-to-be. The Practising Midwife 7(3):22–23

Kelsall J 1992 She can lip read, she'll be all right: improving maternity care for the deaf and hearing impaired. Midwifery 8:178–183

Korman N, Glennester H 1990 Hospital closure. Open University Press, Milton Keynes

Maternity Alliance 1994 Listen to us for a change: a charter for disabled parents and parents to be. In: Maternity group disability working group pack. Maternity Alliance, London

MENCAP 2006 Mencap calls for better supports for parents with a learning difficulty. Online. Available: http://www.mencap.org.uk 27 February 2006

McKay Moffat S 2003 Meeting the needs of women with disabilities. The Practising Midwife 6(7):12–15

McKay-Moffat S, Cunningham C 2006 Services for women with disabilities: mothers' and midwives' experiences. British Journal of Midwifery 14(8):472–477

Middleton A, Hewison J, Mueller R 2001 Prenatal diagnosis for inherited deafness-what is the potential demand? Journal of Genetic Counseling 10(2):121–131

This study assessed the potential uptake of prenatal diagnosis for inherited deafness. It also documented the opinions of deaf and hearing participants towards prenatal testing and termination of pregnancy.

NHS Executive 1999 Once a day; one or more people with learning disabilities are likely to be in contact with your primacy health care team. How can you help them? Department of Health, Weatherby

Oakes P 2003 Sexuality and personal relationships. In: Gates B (ed) Learning disabilities; towards inclusion. 4th edn. Churchill Livingstone, Edinburgh, p 455–470

O'Hara J 2003 Parents with learning disabilities; a study of gender and cultural perspectives in East London. British Institute of Learning Disabilities Publications. British Journal of Learning Disabilities 31:18–24

Rogers J 2005 The disabled woman's guide to pregnancy and birth. Demos Medical Publishing, New York

Ronai C R 1997 On loving and hating my mentally retarded mother. Mental Retardation 35(6): 417–432

Rotheram J 1989 Care of the disabled woman during pregnancy. Nursing Standard 4(10):36–39

Rotheram J 1998 Caring for the minority within the minority. British Journal Midwifery 6(9):596

Rotheram J 2002 Maternity needs of disabled women. Disability Pregnancy and Parenthood International (DPPi) 40:10–11

Royal College of Physicians (RCOP) 1998 Disabled people using hospitals: a charter and guidelines. RCOP, London

Ryan J, Thomas F 1991 The politics of mental handicap. Free Association Books, London

Shackle M 1994 I thought I was the only one. A report of a conference

Disabled people, pregnancy and early parenthood. Part of the Maternity Alliance Working Group Pack. Maternity Alliance, London

Shakespeare T, Gillespie-Sells K, Davies D 1996 The sexual politics of disability, untold desires. Cassell, London

Thomas C, Curtis P 1997 Having a baby: some disabled women's reproductive experiences. Midwifery 13:202–209

Wates M 2003 It shouldn't be down to luck. In: Disabled parents network handbook project. Disabled Parents, London

Wates M, Newman T 2005 Disabled parents and their children: building a better future. Barnados, London

Wates M 1997 Disabled parents: dispelling the myths. National Childbirth Trust (NCT) Publishing, Cambridge

Wates M, Jade R 1999 Bigger than the sky: disabled women on parenting. Women's Press, London. Available from National Library for the Blind. Contact details: Tel: 0161 494 0217 for Braille; tel: 01296 432 339 for audiocassette from Calibre

## HANDOUTS FOR WOMEN

When women with disabilities have shared their experiences in the literature, issues that have recurred have been related to a lack of information on contraception and sexually transmitted infections. This section of the book contains handouts that address those needs. Additionally there is another handout on preconception care as all women are likely to benefit from improving their health and well-being prior to conception. The information on each handout is by necessity only an overview and further information should be offered to women to support that given in the literature or referral made to a specialist advisor.

It is suggested that the information sheet on contraception is given along with further sheets on a specific method(s) as identified during an initial discussion.

Permission is given for individual handouts to be photocopied and given to women as required but must not be copied in bulk or used for publication or commercial use.

## INFORMATION SHEET FOR WOMEN WITH DISABILITY: CONTRACEPTION

Planning to have a family when a couple are in optimum health and when it suits them from a physical, psychological, social and economic standpoint is one key to a successful and satisfying pregnancy and childbirth outcome.

Having effective contraception will aid family planning but not every method of contraception is suitable for every couple at all times in their lives. Many issues have to be taken into consideration when choosing a method. These revolve around reliability, availability, acceptability and suitability of a method.

To accompany this sheet is a series of leaflets that gives information on the methods currently readily available and an overview of how to use those methods to achieve optimum contraceptive reliability, and when they are suitable in relation to the time after having a baby. These methods fall into the categories of hormonal, barrier, intrauterine devices, sterilisation and emergency contraception. The general acceptability of a method is noted and issues of suitability are indicated which may need to be considered depending on individual circumstances. Any additional information and more precise instructions for using a method can be obtained from the local family planning clinic (location and contact details in the telephone book), from GPs or from a nurse or midwife with family planning expertise. Additionally, comprehensive instructions for using a method are usually supplied by manufacturers in the original packaging.

## CONTRACEPTION FOR WOMEN WITH DISABILITY (1)

### Barrier methods

A failure rate means the number of women out of 100 using the method *correctly* for one year who will become pregnant.

#### Male condom (sheath)

A latex tube usually coated in a spermicide—single use. Common makes are Durex and Mates. Some 'fun' designs to encourage use but there may be less contraceptive reliability.

*Reliability*
Failure rate about 2%.

*Availability*
Can be obtained free at family planning clinics (either partner can ask for them and no need to give any personal details or see the doctor), or purchased at varied retail outlets.

*How to use and reduce the risk of method failure*
■ Must be fitted on an erect penis *before* any genital contact is made.
■ Rolled up part of condom should be on the outside before fitting.
■ During fitting the tip of the condom should be squeezed to avoid air getting in otherwise there is more risk of splitting—roll it carefully down the penis (the penis should not go into the tip).
■ Condom must be held on and carefully removed before the erection completely ends.
■ *No* genital or condom contact with female partner after removal.
■ Wrap and dispose of in the dustbin (not down the toilet).

*Acceptability*
■ Need to stop lovemaking to fit condom.
■ Some loss of sensation may occur.

*Suitability and advantages*
■ No medical implications i.e. almost anyone can use them.
■ They usually have a spermicidal lubricant. If this is not enough lubrication then a water-based gel e.g. KY jelly should be used *not* an oil-based one e.g. Vaseline or baby oil as these damage condoms.

■ They offer some protection against sexually transmitted infections and the virus that can cause cervical cancer.
■ Can be used at any time after childbirth.

*Disadvantages and possible risks*
■ Some people are allergic to latex—polyurethane ones available but they are not as strong.
■ Some dexterity is needed to fit them and usually a two-handed process—some people used to one-handed activities in their daily life may manage.
■ Some treatments for thrush may damage condoms e.g. Gyno-Daktarin cream—seek advice if treatment is being used.

#### Female condom

A large tube of polyurethane with an inner ring to aid insertion and an outer ring that remains outside of the body during use—single use.

*Reliability*
Failure rate about 5%.

*Availability*
Purchased at pharmacies.

*How to use and reduce the risk of failure*
■ Must be inserted into the vagina, with the aid of the inner ring, *before* any genital contact with partner.
■ Ensure the outer ring is located outside of the labia (vaginal lips).
■ When the penis penetrates ensure it is not outside of the outer ring.
■ Ensure no spillage of semen when removing the condom from the vagina.

*Acceptability*
■ May be seen as an unattractive piece of 'kit'.
■ Said by some to 'rustle' during use: this may be off-putting.
■ Some people would not use the method as they find touching the genitalia unacceptable.

*Suitability and advantages*
■ No medical implications i.e. almost anyone can use them.

- Offers some protection against sexually transmitted infections and the virus that can cause cervical cancer.
- Can be used any time after childbirth.

*Disadvantages and possible risks*
- Requires considerable dexterity, mobility and leg abduction for insertion—if this is an issue a woman's partner may insert it for her if this is acceptable.
- Unsuitable if either partner has polyurethane allergy.

## Diaphragm (cap)

A dome-shaped latex 'cup' with an outer spring to keep the shape and aid fitting. It fits between the back of the cervix (neck of womb) and behind the pubic bone covering the cervix—reusable.

*Reliability*

Failure rate 2–8% (higher with silicone and non-fitted types).

*Availability*
- Size measured and cap supplied free at family planning clinics and free prescription by some GPs.
- A pack of varied sizes is available over the counter at larger pharmacies i.e. not fitted by a trained professional but most comfortable size chosen by user.

*How to use and reduce the risk of failure*
- No genital contact should occur before the cap is in place.
- A spermicide should always be applied to the cap before use.

- The opposite sides of the spring edges are squeezed together to allow insertion into the vagina.
- Additional spermicide must be inserted into the vagina if the cap has been in place for more than 3 hours.
- Cap must remain in place at least 6 hours after intercourse but removed within 24 hours.
- Care must be taken to avoid damage to the cap e.g. with fingernails during insertion, removal or when washing it before storage.

*Acceptability*
- May be seen as an unattractive piece of 'kit'.
- Some find touching the genital area unacceptable.
- Reliability may not be good enough.

*Suitability and advantages*
- No medical implications i.e. almost anyone can use one.
- Offers some protection against the virus that can cause cervical cancer.
- Can be in place some time prior to intercourse.
- The size of cap used before childbirth needs to be checked from 6 weeks after giving birth—a larger size is often needed.

*Disadvantages and possible risks*
- Latex allergy for either partner (silicone caps available).
- Requires considerable dexterity, mobility and leg abduction for insertion—if this is an issue a woman's partner may insert it for her if this is acceptable.
- Poor skin sensation at the vagina may make self-insertion difficult.
- Can be damaged by oil-based creams e.g. Vaseline, baby oil and some thrush treatments.

## CONTRACEPTION FOR WOMEN WITH DISABILITY (2)

### | Hormonal methods

Failure rate means the number of women out of 100 using the method *correctly* for 1 year who will become pregnant.

#### Combined oral contraceptive (the pill)

Two hormones i.e. oestrogen and progesterone in a daily tablet.

*Reliability*
Failure rate less than 1%.

*Availability*
Free at family planning clinics and on free prescription from GPs.

*How to use and reduce the risk of failure*
■ One tablet daily—take regularly at the same time each day (choose a time you are less likely to forget) for 3 weeks then a pill-free week to enable a withdrawal bleeding (period).
■ If you forget at your usual time you have 12 hours to take it and remain protected e.g. if you usually take it at 6 pm but forget, you must take it by 6 am the following day.
■ If a pill is missed use another method for 7 days e.g. a condom.
■ If you have to take antibiotics you may not be protected during the course and for 7 days afterwards so use another method.
■ Reliability is reduced if you have a bout of diarrhoea—use another method and for 7 days after diarrhoea stops.

*Acceptability*
■ Small and easily swallowed.
■ Once a day and does not interfere with love-making.
■ Religious or cultural beliefs may prevent use.

*Suitability and advantages*
■ Menstruation very regular and often light—less hygiene issues and anaemia.
■ Three consecutive packets can be taken to avoid periods—less hygiene issues and anaemia.
■ Can be taken from 3 weeks after childbirth but *not* suitable during breast-feeding.

*Disadvantages and possible risks*
■ Reduced reliability with some medications e.g. carbamazepine (Tegretol) and St. John's Wort—seek medical advice.
■ Increases the effects of beta blockers (given for high blood pressure); diazepam (Valium); and corticosteroids—seek medical advice.
■ Not suitable for women who are over 35, smokers, or obese women.
■ Deep vein thrombosis (DVT) risk higher when circulation is poor (especially in the lower limbs) or when immobility is an issue.

#### Progesterone oral contraceptive pill (mini pill)

One hormone only i.e. progesterone in a daily tablet.

*Reliability*
Failure rate about 1%.

*Availability*
Free at family planning clinics and free on prescription from GPs.

*How to use and reduce the risk of failure*
■ One tablet daily—take regularly at the same time every day (choose a time that is easy to remember) without a break between packs.
■ Must be taken within 3 hours of the same time i.e. if you usually take it at 6 pm you only have until 9 pm to take it and remain protected against pregnancy.
■ A newer preparation, Cerazette, has a 12-hour 'safety time'.

*Acceptability*
■ Easily swallowed.
■ Less risk factors compared to a combined hormonal contraceptive.
■ Religious or cultural beliefs may prevent use.

*Suitability and advantages*
■ Very reliable if taken promptly every day.
■ Suitable in many cases when combined hormone methods unsuitable e.g. women over 35, smokers, obese women.
■ Periods may be lighter or stop—less hygiene issues and anaemia.
■ Can be taken from 3 weeks after childbirth and suitable during breast-feeding.

## Disadvantages and possible risks

- Some medication *may* reduce reliability (see combined pill above) although less likely.
- Other drug actions may be affected (see combined pill above) although less likely.
- Some side effects possible e.g. weight gain (may affect mobility for some); headaches; fluid retention.
- Irregular periods may occur especially during early packs.
- Unclear if bone density affected by long-term use of progesterone methods.
- Reliability may be reduced if body weight over 70 kg.

## Skin implants (Implanon)

Slow-release progesterone from a semi-rigid rod measuring 40 mm × 2 mm implanted under the skin of the upper arm.

### Reliability

Failure risk minimal.

### Availability

Fitted free of charge at family planning clinics and by some GPs.

### How to use and reduce the risk of failure

- Single 'rod' inserted under local anaesthetic into the skin of the underside of the upper arm.
- Replaced every 3 years.

### Acceptability

- Insertion procedure may be unacceptable.
- May not wish for an obvious sign of contraceptive use.
- Religious or cultural beliefs may prevent use.

### Suitability and advantages

- Useful if remembering to take a tablet is difficult.
- Slow release of hormone means fewer side effects.
- Reliability very high.
- Fertility returns more quickly after removal compared to injected progesterone.
- Suitable in many cases when combined hormone methods unsuitable.
- Periods may stop—less hygiene issues and anaemia.

- Can be used from 3 weeks after childbirth—suitable during breast-feeding.

### Disadvantages and possible risks

- Skin may initially be uncomfortable after insertion.
- In rare cases removal may be difficult.
- Reliability may be reduced by some medication (see combined pill above).
- Irregular periods may occur.
- Unclear if bone density affected by long-term use of progesterone methods.

## Combined hormone skin patch (Evra)

Slow-release oestrogen and progesterone in a skin patch 5 cm × 5 cm.

### Reliability

- Failure rate about 1%.

### Availability

- Available at some family planning clinics (free) and on prescription from GPs.

### How to use and reduce the risk of failure

- One patch placed on the skin at the top or back of an arm or on hip or top of thigh.
- Patch must be changed every week until three have been used then 1 week without a patch when a withdrawal bleed (period) will occur.
- Three cycles can be used i.e. 9 weeks of patches to avoid withdrawal bleeds, followed by 1 patch-free week when a period will occur.

### Acceptability

- May not wish an obvious sign of contraceptive use.
- Religious or cultural beliefs may prevent use.

### Suitability and advantages

- Slow release of hormone through the skin means an overall lower dose at a constant level.
- Useful if taking a daily tablet is difficult.
- Reliable when antibiotics are taken unlike tablets.

### Disadvantages and possible risks

- See combined pill above.
- Skin sensitivity for some women.
- Reliability may be reduced in women over 90 kg.

- Some spotting blood loss may occur during first 3 months.

### Depo Provera
Slow-release progesterone given by injection.

*Reliability*
Failure less than 1%.

*Availability*
Prescribed and injected free at family planning clinics and by GPs.

*How to use and reduce the risk of failure*
- One injection into a large muscle regularly every 11–12 weeks.
- Delay in receiving the next injection will reduce reliability.

*Acceptability*
- Injections may not be liked.
- If side effects felt there will be delay in them going.
- No outward sign of contraception being used.
- Religious or cultural beliefs may prevent use.

*Suitability and advantages*
- Suitable in many cases when a combined hormone method unsuitable.
- Periods may eventually stop or be very light—less hygiene issues and anaemia.
- No risk of forgetting a daily tablet.
- Can be used from 3 weeks after childbirth—suitable during breast-feeding.

*Disadvantages and possible risks*
- Reduced reliability with some medications e.g. carbamazepine (Tegretol) and St. John's Wort—seek medical advice.
- Easy access to a large muscle for injection may be difficult.
- Side effects the same as progesterone pill—weight gain may affect mobility.
- Periods may be heavy initially or irregular.
- Return of fertility may be delayed after stopping contraception.
- Some concerns about bone density with long-term use therefore less suitable for women with a potential to develop osteoporosis.

## CONTRACEPTION FOR WOMEN WITH DISABILITY (3)

### Intrauterine methods

Failure rate means the number of women out of 100 using the method *correctly* for 1 year who will become pregnant.

#### Intrauterine contraceptive devices (coils)

A small plastic device surrounded by a copper thread inserted into the uterus (womb) through the cervix (neck of womb).

*Reliability*
Failure rate less than 1%.

*Availability*
Fitted at family planning clinics and by a few GPs free of charge.

*How to use and reduce the risk of failure*
- Best inserted during or at the end of a period.
- Short lengths of thread attached to the coil hang through the cervix—ideally these should be felt for after each period to ensure coil still in place.
- Replaced approximately every 5 years depending on the type fitted.

*Acceptability*
- Insertion procedure may be unacceptable.
- Religious or cultural beliefs may prevent use.

*Suitability and advantages*
- Useful if taking a daily tablet is difficult.
- Gives long-term protection against pregnancy.
- Infection screening for chlamydia is performed and treatment given if needed prior to insertion which reduces the risk of pelvic inflammatory disease.
- Can be fitted from 12 weeks after childbirth.

*Disadvantages and possible risks*
- Leg abduction needed for insertion which may be difficult when a woman has arthritis/leg spasms.
- May be more painful/not always easy to fit in a woman who has never had a baby as the cervix is usually tightly closed.
- Periods may be heavy and more painful the first 1–3 times.
- Risk of autonomic dysreflexia on insertion in women with spinal cord lesions.

- Women with poor pelvic sensation e.g. when they have a spinal cord lesion, or those with poor understanding may not recognise the pain of pelvic inflammatory disease.

#### Intrauterine system (Mirena)

An intrauterine device like the coil but with a stem of progesterone that is slowly released i.e. two methods in one.

*Reliability*
Failure risk minimal.

*Availability*
Prescribed and inserted at family planning clinics (few GPs).

*How to use and reduce the risk of failure*
- Best inserted during or at the end of a period.
- Short lengths of thread attached to the coil hang through the neck of the womb—ideally these should be felt for after each period to ensure coil still in place.
- Replaced every 5 years.

*Acceptability*
- Insertion procedure may be unacceptable.
- Religious or cultural beliefs may prevent use.

*Suitability and advantages*
- Best inserted during or at the end of a period.
- Gives long-term protection against pregnancy.
- Progesterone increases the reliability—low dose with fewer side effects than other progesterone methods.
- Periods may stop—less hygiene issues and anaemia.
- Fertility may return more readily after removal than with injected progesterone.
- Suitable in many cases when combined hormone methods unsuitable.
- Reliability not affected by medications.
- Can be inserted 12 weeks after childbirth—suitable during breast-feeding.

*Disadvantages and possible risks*
- Leg abduction needed for fitting (see coil above).
- Risk of autonomic dysreflexia during fitting (see above).
- Irregular periods may occur.

## CONTRACEPTION FOR WOMEN WITH DISABILITY (4)

## | Sterilisation

### Female sterilisation (tubal ligation)
The tubes where the ovum (egg) is fertilised before being taken to the uterus (womb) are cut, preventing the sperm reaching the ovum.

*Reliability*
Failure rate about 1 in 200 cases (although much lower with some methods).

*Availability*
Performed on the NHS (waiting list) or paid for through private healthcare.

*How to use and reduce the risk of failure*
- Generally considered a permanent procedure although reversal has been achieved in a few cases but NHS availability of this procedure is low.
- Only a very slight risk of failure.
- Immediate contraception following surgery.

*Acceptability*
- Consent to surgery must be given following clear explanation of the process.
- Some women dislike thinking they are no longer able to have a child.
- Religious or cultural beliefs may prevent use.

*Suitability and advantages*
- Suitability for surgery will depend on individual well-being.
- If surgery is performed via laparoscopic procedure recovery is relatively quick.
- Following recovery from surgery there is little worry of pregnancy occurring.

*Disadvantages and possible risks*
- Risk of any surgical procedure e.g. compromised breathing for someone with high spinal cord damage, or risk of DVT in women with reduced lower limb circulation or mobility.
- Pain of surgery may cause autonomic hyperreflexia in women with spinal cord lesions.
- Very slight chance of method failure.

### Male sterilisation (vasectomy)
The tubes carrying the male sperm are cut to prevent sperm from getting through.

*Reliability*
Failure rate about 1 in 2000 cases.

*Availability*
The same as female procedure.

*How to use and reduce the risk of failure*
- Often performed under local anaesthetic as a hospital day case.
- Three sperm-free semen specimens needed before safety assured.

*Acceptability*
- Male may feel he is less at risk than his partner.
- Religious or cultural beliefs may prevent use.

*Suitability and advantages*
- Suitable for almost everyone.
- Surgery is quick to perform and recovery is faster than for women.

*Disadvantages and possible risks*
- Little risk especially when performed under local anaesthetic.
- Very small chance of method failure.

## CONTRACEPTION FOR WOMEN WITH DISABILITY (5)

### Emergency contraception

These two methods should be used only in an emergency when a method has failed e.g. a split condom, or if unprotected intercourse has occurred. They should not be used as a regular contraceptive method.

Failure rate means the number of women out of 100 using the method *correctly* for 1 year who will become pregnant.

### Hormonal method (morning after pill)

A single tablet of a high dose of progesterone.

*Reliability*
Failure rate from 5 to 42% depending on how soon after unprotected intercourse, or a failed method, it is taken.

*Availability*
- Free at family planning and sexual health clinics, and on prescription from GPs.
- May be purchased through approved pharmacists—costs about £26.

*How to use and reduce the risk of failure*
- Tablet should be taken as soon as possible after the event for the highest reliability but within 72 hours.
- Having a single dose at home 'just in case' may be the answer for immediate use in the event of unprotected intercourse.

*Acceptability*
Very much a personal decision—religious or cultural beliefs may prevent use.

*Suitability and advantages*
Tolerated by most women.

*Disadvantages and possible risks*
- Reduced reliability with some medications e.g. carbamazepine (Tegretol) and St. John's Wort—seek medical advice.
- Some possible short-term side effects e.g. nausea, vomiting, fluid retention.
- Failure rate may be unacceptable.

### Intrauterine device

Either a coil or intrauterine system (Mirena) may be used.

*Reliability*
- Failure rate of the coil less than 1%.
- Failure rate of the Mirena system minimal.

*Availability*
Fitted free at family planning clinics and some GPs.

*How to use and reduce the risk of failure*
- Must be inserted within 5 days or unprotected intercourse or failed method.
- Method can then remain in place for continued protection.

*Acceptability*
- Insertion may not be acceptable.
- Religious or cultural beliefs may prevent use.

*Suitability and advantages*
- Gives immediate and long-term protection against pregnancy.
- Progesterone in Mirena increases the reliability—dose is low with fewer side effects than other progesterone methods.
- Periods may stop with Mirena—less hygiene issues and anaemia.

*Disadvantages and possible risks*
- Leg abduction needed for fitting which may be difficult with arthritis/leg spasms.
- Risk of autonomic dysreflexia in women with spinal cord lesions during fitting.
- First one–three periods may be heavier and more painful.
- Slightly higher risk of pelvic infection as it will be fitted before results of routine infection screening prior to fitting have been obtained (treatment can be given after fitting if needed).
- May be more painful/not always easy to fit in a woman who has never had a baby as the cervix is usually tightly closed.

## SEXUAL HEALTH INFORMATION FOR WOMEN WITH DISABILITY

### Genital tract and sexually transmitted infections

Genital tract infections are a common occurrence and they may or may not be sexually transmitted. They can cause anything from mild discomfort e.g. itching to severe illness. If pregnancy occurs then the health of the baby can be at risk during the pregnancy or the birth. A baby may, in some circumstances, have long-term health problems.

Susceptibility to infections may be related to ineffective hygiene because of incontinence, mobility difficulties or lack of appropriate help at relevant times. Combined hormonal contraceptives and pregnancy alter the natural acid of the vagina and at these times infections can develop even with good hygiene. To minimise the risk of acquiring a sexually transmitted infection a condom should always be used even if this is not the main contraceptive method.

This leaflet gives an overview of the common genital tract infections including if they are sexually transmitted, how to recognise them, the usual treatment and any specific issues that may be relevant because of disability. If you suspect that you have an infection it is important that you seek help from a doctor, genitourinary clinic (phone number and clinic location in the phone book) or health advisor, nurse or midwife as soon as possible to ensure rapid and effective treatment. If an infection is sexually transmitted it is important that your partner(s) is also treated.

### Thrush
#### Cause
Yeast organisms called monilia or candida which may be on the skin and are often present in the bowel, where they rarely causes any problems. If the vagina becomes less acid or the skin becomes moist or soiled for a long time they can grow causing symptoms and treatment is needed.

#### How to recognise it
- Skin may become itchy and inflamed but this may be missed if sensation is poor.
- There may be a thick white discharge.
- There may be a very unpleasant smell.

- Frequent passing of urine with pain (cystitis) but this may not be felt if sensation is poor.

#### Treatment
- Cream can be applied to the skin e.g. Canesten or Gyno-Daktarin for irritation.
- Cream (inserted with a syringe-like applicator) or a pessary (a solid bullet-shaped measure of cream) inserted into the vagina when there is discharge.
- Tablets called metronidazole (Flagyl) to be swallowed.

#### Possible issues
- Poor mobility, dexterity and skin sensation may reduce the ability to self-treat—regular application of skin cream may require a helper; a single-dose pessary can be inserted into the vagina by a helper or health professional.
- Metronidazole
  —May interact with drugs such as steroids and those for arthritis.
  —No alcohol should be taken during treatment.
  —Should be used with caution in people who experience 'pins and needles' because of their condition.

### Bacterial vaginosis (BV)
#### Cause
A vaginal infection caused by one of several organisms that commonly live in the bowel: can be sexually transmitted.

#### How to recognise it
- There may be no symptoms at all.
- There may be an unpleasant 'fishy' smell.
- There may be a watery vaginal discharge which may be missed because of incontinence.
- A burning sensation may be felt around the vaginal entrance unless sensation poor.

#### Treatment
- Antibiotic tablets of metronidazole (Flagyl) or clindamycin to swallow.
- Vaginal cream of clindamycin.

#### Possible issues
See above related to treatment.

## Trichomonas

### Cause

Small organisms with tails: sexually transmitted.

### How to recognise it

- There may be no symptoms.
- There may be a very unpleasant smell and a green/yellow discharge.
- Intercourse may be painful unless sensation is poor.
- Frequent passing of urine with pain (cystitis) but this may not be felt if sensation is poor.
- There may be a general feeling of being unwell.
- Lower abdominal pain unless sensation poor.

### Treatment

- A large single dose tablet of metronidazole (Flagyl) to swallow.
- Sexual partner(s) should be treated.

### Possible issues

See above related to metronidazole.

## Chlamydia

### Cause

Minute parasites that invade cells in the body: sexually transmitted.

### How to recognise it

- Often no symptoms.
- Frequent passing of urine with pain (cystitis) but this may not be felt if sensation is poor.
- Lower abdominal pain which may be missed if sensation poor.

### Treatment

- Antibiotic tablets of tetracycline or doxycycline, or a single large dose of azithromycin to swallow.
- Partner(s) should also be treated.

### Possible issues

- Antibiotic effect may be reduced by some drugs e.g. carbamazepine (Tegretol).
- These antibiotics reduce the reliability of hormonal contraception—use an additional method during treatment and for 7 days afterwards.
- These antibiotics should not be used during pregnancy or breast-feeding.
- If the condition is untreated in pregnancy there is a risk of pre-term birth, small baby and the baby's eyes become infected at birth which can lead to blindness.

## Gonorrhoea

### Cause

Specific bacteria shaped like a pair of coffee beans: sexually transmitted.

### How to recognise it

- No symptoms may be seen in the early stages.
- There may be some vaginal discharge.
- Frequent passing of urine with pain (cystitis) but this may not be felt if sensation is poor.
- Painful intercourse, again, may not be felt if sensation poor.
- Lower abdominal pain in later stages which may be missed if sensation poor.

### Treatment

- Single injection into a muscle of antibiotic (there are several different types).
- Partner(s) should be treated.

### Possible issues

See chlamydia above.

## Syphilis

### Cause

Specific bacteria shaped like spirals: sexually transmitted.

### How to recognise it

- Between 3 weeks and 90 days after infection a single painless ulcer appears on the genital area which disappears rapidly.
- Between 6 weeks and several months later there may be a high temperature, smooth ulcers in the genital area, skin rash, muscle pain, headache and tiredness. Symptoms may eventually disappear but infection remains.
- In the long-term an untreated condition will result in nerve damage, loss of pain sensation and poor muscle coordination.
- A routine blood test offered during pregnancy will help to identify the condition.

### Treatment

- A large single-dose injection into a muscle of penicillin unless allergic when tetracycline can be used.
- Partner(s) should be treated.

*Possible issues*

- The early ulcer symptom may be easily missed by an individual or helper with hygiene.
- Subsequent symptoms e.g. fatigue and muscle pain may be blamed on an existing condition e.g. multiple sclerosis.
- Antibiotic effect may be reduced by some drugs e.g. carbamazepine (Tegretol).
- These antibiotics reduce the effects of hormonal contraception—use an additional method during treatment and for 7 days afterwards.
- Failure to treat during early pregnancy will result in the baby being affected by the disease and if no treatment it will be born with syphilis.

### Herpes simplex virus (HSV)
*Cause*

- There are two types of virus: although not always so; HSV 1 is more common on the face, HSV 2 more common on the genital area. Sexually transmitted or in some cases through skin-to-skin contact.
- The virus remains dormant in the nerve that has been affected.

*How to recognise it*

- Painful blisters on the skin in the genital area or in the vagina especially on initial infection.
- Skin may be highly sensitive and tingling or 'pins and needles' felt.
- Initial infection may cause general flu-like symptoms.
- Recurrent outbreaks.

*Treatment*

- Tablets of antiviral drug acyclovir to swallow.
- Local application of acyclovir ointment.
- Local application of anaesthetic gel to relieve pain.

*Possible issues*

- Painful symptoms may be missed when sensation is poor or they may lead to autonomic hyperreflexia e.g. because of a spinal cord lesion.
- Poor mobility, dexterity and skin sensation may reduce the ability to self-treat—regular application of skin cream may require a helper.
- Lesions may be slow to heal when mobility is impaired or because of incontinence.

- Caesarean section birth is usually recommended during an active episode of infection to avoid infecting the baby.
- Habitual use of condoms reduces the sharing of infection.

### Human papilloma virus (genital warts)
*Cause*

Several strains of virus cause fleshy growths in the genital and/or anal areas; some strains are linked to cancer of the cervix: sexually transmitted.

*How to recognise it*

- Visible fleshy growths (warts) which are painless.
- Cervical cell changes identified by smear test.

*Treatment*

- There are a variety of creams or lotions that are applied to the warts but treatment is usually prolonged.
- Warts may be destroyed by freezing or laser.
- Cervical cell changes require further investigation and specific treatment to prevent cancer developing.

*Possible issues*

- Poor mobility, dexterity and skin sensation may reduce the ability to self-treat warts—regular application of skin cream/lotion may require a helper.
- Compliance with long-term wart treatment.
- Leg abduction needed for cervical smear taking and treatment which may be difficult when there is arthritis or leg spasm.
- Inadequate local anaesthetic resulting in pain during surgical treatment of warts may cause autonomic hyperreflexia in women with spinal cord lesions.
- Habitual use of condoms will reduce shared infection.

### Pelvic inflammatory disease
*Cause*

A variety of viruses and bacteria can lead to the condition; commonly gonorrhoea, chlamydia, and E.coli (a bowel organism).

*How to recognise it*

- Symptoms are not always easily defined.
- There may be signs of vaginal infection (as above).

- Low abdominal pain may be mild to severe.
- In an acute attack there may be a high temperature and general illness.
- There may be deep pain during intercourse.

*Treatment*
- Diagnosis may be difficult requiring surgical investigations and a scan.
- A combination of two or three antibiotics may be given at the same time over a 14-day period.

*Possible issues*
- Failure to recognise symptoms especially for women with reduced/lack of pelvic sensation e.g. due to spinal cord lesion.

- Pain may cause autonomic hyperreflexia in women with spinal cord lesions.
- Untreated condition is likely to result in the tubes of the uterus becoming blocked resulting in infertility.
- Antibiotic effect may be reduced by some drugs e.g. carbamazepine (Tegretol).
- The antibiotic reduces the effects of hormonal contraception—use an additional method during treatment and for 7 days afterwards.

## HEALTH PROMOTION FOR WOMEN WITH DISABILITY

### Preconception care

#### Planning for a family

All women and their partners can do much to improve the outcome of pregnancy and childbirth. These improvements revolve around considering diet and life-style and planning any modifications needed. That planning may need to start 6 months before conception and any modifications needed should be in place at least 3 months prior to trying for a family.

Women with a disability need to bear in mind the same issues as non-disabled women but other factors will need additional consideration. A brief overview is given here of topics common to all women and their partners, with an added focus of information relevant for people with disability.

By necessity only general principles can be included here. If you have specific issues related to your own circumstances you are strongly recommended to speak to your specialist advisor.

#### Timing of pregnancy

In the ideal world all pregnancies should be planned and timed to suit a couple's situation. In reality this happens infrequently. But for women with disability that planning is more likely to be meticulous and carefully considered because of the physical, psychological and social implications having a child is likely to entail.

#### Medical considerations

In some cases, before considering conception some couples may need to know more about how pregnancy and childbirth may affect a woman's condition in the short- and long-term periods; how the condition may influence a pregnancy and perhaps affect a baby; and how she may cope with parenthood. Answers to all questions may not be possible as in some situations little is known, or effects are variable and unpredictable.

Medication taken by a woman for her condition will need to be reviewed prior to conception. Some medication may need to be stopped or changed because of concerns about possible damage to the fetus. Some drugs, for example methotrexate taken for arthritis, need to be stopped at least 6 months before conception, whilst another drug, fluoxetine (Prozac), should be gradually rather than suddenly stopped to avoid withdrawal symptoms in the woman. Medical advice is essential when a couple begin to consider starting a family, and prior to making that decision.

Some conditions have a hereditary origin e.g. some forms of deafness, blindness and degenerative muscle conditions. In these situations advice from a genetic counsellor before planning a family may be invaluable. GPs or specialist medical practitioners are able to refer a couple for genetic screening. The results will offer an indication of the risk that a condition could be inherited by a child. This will help a couple decide (it is *their* choice) whether to go onto start a family or not. No one has any right to make that decision: not doctors, family or friends.

#### Contraception

If a woman has been using hormonal contraception or an intrauterine device (coil) this method should be stopped and a barrier method used e.g. condoms, for 3 months prior to conception to enable the body to adjust. This is now a good time to start folic acid (see below under diet and nutrition). If a progesterone injection has been used conception may take time to be achieved as the effects of the hormone take some time to wear off.

#### Conception

Women need to make a note of the dates of their periods; the first day of bleeding is counted as day 1. If contraception has been stopped as above, it may take several months for the cycle to adjust. If cycles between periods (without contraception) are about 28 days then an ovum (egg) is produced about the middle of the cycle i.e. around day 14. If a cycle is longer e.g. 36 days, then an ovum is produced about 22 days after the last period.

It is difficult to predict the actual day an ovum will be released to plan the most likely time for intercourse to result in pregnancy. As a general guide, intercourse a few days before or around the date the ovum is released would be best (sperm are able to live in a woman's body for several days after entry). Prediction kits are available, from larger chemists and some supermarkets, although they are expensive. They work by giving the results of hormone levels in a specimen of the woman's urine. Even if the timing is right, pregnancy may still not occur as the process has to be highly balanced for success. A couple can do many things to help that balance to be at its best (see below).

### Social and emotional issues

All parents will say that having a baby is a life-changing event: often for the best but sometimes not so good. Each couple need to consider: 'Is it right for me/us at this time?' Factors to take into consideration relate to individual emotional ability to cope e.g. with any worry, anxiety, problems, the responsibility of a new life; relationships e.g. whether it is a supportive relationship; financial and employment implications of having a child; and finally family issues e.g. are they supportive?

For women with disability these factors are often more poignant as they may already have challenges with everyday life and perhaps require additional support or help. Women are likely to be concerned about the affects pregnancy will have on the disability or the disabilities, and perhaps medication, on a baby. Family and friends may have negative attitudes towards a woman having a child because she is disabled. Perhaps because of concerns for her health and well-being but possibly about how they will cope with any extra help and support needed they may have to supply.

All of these issues need to be discussed between the couple and perhaps their family and friends. Plans can be made to arrange for appropriate help, and strategies put into place to meet additional or alternative needs e.g. when extra rest time will need to be scheduled to cope with greater tiredness.

### Diet and nutrition

This is one of the biggest areas that individuals can have a direct impact upon. A well-balanced nutritious diet is recommended, i.e. one that includes portions of food from all of the food groups daily. Ideally this should include five portions of fruit and vegetables per day which is recommended by the Department of Health. This well-balanced diet is not always easy to achieve if an individual has strong food preferences or dislikes, and can be challenging when the opportunity to purchase varied foods is restricted by finances or the ability to shop.

All women are advised to take a folic acid 0.4-mg supplement daily for at least 3 months before conception and during the first 3 months of pregnancy to reduce the likelihood of a baby having a neural tube defect e.g. spina bifida. Women who have such a condition or have had a baby with the condition need to take a dose 10 times greater i.e. 4 mg. Women who take drugs for seizures or spasms e.g. carbamazepine have a higher risk of having a baby with spina bifida and they too are advised to take the higher dose of folic acid. The higher doses can be obtained free on prescription from GPs.

### Substances to avoid

The next important area that an individual and a couple can do a great deal to help themselves is that avoidance of potentially harmful substances for at least 3 months prior to conception.

### Alcohol

There is no known safe level of alcohol during pregnancy: for some women even a little can affect their baby. Therefore it is best to avoid all but an occasional single measure which is:

- One pub measure of spirit.
- 125 ml of wine (not the 150-ml glasses often used as standard now).
- 1/2 pint of normal strength beer or larger (less for stronger brews).
- One standard pub measure of sherry/fortified wine (again not the large glasses).

What is also important is that over indulgence (getting drunk) even before conception (for both men and women) is absolutely avoided as this can damage both ova (eggs) and sperm. This is even more important when medication is being taken as few medicines mix with alcohol.

### Tobacco

It is well known that smoking can have major implications for the health of the smoker and those around them: health and well-being will be so much improved by stopping. If there is a chance that a woman may need an anaesthetic during pregnancy e.g. for caesarean section, there is much less risk during the surgery and afterwards with chest infection.

Avoiding smoking and smoky atmospheres before conception and throughout pregnancy will improve a baby's health and well-being and chances of surviving. Not smoking after the birth is better for the baby when breast-feeding and reduces the chance of cot death.

Most smokers find this a challenge but there is more help and support available to achieve success. People can contact their local support group (details in the phone book) or practice nurse at their GP's surgery.

### Street drugs

Illicit drugs including cannabis (sometimes taken by people to alleviate muscle spasms caused by specific conditions) should be avoided. During pregnancy drugs cross the placenta and may cause miscarriage, low birth weight and result in the baby having withdrawal symptoms for some considerable time after birth. These symptoms not only make the baby unhappy or even distressed, but they also make caring for the baby more challenging because of the distress and often a need for considerable attention. This may be difficult to achieve if a parent's energy levels are reduced.

## Exercise and becoming 'fit'

Not everyone enjoys exercise and if mobility or poor energy levels are an issue then exercise requires even greater motivation. Exercise can improve circulation, strengthen the heart, expand lung capacity and improve general well-being. For someone with a disability improvement in any or all of these factors has the potential to improve general health. That improvement may make the physical challenges that pregnancy, labour and birth bring easier to cope with. Any exercise is beneficial, even just deep breathing exercises, but any exercise that increases breathing and heart rate are enhancing strength. The best professional to give advice to

people with disability is a physiotherapist. GPs or practice nurses should be able to refer women to an NHS physiotherapist, or advice can be obtained through private healthcare. Aquanatal is encouraged.

General health needs to be considered and steps taken where appropriate to obtain optimal well-being. Those steps could include a urine test for infection and blood tests to identify any anaemia. It is not uncommon for women with poor pelvic sensation and those with continence problems to have a urinary tract infection that presents no obvious symptoms. Women who have chronic urinary tract infection or infection in pressure sores are more at risk of anaemia. Identifying any complications in this way enables relevant treatment to be offered ensuring a woman's health is at its best.

## Sexual health

It is not uncommon for women to have genital tract infections and some of these will be sexually transmitted. Non-sexually transmitted infections are more common in women taking hormonal contraception, and when incontinence and personal hygiene are difficult to manage. Women with poor pelvic or lower body sensations may miss symptoms of infection e.g. genital area pain and pain on passing urine.

Sexually transmitted infections are more common when safe sex i.e. condom use, is not habitually practised. Some sexually transmitted infections present few symptoms and can be easily missed.

Untreated infection can lead to pelvic inflammatory disease which often results in the tubes from the uterus that carry the ova (egg) becoming blocked causing infertility. So it is advisable for women to have a check-up at their GP's surgery to ensure that any infection is diagnosed and effectively treated before conception. This is also important because there is a higher risk of miscarriage, of a baby being affected by the infection, and for pre-term birth. Additionally, there are also risks to the mother of becoming unwell during pregnancy or soon after the birth.

# Index